DATE DUE

GAYLORD	PRINTED IN U.S.A.

Complementary/ Alternative Therapies in Nursing

4th Edition

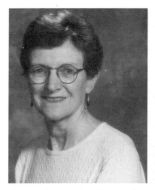

Mariah Snyder PhD, RN, FAAN received her bachelor's degree in nursing from the College of St. Teresa in Winona, MN, her master's degree in nursing from the University of Pennsylvania in Philadelphia, and her doctorate in education from the University of Minnesota. In 2001 Dr. Snyder became a professor emeritus at the University of Minnesota. Complementary therapies/nursing interventions served as the focal point of Dr. Snyder's nursing career. She advanced the knowledge on complementary therapies through research on the use of complementary therapies to promote the health and well-being of elders, nursing and interdisciplinary courses offered on nursing interventions/complementary therapies, and numerous publications presentations on the topic. Dr. Snyder was a founding member of the Center for Spirituality and Healing in the Academic Health Center at the University of Minnesota and the Director of Graduate Studies for the interdisciplinary minor in complementary therapies at the University of Minnesota.

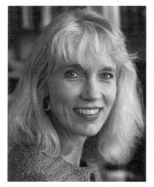

Ruth Lindquist, PhD, RN is an associate professor and Division Head of Adult, Geriatric, and Psychiatric/Mental Health Nursing at the University of Minnesota School of Nursing and a faculty member in the Center for Spirituality and Healing in the Academic Health Center. Her research as a Densford Scholar in the Katharine J. Densford International Center for Nursing Leadership focuses on critical care nurses' attitudes towards and use of complementary/alternative therapies.

Complementary/ Alternative Therapies in Nursing

4th Edition

Mariah Snyder, PhD, RN, FAAN
Ruth Lindquist, PhD, RN, Editors

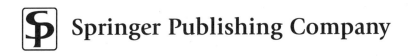

Springer Publishing Company, Inc.
536 Broadway
New York, NY 10012-3955

Acquisitions Editor: Ruth Chasek
Production Editor: Janice G. Stangel
Cover design by Susan Hauley

02 03 04 05 06 / 5 4 3

Library of Congress Cataloging-in-Publication Data

Complementary alternative therapies in nursing / Mariah Snyder, Ruth Lindquist, editors. — 4th ed.
    p. : cm.
  Includes bibliographical references and index.
  ISBN 0-8261-1446-6
  1. Holistic nursing. 2. Nurse and patient. 3. Alternative medicine.
I. Snyder, Mariah. II. Lindquist, Ruth.
  [DNLM: 1. Alternative Medicine—Nurses' Instruction. 2. Holistic Nursing—Nurses Instruction. 3. Nursing Care—Nurses Instruction.
WB 890 C7377 2002]
RT41 d53 2002
610.73—dc21
                                          2001049710

Printed in the United States of America by Maple-Vail.

Contents

Contributors   *ix*

Preface   *xiii*

PART I   Foundations for Practice

1   An Overview of Complementary/Alternative Therapies   3
    Mariah Snyder

2   Self As Healer   16
    Susan Towey and Barbara Leonard

3   Presence   24
    Mariah Snyder, Yueh-hsia Tseng, and Cheryl Brandt

4   Therapeutic Listening   33
    Shigeaki Watanuki, Mary Fran Tracy, and Ruth Lindquist

PART II   Mind-Body Therapies

5   Imagery   43
    Janice Post-White and Maura Fitzgerald

6   Music Intervention   58
    Linda Chlan

7   Humor   69
    Kevin Smith

8   Yoga   81
    Miriam E. Cameron

9   Biofeedback   89
     Marion Good

10   Meditation   101
     Mary Jo Kreitzer

11   Prayer   114
     Mariah Snyder

12   Storytelling As a Healing Tool   124
     Roxanne Struthers

13   Journaling   135
     Mariah Snyder

14   Reminiscence   143
     Mariah Snyder

15   Animal-Assisted Therapy   152
     Jennifer Jorgenson

Part III   Energy Therapies

16   Healing Touch   165
     Alexa W. Umbreit

17   Therapeutic Touch   183
     Janet F. Quinn

18   Reiki   197
     Linda L. Halcón

19   Acupressure   205
     Pamela Weiss

PART IV   Manipulative and Body-Based Therapies

20   Massage   223
     Mariah Snyder and Yueh-hsia Tseng

21   Tai Chi   234
     Kuei-Min Chen

PART V   Biological-Based Therapies

22   Aromatherapy   245
     Jane Buckle

23   Herbal Medicines   259
     Gregory A. Plotnikoff

24   Functional Foods and Nutraceuticals   272
     Bridget Doyle

PARt VI   Lifestyle and Disease Prevention Therapies

25   Exercise   285
     Diane Treat-Jacobson and Daniel L. Mark

26   Groups   297
     Merrie J. Kaas and Mary Fern Richie

27   Progressive Muscle Relaxation   310
     Mariah Snyder, Elizabeth Pestka, and Catherine Bly

Index   321

Contributors

Catherine Bly, BSN, RN
Lutheran Hospital
LaCrosse, Wisconsin

Cheryl Brandt, MS, RN
School of Nursing, College of
   Professional Studies
University of Wisconsin
Eau Claire, Wisconsin

Jane Buckle, PhD, RN
R. J. Buckle Associates LLC
Hunter, New York

**Miriam E. Cameron, PhD, MS,
   MA, RN**
Center for Bioethics and Faculty,
   Center for Spirituality
   and Healing
University of Minnesota
Minneapolis, Minnesota

Linda Chlan, PhD, RN
School of Nursing; Center for
   Spirituality and Healing
University of Minnesota
Minneapolis, Minnesota

Kuei-Min Chen, PhD, RN
Department of Midwifery Nursing
FooYin Institute of Technology
Kaohsiung, Taiwan

**Bridget Doyle, PhD, MPH,
   RD, LD**
Minnesota State Veterans Home
Minneapolis, Minnesota

Maura Fitzgerald, MS, RN, CS
Children's Hospital and Clinics
St. Paul, Minnesota

Marion Good, PhD, RN
Frances-Payne Bolton School
   of Nursing
Case Western Reserve University
Cleveland, Ohio

Linda L. Halcón, PhD, RN
School of Nursing; Center for
   Spirituality and Healing
University of Minnesota
Minneapolis, Minnesota

Jennifer Jorgenson, BSN, RN
University of North Carolina at
    Chapel Hill
Chapel Hill, North Carolina

Merrie J. Kaas, DNSc, RN, CS
School of Nursing
University of Minnesota
Minneapolis, Minnesota

Mary Jc Kreitzer, PhD, RN
Center for Spirituality
    and Healing
University of Minnesota
Minneapolis, Minnesota

Barbara Leonard, PhD, RN
School of Nursing; Center
    for Spirituality and Healing
University of Minnesota
Minneapolis, Minnesota

Daniel L. Mark, MD
Rochester, Minnesota

Elizabeth Pestka, MS, RN, CS
Mayo Medical Center
Rochester, Minnesota

Gregory A. Plotnikoff, MD, MTS
Medical School; Center for
    Spirituality and Healing
University of Minnesota
Minneapolis, Minnesota

Janice Post-White, PhD, RN,
    FAAN
School of Nursing; Center for
    Spirituality and Healing
University of Minnesota
Minneapolis, Minnesota

Janet F. Quinn, PhD, RN,
    FAAN
Haelen Works
Boulder, Colorado

Mary Fern Richie, DSN, RN, CS
Nashville, Tennessee

Kevin Smith, MSN, RN, CNP
School of Nursing
University of Minnesota
Minneapolis, Minnesota

Roxanne Struthers, PhD, RN
School of Nursing
University of Minnesota
Minneapolis, Minnesota

Susan Towey, MS, LP, CNS, LP
Center for Spirituality and Healing
University of Minnesota
Minneapolis, Minnesota

Mary Fran Tracy, PhD, RN,
    CCRN
Fairview-University Medical Center
Minneapolis, Minnesota

Diane Treat-Jacobson, PhD, RN
Vascular Medicine Research
    Program
University of Minnesota
Minneapolis, Minnesota

Yueh-hsia Tseng, PhD, RN
Chung-shan Medical College
Taichung, Taiwan

Alexa Umbreit, MS, RN, C, CHTP
Fairview-University Medical Center
Minneapolis, Minnesota

Shigeaki Watanuki, MS, RN
School of Nursing doctoral
    student
University of Minnesota
Minneapolis, Minnesota

**Pamela Weiss, PhD, MPH, RN,
    Dip. Ac. L. Ac**
Department of Nursing
Augsburg College
Minneapolis, Minnesota

Preface

Nearly two decades have passed since the first edition of this book, then titled *Independent Nursing Interventions*, was published. During this time, interest in complementary/alternative therapies and their use have grown exponentially. Numerous health facilities now provide patients with complementary therapies in addition to biomedical treatments. Funding for the National Center for Complementary/Alternative Medicine (NCCAM) in the National Institutes of Health has increased as well, providing more support for research on complementary therapies, and NCCAM has also funded efforts to augment the content on complementary therapies in health professional curricula.

Because nursing has a tradition of using complementary therapies and has conducted research on a number of the therapies, it is in a prime position to be a leader in the field of complementary therapies. Nursing is concerned with preventing and alleviating health problems, managing symptoms, and viewing healing from a holistic perspective. A holistic philosophy underpins many of the complementary therapies and systems and thus there is congruence with nursing. Empowering persons to assume more responsibility for their own health and well-being is also a concern of nursing. The majority of the therapies included in this book require active participation by the patient, with the patient assuming responsibility for integrating the therapies into their lives.

Not only has interest in complementary therapies increased in the United States, but nurses across the world are seeking ways to increase their knowledge and expertise in the use of these therapies. The third edition of *Complementary/Alternative Therapies in Nursing* has been translated into Chinese and Japanese.

The scope of the field of complementary therapies is very broad and encompasses more than 1,800 therapies and systems of care. The editors faced a major challenge in selecting the therapies to include in the fourth edition. While many therapies that were included in the first edition may have seemed avant-garde at the time, they are quite commonplace today. Some more traditional nursing interventions such as sensation information, validation therapy, and application of heat and cold were deleted so that yoga, acupressure, and herbal preparations could be included. Several factors guided the selection of therapies including the frequency with which it is used by nurses, the availability of a research base to guide practice, and whether it is identified on the NCCAM list of therapies. It is recognized that nurses will use many other complementary therapies in their practice. Thus, there will be a dynamism among the therapies included in subsequent editions.

There has been concern in the biomedical community about the lack of scientific evidence for many complementary therapies, yet a research base does exist for numerous therapies and anecdotal evidence has accumulated over the millennia to support their use. One of the beliefs about complementary therapies, formulated by the Royal College of Nurses, is that where possible nurses should select therapies having a research base. The scientific basis for the use of a therapy, to the extent that it exists, continues to be a focus in the fourth edition. To prompt students, clinicians, and researchers to continue research, each chapter identifies areas in which additional knowledge is needed.

To assist nurses in implementing the therapies in practice settings, specific techniques for each therapy are provided. Although multiple techniques for therapies exist, space only allows for several to be elaborated. Extensive references, including Internet sites, at the end of each chapter provide readers easy access to additional information about the therapy, including other techniques.

While new therapies have been added, a key feature that is present in all editions is the use of a similar format throughout the book. A description of the therapy is followed by the scientific basis for use of the therapy, specific techniques for implementing the therapy in practice, examples of populations and conditions in which the therapy has been used, and areas for future research. Precautions to consider when using specific therapies are noted. Two new chapters have been added: an overview of complementary therapies in nursing and self-care.

As the consumer demand continues to grow for a holistic approach to health care that includes complementary therapies, it is critical that nurses have knowledge about complementary therapies so that they can include selected ones in their practice and provide patients with information about therapies or refer them to resources. This text provides information about the field of complementary therapies and a beginning knowledge about specific therapies for undergraduate and graduate nursing students and nurses practicing in all types of settings.

We wish to thank the many students who have piqued our interest in complementary therapies with their questions and by the examples they have provided of using these therapies in their practice. We wish also to thank our colleagues in the School of Nursing and the Center for Spirituality and Healing of the Academic Health Center at the University of Minnesota who have supported the inclusion of complementary therapies in nursing curricula and have promoted research on these therapies. The increasing interest in complementary therapies has indeed been gratifying.

MARIAH SNYDER, PhD, RN, FAAN
RUTH LINDQUIST, PhD, RN, FAAN

PART I

Foundations for Practice

OVERVIEW

Complementary/alternative therapies (often referenced as complementary/alternative medicine) encompasses more than 1,800 therapies and systems of care (Kreitzer & Jensen, 2000). A brief history of complementary therapies and its place in nursing is provided in chapter 1. The content in Part I addresses the underlying philosophy of complementary therapies. Although it is important for nurses to be competent in a specific therapy before administering it to a patient, it is equally as important that they incorporate the philosophy into their practice. Presence and active listening (chapters 3 and 4) are an integral part of the underlying holistic, caring philosophy of complementary therapies. The content in subsequent chapters may not specifically refer to presence and active listening, but it is understood that these two components will be integrated into the administration of all complementary therapies.

Modeling the holistic, caring philosophy to patients and co-workers is important to the success of complementary therapies. The content in chapter 2 provides nurses with strategies they can use to "take care of self," incorporating self-care practices in their lives to renew their energy and to be more *present* to patients and colleagues.

An Overview of Complementary/ Alternative Therapies

Mariah Snyder

During the past decade complementary/alternative therapies have become an important part of health care in the United States and other countries. Although the term *complementary therapies* will be primarily used in this book, numerous other designations have been used for therapies that have not been a part of the traditional Western medicine system of care. "Complementary" is preferred by some as it conveys a therapy that is used as an adjunct to Western therapies; "alternative" indicates a therapy that is used in place of a Western medicine approach. And both are used by the National Center for Complementary and Alternative Medicine of the National Institutes of Health. More recently the term *integrative medicine* is being used to convey that the care provided is a blend of Western medicine, complementary therapies, and therapies from other systems of health care. Many nursing interventions can be classified as complementary therapies.

This chapter will provide an overview of complementary therapies. Topics include the extent to which complementary therapies are used; the reasons proposed for increased interest in these therapies; definitions, scope, and classification of complementary therapies; the cultural aspects of complementary therapies; and the implications of complementary therapies for nursing.

USE OF COMPLEMENTARY THERAPIES

Interest and the use of complementary/alternative therapies has increased exponentially during the past decade. Eisenberg et al. (1993, 1998) conducted two national surveys to determine the percentage of Americans who used complementary therapies. More than 33% of those surveyed in 1991 used complementary therapies with that number increasing to 42% in 1997. This is believed to be a conservative estimate as the survey inquired only about 16 therapies while multiple others exist. Also, the survey only obtained information from those who spoke English; countless persons from other cultures use complementary therapies on a routine basis. The use of complementary therapies is not limited to adults. Bruener, Barry, and Kemper (1998) found that 70% of a sample of homeless teens reported using complementary therapies.

Currently, third-party payers such as insurance companies pay for a limited number of complementary therapies. The therapies most frequently covered are chiropractic, acupuncture, and biofeedback. In most instances, physician referral is required for reimbursement. Eisenberg et al. (1998) reported that Americans spent more than $22.1 on complementary therapies during a 1-year period and that the majority of the amount was paid for directly by the consumer. Obviously people must feel that complementary therapies produce positive results if they continue to pay for them personally.

What has prompted this rapidly growing interest in complementary therapies? First, the holistic philosophy underlying complementary therapies differs significantly from the dualistic or Cartesian philosophy that for several centuries has permeated Western medicine. According to Fontaine (2000), people believe that Western medicine treats the symptoms with no attention to the underlying cause of the symptoms or to the holistic concerns of the patient. They are seeking care from complementary therapists or facilities because they want to be treated as a whole person and not as a heart attack or fractured hip. Another reason is that they want to be involved in the decision making: They want to be empowered. In a study by Mitzdorf and colleagues (1999), 64% of patients stated that they had too little time for discussing their health concerns with their physicians, and 42% noted that they had little time to ask questions. The increasing pressure of cost containment in health care has reduced the amount of time physicians and nurses spend with their patients. People heal themselves; physicians, nurses, and others provide assistance in this process, but true healing can only come from within the patient. A third reason cited for seeking care from complementary therapies relates to quality of life. Patients have reported they do not want the treatment for a health problem to be worse than the initial health problem. The focus of Western medicine largely has been on curing problems while the philosophy underlying complementary therapies is on harmony within the person and promotion of health. Mitzdorf et al. (1999) found that 82% of patients reported the side effects of medications as a reason for seeking complementary therapies.

The personal qualities of the complementary therapist (whether a nurse, physician, or other therapist) are key in the healing process. Caring, which has received attention in nursing across the years, is a key characteristic. Two therapies that will be covered in subsequent chapters, presence and active listening, convey this caring. Remen (2000), a physician who is involved in cancer care, stated:

> I know that if I listen attentively to someone, to their essential self, their soul, as it were, I often find that at the deepest, most unconscious level, they can sense the direction of their own healing and wholeness. If I can remain open to that, without expectations of what the someone is supposed to *do*, how they are supposed to change in order to be *better*, or even what their wholeness looks like, what can happen is magical. By that I mean that it has a certain coherency or integrity about it, far beyond any way of fixing their situation or easing their pain that I can devise on my own. (p. 90)

This philosophy has been known for ages. Hippocrates stated it was more important to know what sort of person has a disease than to know what sort of disease a person has.

The heightened interest in complementary therapies prompted the National Institutes of Health (NIH) to establish the Office of Alternative Medicine in 1992, which was elevated to the National Center for Complementary/Alternative Medicine (NCCAM) in 1998. What was significant in establishing this NIH office was that consumers lobbied for it rather than health professionals. The purposes of the NCCAM are

1. To facilitate the evaluation of therapies
2. To investigate and evaluate the efficacy of therapies
3. To serve as an information clearinghouse on complementary therapies
4. To support research training

NCCAM has funded research for individual researchers and for centers that explore the efficacy of a number of complementary therapies such as acupuncture and Saint John's-wort. Other centers are exploring the use of complementary therapies in the treatment of specific conditions such as addictive disorders, arthritis, cardiovascular disease, and neurological disorders.

DEFINITION AND CLASSIFICATION

Much debate has ensued on defining complementary therapies. The broad scope of these therapies and the many health professionals and therapists who

are involved in delivering these therapies create challenges for finding a definition that captures the scope of this field. Following a multidisciplinary conference sponsored by NIH, a panel of experts put forth the following definition:

> Complementary and alternative medicine (CAM) is a broad domain of heal-
> ing resources that encompasses all health systems, modalities, and practices
> and their accompanying theories and beliefs, other than those intrinsic to the
> politically dominant health system of a particular society or culture in a given
> historic period. CAM includes all such practices and ideas self-defined by their
> users as preventing or treating illness or promoting health and well-being.
> Boundaries between CAM and between the CAM domain and the domain of
> the dominant system are not always sharp and fixed. (Panel on the Definition
> and Description, CAM Research Methodology Conference, 1997, p. 50)

This definition is broadly inclusive and is not predicated on the Western
medicine system's being the dominant system of care. However, the breadth
of the definition creates problems in identifying the specific therapies that
comprise complementary/alternative therapies. Use of the designation *com-
plementary/alternative* therapies would include more than just medicine
because countless health professionals and therapists other than physicians
are engaged in the delivery of complementary therapies.

The broadness of the definition of complementary therapies also poses
challenges when comparing findings from the various surveys that have been
conducted on the use of complementary therapies (Braun, Halcón, &
Bearinger, 2000). The problem of delimiting the scope of complementary
therapies is furthered by the NIH's designating an overlapping category of in
their classification system. "Overlapping" is used to designate therapies that
the NIH deems can be either complementary/alternative or behavioral
medicine depending on how they are used. Therapies are classified as complementary when used for conditions in which they have not been used previously. For example, if humor were used for a condition on which no
research exists, it would be considered a complementary therapy. Cogan,
Cogan, Walz, and McCue (1987) have found humor useful in promoting
comfort; thus, for promotion of comfort, humor could be considered a part
of behavioral medicine. However, at this point, the scientific knowledge base
for the use of humor with almost all conditions is very limited.

NCCAM has classified the multiple therapies and systems of care into five
categories. According to Kreitzer and Jensen (2000), more than 1,800 therapies have been identified as complementary. The NIH categories and examples of the types of therapies in each category are shown in Table 1.1. Some
of them have been highly publicized and are widely used while others are
not familiar to anyone who has traditionally used Western medicine.

TABLE 1.1   NCCAM Classification for Complementary Therapies and Examples of Therapies

Mind-Body Therapies
  Interventions that employ a variety of techniques to facilitate the mind's capacity to impact physical symptoms and body functions
  Examples: imagery, meditation, yoga, music therapy, prayer, journaling, biofeedback, humor, tai chi, art therapy

Alternative Systems of Care
  Systems of health care that have been developed separate from the Western biomedical approach to care
  Examples: Traditional Chinese Medicine, Ayurvedic, Native American medicine, curanderismo, homeopathy, naturopathy

*Lifestyle and Disease Prevention**
  Practices aimed at preventing illness, identifying and addressing risk factors, and support of the healing processes
  Examples: intuition, chiriography, panchakarm, exercise, stress-management techniques, dietary changes, strategies to promote health

Biological-Based Therapies
  Natural and biological-based practices and products
  Examples: plant-derived preparations (herbs), special diets such as the Pritikin and the Ornish, orthomolecular medicine (nutritional and food supplements), other products such as cartilage

Manipulative and Body-based Systems
  Therapies that are based on manipulation and movement of the body
  Examples: chiropractic medicine, the many types of massage, body work such as rolfing, light and color therapies, hydrotherapy

*Energy Therapies***
  Therapies that focus on energy emanating from within the body (biofields) or energy coming out external sources
  Examples: healing touch, therapeutic touch, Reiki, external qi gong, magnets

* The most recent classification from NCCAM does not include this category.
** The most recent classification combined biofield and bioelectromagnetics into one category.

Table 1.1 describes many therapies that have always been a part of nursing and others that most nurses have not or probably will not use. Nurses often use the term *intervention* to denote therapies used in the delivery of nursing care. The National Intervention Classification project (NIC) has identified more than 400 activities that nurses perform (Iowa Intervention

Project, 1995). Many of the nursing activities included in the NIC project are not specific therapies, however, but rather are management activities and collaborative functions based on physician orders. Therefore, interchanging the terms therapies and interventions as they are currently understood in nursing may not be appropriate at this time.

CULTURAL ASPECTS OF COMPLEMENTARY THERAPIES

Cultural competency—the ability of nurses and other health professionals to provide knowledgeable care to persons of all cultures—is receiving increasing attention in education and practice settings. The vast scope of complementary therapies includes many that are part of the health systems used by people around the globe. More than 70% of the world's population use non-Western health care practices (Kreitzer & Jensen, 2000). The first step in moving toward cultural competency is to gain an awareness of the multitude of therapies used by those to whom nurses provide care (Leonard & Plotnikoff, 2000).

One of the NIH categories for complementary therapies is alternative systems of health care, which differ significantly from Western medicine. Each system is based on a philosophy or theory that guides practitioners in the assessments they make, the diagnoses, and the therapies used. An interesting exploration would be to examine how nursing, which has largely developed within the Western health care system, would function in these other health care systems.

TRADITIONAL CHINESE MEDICINE

Traditional Chinese Medicine (TCM) is the most widely known of the other systems of health care and has been used for more than 3,000 years. The philosophy underlying TCM is that *qi*, energy or a vital life force, flows through the body along channels known as meridians (Kreitzer & Jensen, 2000). Imbalances or blockages in the flow of qi result in disease. Assessment is aimed at identifying the imbalances or blockages and selecting the therapies that would bring about balance or harmony. Multiple concepts exist related to assessment. Many persons have some knowledge about *yin* and *yang*, which comprise the underlying philosophy of TCM. Yin and yang convey that opposing yet complementary phenomena exist and are in a state of dynamic equilibrium. These two concepts, integral to TCM, are used in describing normal physiology and pathological processes (Pelletier, 2000).

Another aspect of assessment focuses on the five phases or elements of TCM: earth, metal, water, wood, and fire. Determining the phase or element that is predominant in a person helps the practitioner to select the correct treatment.

After a diagnosis has been established, and if possible a pattern determined, the treatment is initiated. Treatment of the pathological condition is predicated on the use of opposing measures. For example, if the condition is determined to be cold in nature, heat is used. (Heat and cold are not conceptualized in the same manner in which they are understood in Western health care.) The main therapies used in TCM are acupuncture, moxibustion, cupping and bleeding, herbs, *qi gong*, and Oriental massage. A number of these therapies can be used separately from the total TCM approach to care, but a basic understanding of TCM facilitates their use.

AYURVEDIC MEDICINE

Ayurevdic medicine is more ancient than TCM, having been used for some 5,000 years in India. The term Ayurvedic translates to "the science of life," which is the underlying philosophy of this system of medicine. In Ayurveda, disease results from an imbalance in three fundamental elements of the body: *vata, pitta,* and *kapha.* Vata is the evidence of life in the body; it has many functions such as transmitting sensory impressions to the mind and maintaining the integrity of the body and its proper functioning. Pitta is the primary constituent of the body, its main function being to provide balance and transformation. Kapha's chief function is to promote conservation and stabilization. These are very complex elements and an understanding of them is needed to assess, diagnose, and treat an individual according to the principles of Ayurvedic medicine (Pelletier, 2000). The primary therapies used in Ayurvedic medicine include yoga, herbs, massage, meditation, and diet.

OTHER SYSTEMS

Numerous other systems of care exist here and around the world. Homeopathy and naturopathy are two systems originating from Western medicine that are receiving increasing attention in the United States. Homeopathy was developed by Samuel Hahnemann about 200 years ago and is based on the law of similarities in which a natural substance that causes a disease is used to treat the condition in a person who is ill. Highly diluted mixtures are administered to treat symptoms of a disease (Pelletier, 2000). Naturopathic medicine was developed by Benedict Lust at the beginning of the 20th century. Four principles underlie this system of care: the healing power of nature, healer do not harm, find the cause, and teach the patient (Fontaine, 2000). Great emphasis is placed on the latter principle of helping the patient assume responsibility for his or her health. Naturopathic medicine practitioners use many complementary therapies and also a number of the therapies found in Western medicine; they do not, however, perform surgical procedures.

Indigenous peoples across the globe have developed health care systems. In recent years attention has been given to Native American healers and methods of care. The systems of care vary among the American Indian tribes, but all rely heavily on the use of herbs and natural healing methods. In many instances, Western biomedical practices are intertwined with Native therapies.

Nurses and other health professionals who have been educated in the Western health care system can gain much knowledge about the health beliefs of persons in other cultures by studying the underlying philosophies. Many are based on harmony or balance within the person, which is akin to the holistic philosophy of nursing. While each system has a distinct philosophy, assessment techniques, and therapies, a number of them such as acupuncture, yoga, and meditation are being used separately from the total system.

IMPLICATIONS FOR NURSING

Complementary therapies (although this term was not used) and their basic philosophies have been a part of nursing since its beginnings. In *Notes on Nursing* (1859/1992) Florence Nightingale stressed the importance of creating the environment in which healing could occur and the importance of therapies such as music in the healing process. Complementary therapies provide an opportunity for nurses to demonstrate caring for patients.

While it is indeed gratifying to see that medicine and other professions are recognizing the importance of listening and presence in the healing process, nursing needs to assert that these therapies have been taught in nursing programs and have been practiced by nurses for centuries. It needs to make the public aware that a number of these therapies have been and are an integral part of nursing's armamentarium of therapies. Therapies such as meditation, imagery, support groups, music therapy, humor, journaling, reminiscence, caring-based approaches, massage, touch, healing touch, active listening, and presence have been practiced by nurses throughout time.

Complementary therapies are receiving increasing attention within nursing. Specialty journals such as *AACN Clinical Issues, Journal of Emergency Nursing,* and *Nurse Midwifery* have devoted entire issues to complementary therapies. These articles inform nurses about complementary therapies and how specific therapies can be used in providing care.

Because of the wide use of complementary therapies by patients to whom they provide care, it is critical that nurses possess knowledge about complementary therapies. Milton (1998) noted that "more patients than ever are using these therapies, and they expect nurses to know about them" (p. 500). Nurses need knowledge about complementary therapies to

1. Provide guidance in obtaining health histories and assessing patients
2. Answer basic questions about complementary therapies and to refer patients to reliable sources of information
3. Make referrals to competent therapists
4. Administer a selected number of complementary therapies

Obtaining a complete health history requires that information about the use of complementary therapies be a routine part of the history. Many patients may not volunteer information about using complementary therapies unless they are specifically asked; others may be reluctant to share this information unless the practitioner displays an acceptance of their use. While information about all complementary therapies is needed, it is critical to obtain information about use of herbal preparations. As the number of people using these preparations increases, interactions between certain prescriptive drugs and herbal preparations may pose a threat to health unless complete information is obtained.

As noted by Milton (1998), patients expect nurses to know about complementary therapies. The scope of these therapies makes it impossible for nurses to be knowledgeable about all of them, but knowledge of the more common ones will assist nurses in answering basic questions. Many organizations, professional associations, and individuals and groups have excellent Web sites that provide information about specific therapies. One of the functions of NCCAM is to provide consumer information. A number of Web sites are found in Table 1.2.

Referring patients to competent therapists or helping patients to identify competent therapists is another role for nurses, and it is not an easy task. Because many complementary therapists are not members of one of the health professions, licensure and regulations often do not apply to them, and regulation varies greatly from state to state. Recently the Minnesota legislature passed a bill placing unlicensed complementary and alternative therapies under the auspices of the Department of Health (Alternative Health Care Bill, H.F. 3839). Notably this bill contains a patient bill of rights, one of which is that complementary therapists have to provide clients with a summary of the theoretical approach to their practices and that the patient has a right to complete information about the practitioner's assessment and

TABLE 1.2   Web Sites for Information on Complementary Therapies

Academy of Chinese Culture and Health Science *http://www.acchs.edu*
Alternative Medicine Homepage *http://www.pitt.edu-cbw/internet/html*
Ayurvedic *http://www.ayurvedic.com*
American Holistic Nurses Association *http://www.ahna.org*
Dance of the Deer Foundation *http://www. shamanism.com*
Federal Drug Administration Consumer Line *http://www.fda.gov*
National Center for Complementary/Alternative Medicine *http://nccam.nih.gov*

recommendations. If clients have concerns, they can make them known to the commissioner for complementary and alternative therapies. This law is a beginning in the protection of clients.

The area of practice and a nurse's own preferences will assist in determining those therapies in which they wish to become proficient. As with any treatment or procedure, the nurse must be competent to carry it out. This may require education beyond that received in basic or advanced educational programs. An increasing number of nurses are being certified to administer specific therapies such as healing touch and aromatherapy. Certification conveys to patients and colleagues that the nurse possesses the knowledge and expertise necessary to competently administer the therapy.

EDUCATION

Inclusion of complementary therapies into nursing curricula at all levels is needed if nurses are to be expected to incorporate these therapies into their practices. There has been little discussion about which therapies should be taught to basic nursing programs and which ones should be included in master's curricula. Content is necessary in the philosophy underlying complementary therapies and in specific therapies. Nursing students must learn to view complementary therapies as equally important to knowledge about technology and medications. Now, when the public has a keen interest in complementary therapies, educators have the opportunity to return these therapies to the place they had in nursing in Nightingale's time.

PRACTICE SETTINGS

On an individual basis and in facilities, nurses are incorporating complementary therapies into their practice. Some facilities have developed practice guidelines for the use of specific therapies. In some instances this may mean that only nurses who are certified or who have had additional preparation can administer the therapy. It is critical that not only guidelines for specific therapies be addressed, but also that the philosophy underlying complementary therapies, holism, and a sense of caring for the patient be emphasized. Adding therapies without permeating the facility with the philosophy will often result in nurses' viewing complementary therapies as just another task.

Examples of facilities that have integrated complementary therapies abound. Regions Hospital in St. Paul is one example (Horrigan, 2000). In addition to conventional care, nurses on an 18-bed medical-surgical unit routinely administer massage, aromatherapy, and music therapy. Patients are given opportunities to learn meditation and relaxation techniques, and nurses who have been prepared in other therapies may incorporate these therapies into their care. A second facility in Minnesota, Woodwinds Health Campus, is a new hospital that has as its philosophy an attitude of caring for the whole person. Complementary therapies are an integral part of the care provided in this 78-bed facility.

There has been concern about nurses using complementary therapies. Most states currently do not have specific legislation or guidelines for the use of complementary therapies. Perhaps it is not regulation that is needed, but a set of beliefs such as those put forth by the Royal College of Nursing in England (Buckle, 1997), whose beliefs include the following:

1. We believe that all patients and clients have the right to be offered and to receive complementary therapies either exclusively or as part of orthodox nursing practice.
2. We believe that all patients have the right to expect that their religious, cultural, and spiritual beliefs will be observed by nurses practicing complementary therapies.
3. We believe that all complementary therapies available to patients have the support of the collaborative team.
4. We believe that a registered nurse who is appropriately qualified to carry out a complementary therapy must agree to work to locally accepted protocols for practice and standards of care.

Another belief states that where possible the guidelines used should be based on research, and emphasis is also placed on the need to evaluate the effectiveness of the complementary therapy used. The RCN beliefs provide an excellent resource for facilities and individual nurses to review in establishing guidelines for the use of complementary therapies.

RESEARCH

One of the chief criticisms of complementary therapies is that they lack a scientific basis for use. Few complementary therapies have been studied using the gold standard of Western medicine, the double-blind clinical trial, but research has been conducted outside the United States. For example, scientists in Germany have conducted many studies on herbs. Many of the frequently used complementary therapies have been used for centuries; anecdotal evidence and case studies provide support for their efficacy, yet there is a need for additional studies.

Over the years, nurses have conducted research on a number of the complementary therapies, as can be noted in the references provided for the therapies in this book. Reviews of three therapies—music (Snyder & Chlan, 1999), patient-centered communication (Brown, 1999), and imagery (Feller, 1999)—were highlighted in the *Annual Review of Nursing Research* (Fitzpatrick, 1999). Experience with the administration of complementary therapies places nurses in a prime position for assuming leadership roles on interdisciplinary teams that are investigating complementary therapies. Many challenges exist in conducting research on many complementary therapies because current designs and measurement techniques may not be appropriate for therapies that have a philosophical basis that differs from the traditional Western therapies for which these methods were developed.

REFERENCES

Alternative Health Care Bill. H.F. 3839. Minnesota State Legislature. (2000).

Braun, C. A., Halcón, L. L., & Bearinger, L. H. (2000). Adolescent use of alternative and complementary therapies. *Journal of Holistic Nursing, 18,* 176–191.

Brown, S. J. (1999). Patient-centered communication. In J. F. Fitzpatrick (Ed.), *Annual review of nursing research* (Vol. 17, pp. 85–104). New York: Springer.

Bruener, C., Barry, P., & Kemper, K. (1998). Alternative medicine use by homeless youth. *Archives of Pediatric and Adolescent Medicine, 152,* 1071–1075.

Buckle, J. (1997). *Aromatherapy in nursing.* London: Arnold.

Cogan, R., Cogan D., Walz, W., & McCue, M. (1987). Effects of laughter and relaxation on discomfort levels. *Journal of Behavioral Medicine, 10,* 139–144.

Eisenberg, D. M., Kessler, R. C., Foster, C., Norlock, F. E., Calkins, D. R., & Delbanco, T. L. (1993). Unconventional medicine in the United States. *New England Journal of Medicine, 328,* 246–252.

Eisenberg, D. M., Davis, R. B., Ettner, S. L., Appel, S., Wilkey, S., Van Rommapy, M., & Kessler, R. C. (1998). Trends in alternative medicine use in the United States, 1990–1997. *Journal of the American Medical Association, 280,* 1569–1575.

Feller, L. S. (1999). Guided imagery interventions for symptom management. In J. F. Fitzpatrick (Ed.), *Annual review of nursing research* (Vol. 17, pp. 57–84). New York: Springer.

Fitzpatrick, J.F. (Ed.) (1999). *Annual review of nursing research* (Vol. 17). New York: Springer.

Fontaine, K. L. (2000). *Healing practices, alternative therapies for nursing.* Upper Saddle River, NJ: Prentice-Hall.

Horrigan, B. J. (2000). Regions hospital opens holistic nursing unit. *Alternative Therapies in Health and Medicine, 6*(4), 92–93.

Iowa Intervention Project. (1995). Validation and coding of the NIC taxonmy structure. *Image: Journal of Nursing Scholarship, 27,* 43–49.

Kreitzer, M. J., & Jensen, D. (2000). Healing practices: Trends, challenges, and opportunities for nurses in acute and critical care. *AACN Clinical Issues, 11,* 7–16.

Leonard, B. J., & Plotnikoff, G. A. (2000). Awareness: The heart of cultural competence. *AACN Clinical Issues, 11,* 51–59.

Milton, S. (1998). Using alternative and complementary therapies in the emergency setting. *Journal of Emergency Nursing, 24,* 500–508.

Mitzdorf, U., Beck, K., Horton-Hausknecht, J., Weidenhammer, W., Kindermann, A., Takaxc, M., Astor, G., & Melchart, D. (1999). Why do patients seek treatment in hospitals of complementary medicine? *Journal of Alternative and Complementary Medicine, 5,* 463–473.

Nightingale, F. (1936/1992). *Notes on nursing.* Philadelphia: Lippincott.

Panel on Definition and Description, CAM Research Methodology Conference. (1997). Defining and describing complementary and alternative medicine. *Alternative Therapies in Health and Medicine, 3*(2), 49–57.

Pelletier, K. R. (2000). *The best in alternative medicine: What works? What does not?* New York: Simon & Schuster.

Remen, R. N. (2000). *My grandfather's blessings.* New York: Riverhead Books.

Snyder, M., & Chlan, L. (1999). Music therapy. In J. F. Fitzpatrick (Ed.), *Annual review of nursing research* (Vol. 17, pp. 3–25). New York: Springer.

2

Self As Healer

Susan Towey and Barbara Leonard

As nursing students or practitioners of complementary/alternative therapies, the process of developing an authentic self is as integral as learning the technical skills for administering various complementary therapies. An individual's explorations of self-knowledge, self-awareness, consciousness, and spiritual development are an ongoing dialogue between the inner and outer aspects of one's being. The self as healer is a "both/and" concept rather than an "either/or" concept. A nurse must balance being in the moment and being fully present to a patient with walking the path of the self-healing journey. This is a lifelong unfolding process. Nurses integrating complementary therapies into their practice need to embark on the integrative path of personal inner and outer development as part of their educational journey. The student and the professional need to intentionally create personal ways to facilitate self-awareness and self-care methods.

Self-awareness and self-care are an integral part of reflective holistic nursing practice. In its code of ethics, the American Holistic Nurses Association states that "the nurse has a responsibility to model healthy behaviors. Holistic nurses strive to achieve harmony in their own lives and to assist others who are striving to do the same" (American Holistic Nurses Association, 1992, p. 275). Quinn (as cited in Horrigan, 1996) notes that nurses need to do their own work to become a healing energy for their patients. They need to become whole persons, live authentic lives, and become healed. The physical, emotional, and spiritual health of the practitioner-healer is experienced in the relationship with the patient. Commitment to the use of self as an "instrument of healing" and understanding it is the core concept of this chapter.

How do nurses care for themselves as instruments of healing as they care for patients? Metaphors used in the reductionistic biomedical health-care system help us understand the issues of self as healer. Just as instruments used in surgical procedures are washed and sterilized before being used for another procedure, professionals who are instruments of healing must identify models of self-care, interventions, and therapies that will ensure the cleansing of self in order to provide a personal energy field and space that facilitates healing for self and patients. In the literature on energy healing therapies, Brennan (1987) describes the human energy field as the "manifestation of universal energy that is intimately involved with human life" (p. 41). Energetic healing is a metaphor for healing that occurs at the quantum and electromagnetic levels of a person (Slater, 1995). Barbara Dossey, a leader in holistic nursing, stated that self-care includes activities that promote self-awareness and facilitate being an instrument of healing (Horrigan, 1999).

SELF-CARE

Becoming a healer is a very individual process, one that grows from the inside (Brennan, 1987). Each person is unique and must assess her or his individual strengths and talents. This assessment will help individuals strive toward wholeness in their journeys. There are multiple ways of creating a plan for self-care and intentional personal healing. Interventions need to be explored that help a person increase knowledge about self, become more aware of self including transpersonal (non-local) experiences, and accept the paradoxical mysteries in life.

Several concepts and techniques that are widely accepted as important in self-care are

- A balanced diet appropriate to current health needs
- Exercise appropriate to the individual
- Adequate sleep and rest
- Social support systems
- Stress management skills
- Meditation and prayer
- An active sense of humor (Towey, 1995, p. 11)

Many of the therapies included in this book can be used in self-care. Santorelli (1999) suggested use of mindfulness meditation, a mind-body intervention, to heal the self. Nature is another therapy frequently used in self-healing. Spending time in an outdoor, natural environment is innately renewing, restorative, and healing. According to Lewis (1996), "as we garden, tramp through field or forest, stroll in city parks, or rest beneath a tree, we may come to an unexpected door that opens inward to self" (p. xix). Two other interventions that can be used in self-care—spiritual direction and dreams—will be discussed.

SPIRITUAL DIRECTION

Spiritual direction is a time-honored, privileged relationship with a mentor who serves as a witness to the action of the holy in the life of a person seeking direction on their spiritual journey. Spiritual direction is sometimes referred to as spiritual friendship. Here, friendship is understood not as one who shares mutuality with another, but as one who shares with a professional person. A director is not a go-between, but one who has succeeded in reaching God (the term that will be used to designate a higher being) and can point the way.

Some form of spiritual direction can be found in most of the major religions of the world. Among traditional Native Americans, a medicine man or woman guides a vision quest, interprets dreams, and facilitates healing. They are typically elders who are recognized by their communities as having spiritual gifts. In the Christian tradition, spiritual direction has existed in various forms since antiquity. After the Reformation and before the most recent 30 years, spiritual direction was almost exclusive to monastic and religious life; lay persons rarely sought direction.

The modern spiritual director is a professional person who has received education in the art and practice of spiritual direction. Most directors receive ongoing direction and supervision and adhere to the ethics of the profession as specified by Spiritual Directors International. The credentials of a spiritual director are important, and they frequently collaborate with other professional persons who are providing care to the directee.

A nurse would seek spiritual direction primarily to reflect with another on the meaning of life experiences. Direction differs from psychotherapy or pastoral counseling in its focus (Edwards, 1980). In direction, the focus is on the inward movement of the spirit and not on problem solving or developing insight into one's problems. In the course of direction a person's life is frequently transformed as the holy or spiritual is experienced more deeply. The circumstances of one's life may appear unchanged, but the inner transformation will be evident in all aspects of life including professional work, personal relationships, and the environment. Problems may be solved as a side benefit but not as the primary focus. The goal of spiritual direction is discerning the holy in one's life and building a relationship with the sacred or spiritual.

Spiritual direction is about reflection on one's life in all of its complexity. At the heart of direction is one's unique relationship with God. For example, persons who come to direction in times of transition or crisis ask deep spiritual questions about the meaning of life. A director listens to those questions with empathetic reverence, never trying to fix the person or the problem. Rather, the director seeks to illuminate how God is working in and through these stressful circumstances to bring life to the person who is seeking direction. All of one's life experiences can be brought to direction but always at the discretion of the person seeking direction (Birmingham & Connolly, 1994). One's prayer life and dreams are frequently shared with the director. Prayer, meditation, and dreams provide precise spiritual information that is uncensored by the ego. They may reveal information that has direct applicability to one's circumstances.

DREAMS

The ancients asserted the relationship of health and dreams. Greek temples served as places to receive a dream. The given dream would reveal the nature of a person's illness or need, enabling the physician to prescribe treatment. In the West, until the 5th century dreams were respected by all religions as revealing the divine. After the 5th century, Christians were admonished to ignore dreams as they were thought to be linked with the occult. This thinking prevailed in the West until the 20th century but changed with the discovery of a mistranslation of scripture from the Greek to Latin 15 centuries earlier. Fortunately, dreams are once again recognized for their importance to human health (Kelsey, 1974). In the 20th century, Jungian psychology has contributed greatly to the restoration of dreams as a part of health and healing.

Dreams serve many functions for the psyche in healing and the maintenance of health. They give emotional compensation, reveal truths about life situations the ego resists, provide warnings, and uncommonly provide what Jung call archetypal understanding (Kelsey, 1974). An example of emotional healing occurred through a dream a woman had following her husband's death. She was in deep grief until her husband appeared to her in a dream, reassuring her that he was happy and wanted her to be as well. It freed her to move on with her life. While experts claim that few dreams are prophetic, dreams are specific to the individual. When interpreting them, the adage that only the dreamer knows for sure is correct. The meaning of the dream is for the person to interpret and not for someone else to do so although another person's insights may be helpful. For example, one dreamer with a recent diagnosis of cancer saw herself riding a bicycle, hitting a bump in the road, falling off of the bicycle, and then dusting herself off and riding on happily. A trusted friend helped her to see the relationship between the bump in the road and her cancer. The dream reassured her that she would be able to continue her journey.

All humans and many animals dream, but unless they are recorded, dreams are not remembered. A time-tested way to remember dreams is to jot them down even in the middle of the night (a pad and pencil at the bedside aids this process). When one awakens, the dream fades quickly and cannot be recalled unless it recurs. The process of interpreting the dream is done by rewriting the dream in as much detail as possible without editing it. One notes the words, the feeling state, and the sequence of the events in the dream. Once the dream is recorded without editing, interpretation can begin. Words may be looked up in the dictionary, and the dream can be meditated upon for further understanding. Dreams provide a unique opportunity to understand one's self, one's needs, and how to change one's life. They are amazingly accurate and are always given for the good of the dreamer (Guiley, 1998; Kelsey, 1978).

THE TRANSFORMATIONAL JOURNEY

Healing is a key element of the transformational journey. Keegan (1994) defines healing as the integration of the totality of humankind in body, mind, and spirit. Therefore, the healer is one who is capable of producing and catalyzing integration within self and patients. Keegan further notes that "the spiritual journey involves the process an individual undergoes in the search of the meaning and purpose of life" (p. 4).

The initiation of a healer in ancient cultures was a rigorous process that included a personal journey of inner development and transformation that were part of the process of becoming healer. For centuries, cultures have treated inner transformation as a necessary and desirable aspect of life. The invisible aspects of healing are a part of past and present cultures. The universal aspects of shamanism work with inner aspects of healing through the use of altered states of consciousness (Grof & Grof, 1990). Like the Greek mythological figure Chiron, shamans, as wounded healers, have the gift for healing others while remaining unable to heal themselves. A nurse's transformational healing journey is a living mythology of both the woundedness of Chiron and current knowledge about one's ability and need to connect with the inner healer (Santorelli, 1999).

In keeping with Taoist philosophy, Mindell (as cited in Bodian, 1991) believed a person's path unfolds each moment in ways that are meant to happen, and that the task is to learn to follow this unfolding process. Trusting in this process may help reveal a deeper significance. The journey to becoming a healer is very personal, and the strategies and methods used to work with these inner dimensions of the self are an individual responsibility of discernment.

As the 21st century begins, the rapid transformation of health care systems and health profession education has placed great demands on the time, energy, spirit, and health of health care professionals and students. Nurses and other health care employees are often caught in the cross-fire of mergers, downsizing, redesign, and other changes that create uncertainty and anxiety in the work environment (Disch & Towey, 1998). The current national nursing shortage is making work environments more stressful, and professionals must rapidly acquire new information in order to accomplish their work. Limits of time and economic resources in health care create many challenges to health professionals (Buerhaus, 1996). The paradox of the 21st century requires new perspectives in education that incorporate self-healing practices. The challenge for health professional education is creating models that include content on healing, caring relationships with patients and with colleagues (Pew-Fetzer, 1994).

Viewing time as an enemy creates stress that is not conducive to a healing environment in the workplace (Lofy, 2000). Bailey (1999) identifies the dimensions of the loss of quality relationships with each other as one more unhealthy factor in workplaces. Time spent with self or another person is an integral part of healing: In the midst of a person's busy and chaotic life, longings surface for time to listen to the voice of inner wisdom. Silence may help reduce stress (Rubin, 2000), yet silent reflection is often difficult to attain without intentionally setting aside time for quiet. Uncertainty is another stressor in current health care settings. Finding ways to maintain hope, develop resiliency, and nurture supportive interpersonal relationships may be helpful in the face of uncertainty (Towey, 1995).

Increased awareness is an integral part of the transformational journey of the healer. The science of unitary consciousness (Watson, 1995) and health as expanding consciousness (Newman, 1994) are nursing models that describe the evolution of consciousness in health and healing. Newman's "pattern recognition" and Watson's "unitary-transformative" models provide descriptions of phenomena of the unseen world of human and spiritual energy systems.

The Dalai Lama (1999) described the ethics he believes are needed for the 21st century. In addition to restraint, virtue, and compassion, he also identifies the need for discerning the truth in the unseen world, which takes a healthy level of spiritual development, discipline, and practice.

FUTURE RESEARCH

Watson (1995) described a research methodology that incorporates a creative combination of unfolding and evolving approaches for studying nursing problems. This model may be an excellent one for studying complementary therapies, the complexity of physical and nonphysical phenomena, and non-local and transcendent consciousness. Future research that may contribute to knowledge about self care and the nurse as healer includes:

- Qualitative studies of the transformational journeys of healers
- Studies of the effects of the energy field of the healer on the patient and colleagues
- A survey of healers to identify their self-care methods
- Identification of core methods of self-care
- Studies of the outcomes of changes in practitioners who practice med-itation

REFERENCES

American Holistic Nurses Association. (1992). Code of ethics for holistic nurses. *Journal of Holistic Nursing, 10*(3), 275–276.

Bailey, J. (1999). *The speed trap: How to avoid the frenzy of the fast lane.* San Francisco: HarperCollins.

Birmingham, M., & Connolly, W. J. (1994). *Witnessing to the fire: Spiritual direction and the development of directors. One center's experience.* Kansas City, MO: Sheed & Ward.

Bodian, S. (1991). *Timeless visions, healing voices: Conversations wih men and women of the spirit.* Freedom, CA: The Crossing Press.

Brennan, B. (1987). *Hands of light: A guide to healing through the human energy field.* New York: Bantam Books.

Buerhaus, P. (1996). Understanding the economic environment of health care. In J. M. Disch (Series Ed.), *AONE Leadership Series: The managed care challenge for nurse executives* (pp. 1–15). American Hospital Publishing.

Dalai Lama, (1999). *Ethics for the new millennium.* New York: Riverhead.

Disch, J., & Towey, S. (1998). Unit III case study: The healthy work environment as core to an organization's success. In D. Mason & J. Leavitt (Eds.), *Policy and politics in nursing and health care* (pp. 332–346). Philadelphia: W. B. Saunders.

Edwards, T. (1980). *Spiritual friend: Reclaiming the gift of spiritual direction.* New York: Paulist Press.

Grof, S., & Grof, C. (1990). *The stormy search for the self.* New York: Tarcher-Putnam.

Guiley, R. (1998) *Dreamwork for the soul: A spiritual guide to dream interpretation.* New York: Berkley.

Horrigan, B. (1996). Janet Quinn, RN, PhD on therapeutic touch and a healing way. [Interview] *Alternative Therapies in Health and Medicine, 2*(4), 68–75.

Horrigan, B. (1999) Barbara Dossey, RN, MS on holistic nursing, Florence

Nightingale, and the healing rituals. [Interview] *Alternative Therapies in Health and Medicine, 5*(1), 79–86.

Keegan, L. (1994). *The nurse as healer.* Albany, NY: Delmar.

Kelsey, M.T. (1974). *God, dreams & revelation: A Christian interpretation of dreams.* Minneapolis, MN: Augsburg Publishing House.

Kelsey, M.T. (1978) *Dreams: A way to listen to God.* New York: Paulist Press.

Lewis, C. (1996). *Green nature/human nature: The meaning of plants in our lives.* Urbana and Chicago: University of Illinois Press.

Lofy, M. (2000). *A matter of time: Power, control, and meaning in people's everyday experience of time.* Unpublished doctoral dissertation, the Fielding Institute, Santa Barbara, CA.

Newman, M. (1994). *Health as expanding consciousness.* New York: National League for Nursing.

Rubin, A. (2000). *The power of silence: Using technology to create free structure in organizations.* Unpublished master's thesis, the Fielding Institute, Santa Barbara, CA.

Santorelli, S. (2000). *Heal thyself: Lessons on mindfulness in medicine.* New York: Bell Tower.

Slater, V. (1995). Toward an understanding of energetic healing, Part I: Energetic structures. *Journal of Holistic Nursing, 13*(3), 209–224.

Towey, S. (1995). Personal and professional skills for living with uncertainty. *Creative Nursing, 2*(1), 9–11.

Tresolini, C. P., and the Pew-Fetzer Task Force (1994). *Health professions education and relationship-centered care.* San Francisco: Pew Health Professions Commission.

Watson, J. (1995). Nursing's caring-healing paradigm as exemplar for alternative medicine? *Alternative Therapies in Health and Medicine, 1*(3), 64–69.

3

Presence

Mariah Snyder, Yueh-hsia Tseng,
and Cheryl Brandt

Presence is a complementary therapy that is integral to the administration of all complementary therapies, though it can be used independently of other therapies. Presence is closely related to the therapy of active listening, and the two therapies share many characteristics. Although recognized for centuries within nursing, research on presence has been initiated only recently. This research has largely been conducted in conjunction with the concept of caring.

DEFINITION

Two of the pioneers in this field, Paterson and Zderad (1976), described presence as the process of being available with the whole of oneself and open to the experience of another through a reciprocal interpersonal encounter. Gardner (1992) expanded on this definition by adding specifics related to physical and psychological presence. She defined presence as "the physical *being there* and the psychological *being with* a patient for the purpose of meeting the patient's health care needs" (p. 191). According to Liehr (1989), the nurse needs to be genuinely engaged with the patient for true presence to occur. True presence requires the nurse to be sensitive to the patient's emotions, particularly anger, joy, fear, and pain and for the nurse to accept herself or himself and bring this into the encounter.

Benner (1984) chose the verb *presencing* to denote the existential practice of being with a patient. Presencing is one of the eight competencies Benner identified as constituting the helping role of the nurse. This view of presence in nursing is supported by Parse (1992) who characterized presence as "the primary mode of nursing practice" (p. 40).

Presence is reciprocal: The interaction must be meaningful to both the patient and the nurse. According to Pettigrew (1990), nurses must be willing to be involved in the interaction, and the interaction must be deemed meaningful by the patient for presence to produce positive patient outcomes. This transactional characteristic of presence was emphasized by McKivergin and Day (1998): in presence, the nurse is available to the patient with the wholeness of her or his unique individual being. Presence can be characterized as a process that consists of an exchange in which meaningful awareness on the part of the nurse helps to bring integration and balance to the life of the patient (Snyder, Brandt, & Tseng, 2000).

Several classifications of presence have been developed (McKivergin & Daubenmire, 1994; Osterman & Schwartz-Barcott, 1996). The continuum in both classifications extends from merely being physically present with the patient to being available with the wholeness of self. Table 3.1 describes the categories of presence and provides example of each type of presence. It is only the transcendent (Osterman & Schwartz-Barcott, 1996) or therapeutic presence (McKivergin & Daubenmire, 1994) that constitutes the complementary therapy designated as presence.

SCIENTIFIC BASIS

Paterson and Zderad (1976) recognized presence as an integral component of their theory of humanistic nursing. Presence implies an openness, a receptivity, readiness, or availability on the part of the nurse. Many nursing situations require close proximity to another person, but that in itself does not constitute presence. In order to experience the lived dialogue of nursing, the nurse responds with an openness to a "person-with-needs" and with an "availability-in-a-helping way" (Paterson & Zderad, 1976). Reciprocity often emerges through the dialogue.

Presence is closely aligned with caring. It involves the nurse as "co-participant" in the caring process (Watson, 1985). Caring requires the nurse to be keenly attentive to the needs of the patient, the meaning the patient attaches to the illness or problem, and how the patient wishes to proceed. According to Watson, "a truly caring nurse/artist is able to destroy in the consciousness of the recipient the separation between him or herself and the nurse" (p. 68). The use of presence assists the patient to healing, discovery, and finding meaning.

The body of knowledge documenting patients' perceptions of the value of presence is evolving. Much of the research on presence is found within studies on caring. Presence was one of the major constructs of caring identified by Leininger (1984) in her multicultural studies of caring.

TABLE 3.1   Examples of Use of the Various Types of Presence

Types of Presence	Example
Presence/partial presence (Osterman & Schwartz-Barcott, 1996); physical presence (McKivergin & Daubenmire, 1994)	Routine tasks such as taking vital signs and administering medications; nurse enters a patient's room to check the blood pressure, doing so deftly but failing to notice the tears slipping from the patient's eyes; nurse is absorbed in own thoughts.
Full presence (Osterman & Schwartz-Barcott, 1996); psychological presence (McKivergin & Daubenmire, 1994)	Nurse enters patient room to check ventilator. The nurse greets the patient by name and uses personalized ways of interacting with the patient. The nurse is attentive to nonverbal responses of the patient and will occasionally touch the patient. Needs are assessed and a plan of care is developed in conjunction with the patient.
Transcendent presence (Osterman & Schwartz-Barcott, 1996); therapeutic presence (McKivergin & Daubenmire, 1994)	The nurse uses centering before entering the patient's room. The nurse greets the patient by name while simultaneously holding the patient's hand or arm. The nurse uses all of her personal resources of body, mind, emotions, and spirit in being present and available to the patient. The nurse is attentive to responses of the patient and directs attention to specific concerns. All of these can be done while simultaneously regulating the IV or doing other care activities.

Note: From "Use of Presence in the Critical Care Unit," by M. Snyder, C. Brandt, and Y. Tseng, 2000, *AACN Clinical Issues: Advanced Practice in Acute and Critical Care,* 11(1), pp. 27–33. Copyright 2000 by Lippincott. Reprinted with permission.

Nurse researchers have sought to elicit patients' views of the caring behaviors of nurses. Brown (1986) asked 50 adult patients to describe experiences in which they felt that nurses had truly cared for them as persons. Eight themes were identified: recognition of individual qualities and needs; reassuring presence; provision of information; demonstration of professional expertise; assistance with pain management; time spent with the patient;

promotion of autonomy; and use of surveillance. While all of these themes have some association with presence, two (reassuring presence and time spent) are integral components of presence. Presence was also validated as a caring behavior in a study by Hegedus (1999).

Similar findings have been reported in other studies. In a qualitative study by Riemen (1986) of patients' perceptions of nurses' behaviors, noncaring actions included having minimal contact with the patient and being physically present but emotionally distant. Availability, kindness, and consideration were desired characteristics identified by patients in a study by Cronin and Harrison (1988). Engaging in a reciprocal process with the nurse was one of the caring behaviors identified by patients who had been discharged from a critical care unit (Burfitt, Greiner, Miers, Kinney, & Branyon, 1993).

Studies on the expert practice of critical-care nurses have demonstrated the importance of presence. Minick (1995) found that connectedness with the patient was important not only as a caring behavior but also because it assisted the nurse in the early identification of postoperative problems. Presence may help nurses to be more attentive and to detect subtle changes that may not be evident in the absence of therapeutic presence. Nurses who lacked this connectedness were perceived by their patients as detached. Hanneman (1996) explored the effects of expert nurses on care outcomes and she found that these nurses displayed two characteristics: presence with and focused assessment of a patient's situation. Use of presence included attentiveness to the patient that was grounded within the care situation.

Mohnkern (1992) queried 15 nurses to identify the antecedents, defining attributes, and consequences of presence. Antecedents to presence included a patient who trusts the nurse and has a need to have her or his life processes facilitated; and a nurse who possesses a sense of mission, has an altruistic desire to help the patient, and is willing and strong enough to be open to the experience of the patient. Attributes of presence identified by Mohnkern were physical closeness between the nurse and the patient, a metaphysical connection between the nurse and patient in which energy is exchanged, and the nurse using a range of skills to facilitate the patient's experience. Perspectives of patients were not reported.

The importance of presence in care has been recognized for centuries. Documentation of why it plays a role in health outcomes is slowly evolving.

INTERVENTION

The description of presence related by Mitch Albom (1997) in *Tuesdays With Morrie* succinctly captures the essential elements of presence. Albom is reporting how Morrie, a man with advanced amyotrophic lateral sclerosis, viewed presence:

> I believe in being fully present. That means you should be with the person you're with. When I'm talking with you now, Mitch, I try to keep focused only on what is going on between us. I am not thinking about something we said last week. I am not thinking about what's coming up this Friday. I am not thinking about doing another Koppel show, or about medications I'm taking. I am talking to you, I am thinking about you. (pp. 135–136)

CENTERING

Presence entails conscious attention to the upcoming interaction with the patient. The nurse must be available with the whole of self and be open to the experience of the patient. This process is called *centering*, a meditative state (Egan, 1998). The nurse takes a short time, sometimes only 10 or 20 seconds, to eliminate distractions, so that the focus can be on the patient. Some persons find that taking a deep breath and closing the eyes helps in freeing the self of distractions and becoming centered. This may be done outside the room or setting in which the encounter will occur. Centering allows the nurse to be open to the personal and care needs of the patient. Centering may also be as simple as the nurse's pausing before contact with the patient and repeating the patient's name to help focus attention on that person.

TECHNIQUE

Table 3.2 lists the key components of presence and the skills necessary for practicing presence. Sensitivity to the other requires the nurse to be an excellent listener and observer. (Active listening is addressed in chapter 4.) Good observation skills assist nurses in identifying nuances in expression and communication that may reveal the real concerns of the patient. Presence often means periods of silence in which subtle interchanges occur. Continuing attentiveness on the part of the nurse is a critical aspect of this therapy. Through presence, a connectedness with the patient occurs. Both the nurse and the client experience a sense of union or joining for a moment in time.

Little is known about the length of a therapy session or when therapeutic presence should be used. Often the nurse identifies this in an intuitive manner: It just seems like this patient truly needs me now. Because of the intense nature of the interaction, the length of time the nurse is present to the patient may seem greater though only a minute or a two may have passed. Presence

TABLE 3.2   Presence: Key Components and Necessary Skills

Key Components	Necessary Skills
Whole person to whole person interaction	Centering
Intersubjectivity	Sensitivity and openness
Direction of self toward other	Communication and active listening
Attentiveness	
Accountability	

Note: From "Use of Presence in the Critical Care Unit," by M. Snyder, C. Brandt, and Y. Tseng, 2000, AACN *Clinical Issues: Advanced Practice in Acute and Critical Care, 11*(1), pp. 27–33. Copyright 2000 by Lippincott. Reprinted with permission.

is often used in conjunction with another therapy or treatment. However, identifying when a patient needs someone to *just be present* for a few minutes may be the most effective therapy.

MEASUREMENT OF EFFECTIVENESS

Measuring outcomes of presence interventions will involve both the client and the nurse because of the reciprocal interaction in presence. Comments from the patient about feeling cared for, being able to express concerns, and feeling understood are some outcome measures that can be used. The consequences of presence identified by Mohnkern (1992) included improved psychosocial, spiritual, and emotional functioning; improved physical functioning or a peaceful death; and an appreciation of more interaction with the nurse. According to Mohnkern, one consequence noted by nurses was an affirmation of their role as nurses. Because of the intangibles that often occur with the use of presence, finding words or indices to measure presence may be difficult.

PRECAUTIONS

The major precaution in the use of presence is to take one's cue from the patient and not force a presence encounter. A true presence encounter considers the wants and needs of the patient and is not for the nurse's primary benefit. If the nurse is "available with the whole of oneself and open to the experience" of the client, as the definition states, the nurse will be attentive to the patient and act in accordance with the wishes and needs of the patient.

One negative consequence of presence identified by Mohnkern (1992) was nurses reporting that colleagues were critical about the time they spent with patients and families. Certainly this should not be a deterrent to the use of presence, but rather a concern that should be discussed and resolved by nursing staff.

USES

Presence can be used in any nursing situation. Persons struggling with a new diagnosis, an exacerbation of a condition, or with a loss are especially in need of moments of presence. Moch (1995) included presence as part of a psychosocial intervention for women diagnosed with breast cancer and found the intervention to be helpful to these women. Presence is of particular value with hospice patients (Raudonis, 1993; Zerwekh, 1995).

Presence is also needed with patients in critical care settings (Snyder et al., 2000). Patients and their families often feel lost in high-tech critical-care settings. The use of presence helps prevent critical-care nurses being viewed by their patients as emotionally distant and being there "only because it is part of their job" (Riemen, 1986, p. 32). Marsden (1990) noted that the use of technology in critical-care units may be dehumanizing unless nurses practice in more than a perfunctory, technically competent but detached manner. Research suggests that incorporating the therapy of presence in critical-care settings can go a long way to making this a less traumatic experience for patients (Mohnkern, 1992).

FUTURE RESEARCH

Nurses often chart assessments and specific treatments but rarely document the use of presence and the outcomes of this therapy. Those seeking complementary therapies have noted that caring practitioners are one of the reasons they seek and use these therapies. Despite the challenges in identifying and documenting outcomes of presence, current interest in complementary therapies provides an opportunity for nursing to validate the positive outcomes from the use of presence. Areas in which research is needed include the following:

1. While every patient could benefit from presence, large caseloads often place restrictions on nurses' time. What are assessments that would alert nurses to patients who most need the therapy of presence?
2. What are some effective strategies for increasing the use of presence by nurses and other health professionals?

3. With the advent of telemedicine, how can presence be introduced into these contacts with patients? Is physical presence essential or is presence a non-local phenomenon like prayer?

REFERENCES

Albom, M. (1997). *Tuesdays With Morrie*. New York: Doubleday.

Benner, P. (1984). *From novice to expert: Excellence and power in clinical nursing practice*. Menlo Park, CA: Addison-Wesley.

Brown, L. (1986). The experience of care: Patient perspectives. *Topics in Clinical Nursing, 8*, 56–62.

Burfitt, S. N., Greiner, D. S., Miers, L. J., Kinney, M. R., & Branyon, M. E. (1993). Professional nurse caring as perceived by critically ill patients: A phenomenologic study. *American Journal of Critical Care, 2*, 489–499.

Cronin, S. N., & Harrison, B. (1988). Importance of nurse caring behaviors as perceived by patients after myocardial infarction. *Heart and Lung, 17*, 374–380.

Egan, E. C. (1998). Therapeutic touch. In M. Snyder & R. Lindquist (Eds.), *Complementary/alternative therapies in nursing* (pp. 49–62). New York: Springer.

Gardner, D. L. (1992). Presence. In G. M. Bulechek & J. C. McCloskey (Eds.), *Nursing interventions: Essential nursing treatments* (2nd ed., pp. 191–200). Philadelphia: W. B. Saunders.

Hanneman, S. K. (1996). Advancing nursing practice with a unit-based clinical expert. *Image: Journal of Nursing Scholarship, 28*, 331–337.

Hegedus, K. S. (1999). Providers' and consumers' perspective of nurses caring behaviors. *Journal of Advanced Nursing, 30*, 1090–1096.

Leininger, M. M. (1984). *Care: The essence of nursing*. Thorofare, NJ: Slack.

Liehr, P. R. (1989). The core of true presence: A loving center. *Nursing Science Quarterly, 2*(1), 7–8.

Marsden, C. (1990). Ethical issues in critical care. *Heart and Lung, 19*, 540–541.

McKivergin, M., & Daubenmire, J. (1994). The essence of therapeutic presence. *Journal of Holistic Nursing, 12*(1), 65–81.

McKivergin, M., & Day, A. (1998). Presence: Creating order out of chaos. *Seminars in Perioperative Nursing, 7*, 96–100.

Minick, P. (1995). The power of human caring: Early recognition of patient problems. *Scholarly Inquiry for Nursing Practice: An International Journal, 9*, 303–317.

Mohnkern, S. M. (1992). *Presence in nursing, its antecedent, defining attributes, and consequences*. Doctoral dissertation, University of Texas, Austin.

Moch, S. D. (1995). *Breast cancer: Twenty women's stories*. New York: National League for Nursing Press.

Osterman, P., & Schwartz-Barcott, D. (1996). Presence: Four ways of being there. *Nursing Forum, 31*, 23–30.

Parse, R. R. (1992). Human becoming: Parse's theory of nursing. *Nursing Science Quarterly, 5,* 35–42.

Paterson, J. G., & Zderad, L. T. (1976). *Humanistic nursing.* New York: John Wiley.

Pettigrew, J. (1990). Intensive nursing care: The ministry of presence. *Critical Care Nursing Clinics of North America, 2,* 503–508.

Raudonis, B. M. (1993). The meaning and impact of empathic relationships in hospice nursing. *Cancer Nursing, 16,* 304–309.

Riemen, D. J. (1986). Noncaring and caring in the clinical setting: Patients' descriptions. *Topics in Clinical Nursing, 8,* 30–36.

Snyder, M., Brandt, C. L., & Tseng, Y. (2000). Use of presence in the critical care unit. *AACN Clinical Issues, 11,* 27–33.

Watson, J. (1985). *Nursing: Human science and human care, a theory of nursing.* Norwalk, CT: Appleton-Century-Crofts.

Zerwekh, J. V. (1995). A family caregiving model for hospice nursing. *Hospice Journal, 10,* 27–44.

4

Therapeutic Listening

Shigeaki Watanuki, Mary Fran Tracy,
and Ruth Lindquist

Therapeutic listening is an integral part of nurse-client relationships. Listening is one of the most effective therapeutic techniques available (Sundeen, Stuart, Rankin, & Cohen, 1998), and the theoretical underpinnings of therapeutic listening can be traced back to counseling psychology and psychotherapy. Rogers (1957) used counseling and listening to foster independence and promote growth and development of clients and emphasized that empathy, warmth, and genuineness with clients were necessary and sufficient for therapeutic changes to occur. In nursing, Travelbee (1971) described the nurses' conscious use of self and the directing of their full awareness to clients as foundational to the establishment of therapeutic relationships.

DEFINITION

Listening is an active and dynamic process of interaction that requires intentional effort to attend to a client's verbal and nonverbal cues. A variety of modifiers are used with the word *listening*, including active, therapeutic, empathic, and holistic. The choice of modifier seems to depend more on the authors' paradigm than on differences in the descriptions of listening (Fredriksson, 1999). Unless active listening was explicitly used by researchers in the articles reviewed, the term therapeutic listening is used here to focus on the formal, deliberate actions of listening for therapeutic purposes (Lekander, Lehmann, & Lindquist, 1993). Therapeutic listening is defined as "an interpersonal, confirmation process involving all the senses in which the therapist attends with empathy to the client's verbal and nonverbal messages to facilitate the understanding, synthesis, and interpretation of the client's situation" (Kemper, 1992, p.22).

Empathy is a concept related to therapeutic listening in that therapeutic listening has been viewed as a measurable dimension of empathy (Olson & Iwasiw, 1987). Empathy involves intellect, internal motivation to relate to another, subjective feelings, and communication (Rogers, 1957; Morse et al., 1992). Basic empathy develops in the process of becoming adult; therapeutic empathy develops through training and builds on basic empathy (Alligood, 1992).

SCIENTIFIC BASIS

In nursing, medical, and counseling psychology literature, listening tends to be addressed anecdotally rather than scientifically. Only a limited number of systematic studies of listening can be found in the literature (Fredriksson, 1999).

In a study of client outcomes, client distress was inversely associated with nurse-expressed empathy and client-perceived empathy (Olson & Hanchett, 1997). Communication training for nurses and other health care providers was found to have positive effects on clients' well-being. Clients in a cancer center who were cared for by nurses trained in therapeutic listening showed significantly less anxiety and hostility than those cared for by untrained nurses (La Monica, Wolf, Madea, & Oberst, 1987). Clients of a community mental-health center who perceived that the practitioner used skills of empathy, listening, openness, and genuineness were more satisfied with the care received (Sheppard, 1993). In another study, a 6-hour communication-skills training module attended by 26 RN graduates was effective in improving their skills. An analysis of the students' audiotaped verbal responses to clinical vignettes revealed that active listening scores increased significantly, while attempts to suppress or discount clients' feelings decreased significantly when compared to pretraining scores (Olson & Iwasiw, 1987).

Several other studies did not support the effectiveness of training programs. Empathy scores based on clients' perception and nurses' self-report did not improve as a result of training programs although the level of patient distress decreased (La Monica et al., 1987). The level of patient satisfaction did not significantly improve after a health-system-wide communication-training program for physicians, although their self-assessed scores of confidence and communication style improved significantly (Brown, Boles, Mullooly, & Levinson, 1999). These inconclusive results point to the complexities of disentangling relationships between empathic interpersonal and therapeutic listening skills and client outcomes. Problems with studies of therapeutic listening include the lack of a clear theoretical framework, limitations in design and measurement sensitivity, and deficiencies of sample size, which contribute to inconclusive results (Kruijver, Kerkstra, Francke, Bensing, & van de Wiel, 2000).

The helping styles of psychotherapists, crisis intervenors, and untrained individuals were compared with those of nursing school seniors who were completing a course in interpersonal relationships. The students were similar to trained psychotherapists in their use of empathic listening as evidenced by statements reflecting affect and content (Ryden, McCarthy, Lewis, & Sherman, 1991). Reid-Ponte (1992) found that primary nurses with more education or with longer professional experience were rated by the clients as less empathic, perceiving, feeling, and listening than nurses with less education or shorter professional experience. This may reflect the realities of busy clinical settings or the fact that experienced nurses use intuition rather than therapeutic listening to elicit clients' feelings and needs.

Biophysiological instruments can be useful in capturing the process changes of clients and nurses. Electroencephalography (EEG) changes were observed during client-centered interviews conducted by a nurse trained with Rogers' psychotherapy techniques (Minamisawa & Mitoh, 1997). An increased frequency of the nurses' alpha wave activity (implying a relaxed state) was observed when the nurse perceived that she established empathic rapport and active presence with her client. The client's EEG pattern also showed occasional increased frequency of alpha wave activity at about the same time as that of the nurse interviewer.

Qualitative methodologies provide rich understanding of the nature of therapeutic listening and explore the meaning and experience of being listened to in the context of real-world settings. Self-expression opportunities that enable clients to be listened to and understood can promote clients' self-discovery, meaning reconstruction, and healing (Myers, 2000; Sandelowski, 1994). Phenomenological methods have been used to explore and deeply understand what participants say in relation to the meaning of their experience (Hirose, 1999).

INTERVENTION

Therapeutic listening enables clients to better understand their feelings and to experience being understood by another caring person. There are multiple levels of listening that range from simple acknowledgement of what the client says to the deepest level of entering an intuitive relationship with the client (Rowan, 1986). Effective engagement in therapeutic listening requires nurses to be aware of verbal and nonverbal communication that conveys explicit and implicit messages. When words contradict nonverbal messages, communicators rely more often on nonverbal cues; facial expression, tone of voice, and silence are as important as words in determining the meaning of a message (Kacperek, 1997; Mehrabian, 1971).

GUIDELINES

Therapeutic listening is more than simply hearing the words being said; it requires the receiver to tune into the client and to use all the senses in analyzing, inferring, and evaluating the stated and underlying meaning of the client's message. Therapeutic listening requires concentration and an ability to differentiate between what is actually being said and what one wants or expects to hear. Schlesinger (1994) cautions listeners to avoid making assumptions that might lead them to hear what they think the client ought to say. It may be difficult to listen accurately and interpret messages they find difficult to relate to (Egan, 1990) or to listen to information that they may not want to hear. The brain is capable of processing information much more rapidly than the rate at which the average person talks (Davis, 1984), leaving the listener with free brain time during which it is easy to become distracted or to start formulating a response rather than to stay focused on the message. Many techniques can be used to maximize the effectiveness of therapeutic listening (Koshy, 1989). Table 4.1 presents selected techniques for this type of intervention.

MEASUREMENT OF OUTCOMES

Inclusion of multiple quantitative measures such as self-report, behavioral observation, physiological measures, and qualitative methods provide a rich and full approach to the study of therapeutic listening. Challenges include the isolation of therapeutic listening as an independent variable and the complexity of a multivariate design (Bennett, 1995). Nurse outcomes (knowledge, skills, attitudes, or behavioral change) and client outcomes need to be considered in study design (Kruijver et al., 2000).

Positive changes in psychological variables such as anxiety, depression, hostility, or nursing-care satisfaction are potential client outcomes of therapeutic listening. It may also be useful to examine physiological measures (heart rate, blood pressure, respiratory rate, temperature, oxygen saturation, EEG) as outcomes of therapeutic interchange. Outcomes may also include clinical variables such as length of stay, compliance, morbidity, and cost.

TABLE 4.1   Therapeutic Listening Techniques

Active Presence: Active presence involves focus on the client to interpret the message that he/she is trying to convey, recognition of themes, and hearing what is left unsaid.

Accepting Attitude: An accepting attitude will allow clients to feel comfortable expressing themselves. This can be demonstrated by short affirmative responses or gestures.

Clarifying Statements: Clarifying statements and summarizing can help the listener verify message interpretation and create clarity. Encourage specificity rather than vague statements to facilitate communication. Rephrasing and reflection can assist the client in self-understanding.

Use of Silence: Use of silence can encourage the client to talk, facilitate the nurse to focus on listening rather than formulating responses, and reduce the use of leading questions.

Tone: Tone of voice can express more than the actual words through empathy, judgment, or acceptance. Match the intensity of the tone appropriately to the message received to avoid minimizing or overemphasizing.

Nonverbal: Clients relaying sensitive information may be very aware of the listener's body language and will be viewed as either accepting of the message or closed to it, judgmental, and/or disinterested. Eye contact is essential to convey true interest. Maintaining a conversational distance and judicious use of touch may increase the client's comfort. Cultural and social awareness is important to avoid undesired touch.

Environment: Distractions should be eliminated to encourage the therapeutic interchange. Therapeutic listening may require careful planning to provide time for undivided attention or may occur spontaneously. Some clients may feel very comfortable having family present while others may feel inhibited when others are present.

PRECAUTIONS

Therapeutic listening has at its heart the intent to be helpful, so few precautions seem warranted. However, sensitivity and awareness to cultural variations of communication styles are vital to the effectiveness of the intervention, because there may be cultural differences in meanings of certain words or in nonverbal communication including silence, touch, smile, or presence (Seidel, Ball, Dains, & Benedict, 1995). Maintaining boundaries during therapeutic listening is important; empathy may be demonstrated without crossing professional therapeutic boundaries. Referrals for professional counseling may be indicated in cases including psychiatric crises. Ethical dilemmas may result if there are conflicts in keeping clients' confidentiality versus the professional responsibility for taking action based on sensitive information shared in the therapeutic exchange.

USES

There is potentially an unlimited number of situations where therapeutic listening would be an appropriate intervention to promote positive outcomes of care. Examples noted in the literature include increasing client satisfaction among community-dwelling mentally impaired individuals (Sheppard, 1993); promoting empathic understanding among clients with cancer (Hirose, 1999); improving empathic and therapeutic skills in nursing students (Olson & Iwasiw, 1987); understanding the lived experience of loss and grief (Gibbons, 1993). Other opportune situations would include client crisis, perioperative settings, palliative care, dying process, addressing complex family dynamics in critical care, personnel management, and anxiety disorder among adolescents.

FUTURE RESEARCH

There are many potentially interesting scientific and scholarly research questions to pursue in this area.

- Can therapeutic listening via phone or other interactive technology be effective at a distance?
- How could systematic therapeutic listening contribute to client and family satisfaction?
- Can client outcomes be improved using therapeutic listening on a regular basis?
- What are the psychosocial or spiritual effects of therapeutic listening?
- How do multicultural differences manifest in the processes and effectiveness of therapeutic listening?

REFERENCES

Alligood, M. R. (1992). Empathy: The importance of recognizing two types. *Journal of Psychosocial Nursing & Mental Health Services, 30*(3), 14–17.

Bennett, J. A. (1995). Methodological notes on empathy: Further considerations. *Advances in Nursing Science, 18*(1), 36–50.

Brown, J. B., Boles, M., Mullooly, J. P., & Levinson, W. (1999). Effect of clinician communication skills training on patient satisfaction: A randomized, controlled trial. *Annals of Internal Medicine, 131,* 822–829.

Davis, A. J. (1984). *Listening and responding.* St. Louis, MO: Mosby.

Egan, G. C. (1990). *The skilled helper: A systematic approach to effective helping* (4th ed.). Pacific Grove, CA: Brooks/Cole.

Fredriksson, L. (1999). Modes of relating in a caring conversation: A research synthesis on presence, touch and listening. *Journal of Advanced Nursing, 30,* 1167–1176.

Gibbons, M. B. (1993). Listening to the lived experience of loss. *Pediatric Nursing, 19,* 597–599.

Hirose, H. (1999). Classifying the empathic understanding of the nurse psychotherapist. *Cancer Nursing, 22,* 204–211.

Kacperek, L. (1997). Non-verbal communication: The importance of listening. *British Journal of Nursing, 6,* 275–279.

Kemper, B. J. (1992). Therapeutic listening: Developing the concept. *Journal of Psychosocial Nursing and Mental Health Services, 30*(7), 21–23.

Koshy, K. T. (1989). I only have ears for you... Active listening. *Nursing Times, 85*(30), 26–29.

Kruijver, I. P. M., Kerkstra, A., Francke, A. L., Bensing, J. M., & van de Wiel, H. B. M. (2000). Evaluation of communication training programs in nursing care: A review of the literature. *Patient Education and Counseling, 39,* 129–145.

La Monica, E. L., Wolf, R. M., Madea, A. R., & Oberst, M. T. (1987). Empathy and nursing care outcomes. *Scholarly Inquiry for Nursing Practice, 1,* 197–213.

Lekander, B. J., Lehmann, S., & Lindquist, R. (1993). Therapeutic listening: Key nursing interventions for several nursing diagnosis. *Dimensions of Critical Care Nursing, 12,* 24–30.

Mehrabian, A. (1971). *Silent messages.* Belmont, CA: Wadsworth.

Minamisawa, H., & Mitoh, T. (1997). Relating EEG changes and I-thou feelings during nursing interview. *Journal of Neuroscience Nursing, 29,* 32–38.

Morse, J. M., Anderson, G., Bottorff, J. L., Yonge, O., O'Brien, B., Solberg, S. M., & McIlveen, K. H. (1992). Exploring empathy: A conceptual fit for nursing practice? *Image: Journal of Nursing Scholarship, 24,* 273–280.

Myers, S. (2000). Empathic listening: Reports on the experience of being heard. *Journal of Humanistic Psychology, 40*(2), 148–173.

Olson, J. K., & Hanchett, E. (1997). Nurse-expressed empathy, patient outcomes, and development of a middle-range theory. *Image: Journal of Nursing Scholarship, 29,* 71–76.

Olson, J. K., & Iwasiw, C. L. (1987). Effects of a training model on active listening skills of post-RN students. *Journal of Nursing Education, 26,* 104–107.

Reid-Ponte, P. (1992). Distress in cancer patients and primary nurses' empathy skills. *Cancer Nursing, 15,* 283–292.

Rogers, C. R. (1957). The necessary and sufficient conditions of therapeutic personality change. *Journal of Consulting Psychology, 21*, 95–103.

Rowan, J. (1986). Holistic listening. *Journal of Humanistic Psychology, 26*(1),
83–102.

Ryden, M. B., McCarthy, P. R., Lewis, M. L., & Sherman, C. (1991). A behavioral
comparison of the helping styles of nursing students, psychotherapists, crisis
interveners, and untrained individuals. *Archives of Psychiatric Nursing, 5*, 185–188.

Sandelowski, M. (1994). We are the stories we tell: Narrative knowing in nursing
practice. *Journal of Holistic Nursing, 12*, 23–33.

Schlesinger, H. J. (1994). How the analyst listens: The pre-stages of interpretation.
International Journal of Psycho-Analysis, 75, 31–37.

Seidel, H. M., Ball, J. W., Dains, J. E., & Benedict, G. W. (1995). Cultural awareness. In H. M. Seidel, J. W. Ball, J. E. Dains, & G. W. Benedict (Eds.), *Mosby's
guide to physical examination* (3rd ed., pp. 34–56). St. Louis, MO: Mosby.

Sheppard, M. (1993). Client satisfaction, extended intervention, and interpersonal
skills in community mental health. *Journal of Advanced Nursing, 18*, 246–259.

Sundeen, S. J. Stuart, G. W., Rankin, E. A. D., & Cohen, S. A. (1998). *Nurse-client
interaction: Implementing the nursing process* (6th ed.). St. Louis, MO: Mosby.

Travelbee, J. (1971). *Interpersonal aspects of nursing* (2nd ed.). Philadelphia: Davis.

PART II

Mind-Body Therapies

OVERVIEW

In reality, all complementary therapies could be placed in this category. According to the National Center for Complementary/Alternative Medicine (NCCAM), mind-body therapies encompass therapies that promote the mind's capacity to have an impact on the functioning of the body. This definition does not mention that the reverse is also true: that therapies that affect the body can have an impact on the mind. And the definition does not make reference to the spiritual realm that is a part of a holistic perspective. The more encompassing perspective, mind-body-spirit, will be focused on in this book.

Mind-body therapies stand in opposition to the long-standing beliefs that underlie Western biomedicine in which the body and mind are examined separately. This separation was based on the philosophy of René Descartes. Nursing care has been based on a holistic philosophy. Florence Nightingale documented the impact that therapies such as music have on the whole person (Nightingale, 1936/1992). Despite the literature on holistic philosophy and the emphasis that has been given to holistic assessments, in actuality the biomedical model has often predominated in nursing until recently. It is encouraging to see that nursing, medicine, and other health professions are shifting away from the dichotomy of mind and body and are viewing persons from a holistic perspective.

An emerging body of research provides the basis for the use of mind-body therapies. From Herbert Benson's work in the 1960s on the effect of transcendental meditation on blood pressure to the increasing number of psychoneuroimmunological studies, the interconnectedness of the mind and body is being documented. Measurement is needed of multiple outcomes (physiological, psychological, and spiritual) in studies in which complementary therapies are tested.

41

Many, many therapies are classified as mind-body therapies. Nurses have and continue to use many of these therapies such as imagery, music, reminiscence, and humor. Many other mind-body therapies such as internal qi gong, soul retrieval, sweat lodges, and body psychotherapy are less familiar to nurses. The therapies chosen for inclusion in this section are ones that nurses frequently use and ones on which nurses have conducted research.

REFERENCE

Nightingale, F. (1936/1992). *Notes on nursing*. Philadelphia: Lippincott.

5

Imagery

Janice Post-White and Maura Fitzgerald

Imagery is a mind-body intervention that uses the power of the imagination to affect change in physical, emotional, or spiritual dimensions. Throughout our daily lives we constantly see images, experience sensations, and make impressions: a picture makes us angry or sad, a smell transports us to a moment in the past, a sound makes the muscles in our neck tighten. A billboard featuring a cool glass of lemonade makes our mouth water, and a fondly remembered song on the radio takes us back to a carefree youth. Images evoke physical and emotional responses and help us to understand the meaning of events.

Imagery is described as "the world's oldest and greatest healing resource" (Achterberg, 1985, p. 3), and is used in many ancient healing traditions to affect cure, alleviate suffering, and facilitate spiritual transformation. Throughout time, healers and shamans used imagery to access the patients' subconscious minds and belief system in order to open communication among the body, mind, and spirit.

Imagery is commonly used in modern health care, most often in the form of guided imagery, clinical hypnosis, or self-hypnosis. In the mid-1950s, the American Medical Association and the American Psychiatric Association recognized hypnosis as a therapeutic tool. Nurses, physicians, psychologists, and others use it in their practices for treatment of acute and chronic illness, relief of symptoms, and enhancement of wellness. Imagery has become standard therapy to alleviate anxiety and promote relaxation in adults and children, and has been successfully used to relieve pain, reduce nausea and vomiting associated with chemotherapy, prevent allergic responses, and lower high blood pressure. Imagery is a hallmark of current stress-management programs and is used to promote deep relaxation, gain psychological insight, and progress on a chosen spiritual path.

DEFINITION

Imagery is the formation of a mental representation of an object, place, event, or situation that is perceived through the senses. Imagery is based on the individual's own imagination and cognitive processing. However, it can be practiced as an independent activity (self-hypnosis) or guided by a professional (guided imagery).

Imagery can be active or passive. For adults and adolescents, physical and mental relaxation tends to facilitate imagery. Younger children often do not need to assume a relaxed state. Imagery may be receptive, with the individual perceiving messages from the body; or it may be active, with the individual cognitively evoking thoughts or ideas. Active imagery can be outcome- or end-state oriented, when the individual envisions a goal such as being healthy and well; or it can be process-oriented, where the mechanism of the desired effect is imagined such as envisioning a strong immune system fighting a viral infection or tumor.

Images employ all six senses—visual, aural, tactile, olfactory, proprioceptive, and kinesthetic. Although imagery is often referred to as "visualization," it includes imagining through any sense and not just being able to see something in the mind's eye. While inducing imagery, the individual often imagines seeing, hearing, smelling, tasting, or touching something in the image.

SCIENTIFIC BASIS

Imagery is thought to modify disease and reduce symptoms by reducing the stress response, which is mediated by psychoneuroimmune interactions. The stress response is triggered when a perceived or real situation or event threatens physical or emotional well-being or when the demands of the situation exceed available resources. One of the goals of imagery is to reframe stressful situations from negative responses of fear and anxiety to positive images of healing and well-being (Dossey, 1995). Imagery also can be used to increase emotional awareness and restructure the meaning of a situation. Emotional responses to situations trigger the limbic system and signal physiologic changes in the peripheral and autonomic nervous systems, resulting in the characteristic fight-or-flight stress response. Over time, chronic stress results in adrenal and immune suppression and may be the most harmful to cellular immune function, impairing the ability to ward off viruses and control tumor cells (Pert, Dreher, & Ruff, 1998). Converting negative responses into positive images and meaning reduces the physiologic stress response of the body.

Extensive rat model research by Ader and Cohen in the 1970s confirmed that the immune system can be *conditioned* by expectations and beliefs (Ader, Felten, & Cohen, 1991). Subsequent research in psychoneuroimmunology attempted to explain the *mechanisms* of how the brain and body communicate through cellular interactions. Receptors for neuropeptides, neurohormones, and cytokines reside on neural and immune cells and induce biochemical changes when activated. Serotonin and dopamine are two neurotransmitters that increase with stress and activate hypothalamic activity through receptor signaling (Black, 1995).

A cascade of signaling events in response to perceived stress results in the release of corticotropin releasing hormone (CRH) from the hypothalamus, adrenocorticotropin releasing hormone (ACTH) from the pituitary, norepinephrine and epinephrine from the adrenal medulla and peripheral sympathetic nerve terminals, and immunosuppressive cortisol from the adrenal cortex. These interactions are bidirectional, and changes in one system will influence the others.

Although immune responses to emotional states are extremely complex, it can be said in general that acute stress activates cardiac sympathetic activity and increases plasma catecholamines and natural killer cell activity, whereas chronic stress (or inescapable or unpredictable stress) is associated with suppression of NK cells and interleukin 1B, and an elevated blood pressure (Cacioppo et al., 1998). The degree of response also varies. Cacioppo and colleagues hypothesize that persons who have large physiologic responses to everyday stressors have "high stress reactivity" and are at greater risk for disease susceptibility, even when coping, performance, and perceived stress are comparable. And although genetic factors remain to be studied, baseline levels of neuroendocrine activity are likely to be regulated by genes and may determine the degree of natural resistance to disease, independent of external stimuli and stressors (Bonneau, Mormede, Vogler, McClearn, & Jones, 1998). The incredible heterogeneity in individual responses to stressful situations may determine not only how the individual responds, but also which interventions are more effective for individual adaptation.

INTERVENTION

TECHNIQUES

Imagery may be practiced independently, with a coach or teacher, or with a videotape or audiotape. The most effective imagery intervention is one that is specific to the individual's personality, to their preferences for relaxation and specific settings, their developmental age, and to the desired outcomes. An example of the steps of a general imagery session is outlined in Table 5.1.

Imagery sessions for adults and adolescents are usually 10 to 30 minutes in length, whereas most children tolerate 10 to 15 minutes. The session typically begins with a relaxation exercise or a focused "centering" for children. Breathing during imagery is slow and expansive, which facilitates relaxation as the breath moves lower into the chest and the abdominal muscles are used more than the chest muscles. Relaxation helps makes the mind more susceptible to new information (Benson, 1993), but is not required for imagery. Some children use active imagery very successfully and may use their bodies to demonstrate or respond to their image.

Once in a relaxed or "altered" state, the practitioner suggests an image of a relaxing, peaceful, or comforting place or introduces a predetermined and agreed upon image suggested by the client. Scenes commonly used to induce relaxation include watching clouds float by or a sunset, sitting on a warm beach or by a fire on a snowy evening, or floating through water or space. The scene used is often one that the client has actually experienced previously and found to be relaxing. Children may prefer active images that involve motion, such as flying or playing a sport.

For active imagery, the practitioner guides the imagery, using positive suggestions to alleviate specific symptoms or conditions (outcome or end-state imagery) or to rehearse or walk through an event (process imagery). Images do not need to be anatomically correct or vivid. Symbolic images may be the most powerful healing images because they are drawn from individual beliefs, culture, and meaning. For example, a 54-year-old woman with metastatic breast cancer watched her Alaskan husky dogs devour their breakfast and then used imagery to envision them scouring her body for tumor cells.

The ability to use guided imagery for therapeutic purposes is related to the individual's hypnotic ability or the ability to enter an altered state of consciousness and to become involved or absorbed in the imagery (Kwekkeboom, Huseby-Moore, & Ward, 1998). Some individuals have naturally high hypnotic abilities. These individuals recall pictures more accurately, generate more complex images, have higher dream recall in the waking state, and make fewer eye movements in imagery than poor visualizers.

Imagery has been used extensively in children and adolescents as well as with adults. Children as young as 4 (Olness & Kohen, 1996) who have language skills that are adequate to understand the suggestions can benefit from imagery. Young children often are better at imagery because of their natural active use of their imaginations. It has been found that hypnotizability rises through early childhood, peaking somewhere between ages 7 to 14 and then leveling off into adolescence and adulthood (Olness & Kohen, 1996).

TABLE 5.1 General Guided Imagery Technique

General guided imagery technique

1. *Achieving a relaxed state*
   a. Find a comfortable sitting or reclining position (not lying down).
   b. Uncross any extremities.
   c. Close your eyes or focus on one spot or object in the room.
   d. Focus on breathing with abdominal muscles; with each breath say to yourself "in" and "out."
      Notice your breath as it moves in and out. With your next breath let the exhalation be just a little longer and notice how the inhalation that follows is deeper. And as you notice that, let your body become even more relaxed.
   e. Feel your body becoming heavy and warm from the top of your head to the tips of your fingers and toes.
   f. If your thoughts roam, bring your mind back to thinking of your breathing and your relaxed body.

2. *Specific suggestions for imagery*
   a. In your mind, go to a place you enjoy and feel good.
   b. What do you see, hear, taste, smell, and feel?
   c. Take a few deep breaths and enjoy being there.
   d. Now imagine yourself the way you want to be. (Describe the desired goal specifically.)
   e. Imagine what steps you will need to take to be the way you want to be.
   f. Practice these steps now—in this place where you feel good.
   g. What is the first thing you are doing to help you be the way you want to be?
   h. What will you do next?
   i. When you reach your goal of the way you want to be, feel yourself, touch yourself, embrace yourself, listen to the sounds surrounding you.

3. *Summarize process and reinforce practice*
   a. Remember that you can return to this place, this feeling, this way of being, anytime you want.
   b. You can feel this way again by focusing on your breathing, relaxing, and imagining yourself in your special place.
   c. Come back to this place and envision yourself the way you want to be every day.

4. *Return to present*
   a. When you are ready you may return to the room we are in.
   b. You will feel relaxed and refreshed and be ready to resume your activities.
   c. You may open your eyes and tell me about your experience when you are ready.

When doing imagery with children, techniques must be modified to suit their developmental and cognitive age and their personal preferences. Adjustments may include reducing the length of time and modifying the types of imagery used. Children often do not like to close their eyes. Preschool and school-age children most often imagine in an active state; therefore muscle relaxation is not necessarily a goal. For example, a group of 9 to 12-year-old boys with sickle cell disease were being taught guided imagery as a pain control technique. When asked what special place they would like to go to, they requested a trip to a local amusement park and a ride on the roller-coaster. During the imagery many of them were physically and vocally active, swaying from side to side and moving their arms up and down. At the end of the visualization they all reported feeling like they were in the park (absorption) and gave examples of things they felt, saw, heard, or smelled. Recognizing individual and developmental preferences for settings, situations, and relaxation or stimulation can improve the effectiveness of the imagery and reduce time and frustration with learning imagery. Practicing imagery oneself is extremely helpful in guiding others.

MEASUREMENT OF OUTCOMES

Evaluating and measuring outcomes are important to determining the effectiveness and value of imagery in clinical practice. Clinical outcomes of imagery include physical signs of relaxation, less distress, lower anxiety and depression, a sense of meaning, purpose, and competency and positive changes in attitude or behavior (Post-White & Johnson, 1991). Health service benefits may reduce costs and morbidity and improve functional performance and quality of life.

The outcomes measured should reflect the client situation and the conceptual framework of the rationale for using imagery. If imagery is used to facilitate relaxation and progression during the birthing experience, outcomes might include level of pain, medications used, perceived helpfulness, and progression of labor. If imagery is used to control symptoms in clients undergoing chemotherapy for cancer, expected outcomes might include reduced nausea, vomiting, and fatigue and enhanced body image, positive mood states, and functional abilities. Imagery is often used to reduce the stress response and promote relaxation. Outcomes of relaxation include increased oxygen saturation levels, lower blood pressure and heart rate, warmer extremities, reduced muscle tension, greater alpha waves on EEG, as well as lower anxiety.

One of the most difficult conclusions to make is whether the outcomes are the result of imagery solely or a combination of interventions. Learning and practicing imagery often changes other health-related behaviors, such as getting more sleep, eating a healthier diet, stopping smoking, or exercising regularly.

The therapist's presence, attention, and compassion also may be an intervention independent of the imagery process. Because the ability to generate images and become involved in them as if they were real may moderate the effects of imagery on outcomes (Kwekkeboom et al., 1998), it is important to assess the ability to image. Several instruments can be used to measure the effectiveness of the ability to image (Achterberg & Lawlis, 1984) and absorption (Tellegen, 1993).

PRECAUTIONS

The physical and emotional risks of mind-body techniques are virtually nonexistent as long as they are not used in place of conventional medicine (Goleman & Gurin, 1993). There are few reports of adverse events with imagery. Kwekkeboom and colleagues (1998) reported increased anxiety in 3 of 15 subjects using imagery specifically to reduce anxiety associated with a stressful task. However, the authors also acknowledge that the imagery exercise was perceived as pleasant, despite the inability to relieve anxiety. Some individuals have anecdotally reported airway constriction or difficulty breathing when they focus on breathing techniques. Using another centering method such as focusing on an object in the room or repeating a mantra can reduce this distressing response and still induce relaxation.

The expertise and training of the nurse should guide judgment in using imagery to achieve outcomes in practice. Imagery techniques can be applied quite easily to managing symptoms (pain, nausea, vomiting) and facilitating relaxation, sleep, or anxiety reduction. Advanced techniques such as age regression and management of depression require further training.

USES

Imagery has been used therapeutically in a variety of conditions and populations (Table 5.2). Pain and cancer are two conditions in which imagery has been found to be helpful in both adults and children. Evidence for effectiveness of imagery in these conditions will be discussed here.

Pain

Whether pain is from cancer, other illness, side effects of treatment, injury, or physical stress on the body, emotional factors contribute to pain perception,

TABLE 5.2   Conditions for Which Imagery Has Been Tested in Children and Adults

Clinical Conditions	Selected Sources
Children	
Asthma	Hackman, Stern, & Gershwin (2000)
Burn-dressing change	Foertsch, O'Hara, Stoddard, & Kealy (1998)
Cancer	Steggles et al. (1997)
Cardiac catheterization	Pederson (1995)
Emotional and behavioral disorders	Olness & Kohen (1996)
Managing procedural pain (lumbar puncture, bone marrow biopsies)	Broome, Rehwaldt, & Fogg (1998); Liossi & Hatira (1999); Stevens et al. (1994)
Nausea and vomiting	Keller (1995)
Pain	Broome et al. (1998); Lambert (1999)
Adults	
Phobias, anxiety	Thompson & Coppens (1994); Baider, Uziely, & DeNour (1994); Walker (1998)
Childbirth/postpartum care	Rees (1995)
Depression & fatigue in HIV	Eller (1995)
Anxiety and pain medication use following coronary artery bypass surgery	Ashton et al. (1997)
Psoriasis	Zachariae et al. (1996)
Nausea and vomiting	Burish & Jenkins (1992); Troesch et al. (1993)
5-year survival in lymphoma	Ratcliffe et al. (1995)
Immune response in healthy volunteers; immune response in breast cancer	Johnson et al. (1996); Post-White et al. (1996); Richardson et al. (1997); Walker et al. (1996)
Cancer pain	Wallace (1997); Syrjala et al. (1995)
Comfort during cancer therapy	Kolcaba & Fox (1999)

and mind-body interventions such as imagery can help make the pain more manageable. Stress, anxiety, and fatigue decrease the threshold for pain, making the perceived pain more intense. Imagery can break this cycle of pain-tension-worry-anxiety-pain. Relaxation with imagery decreases pain directly by reducing muscle tension and related spasms and indirectly by lowering anxiety and improving sleep, which influence pain perception. Imagery also is a distraction strategy; vivid, detailed images using all senses tend to work best for pain control. In addition, the cognitive reappraisal/restructuring used with imagery can increase a sense of control and power over the ability to reframe the meaning of pain. While highly hypnotizable persons benefit more readily than others, practically all patients can learn to better manage their pain and pain-related stresses through simple imagery exercises (Spira & Speigel, 1992).

Guided imagery has been used extensively in children to alleviate pain and anxiety (Lambert, 1999; Rusy & Weisman, 2000; Steggles, Damore-Petingola, Maxwell, & Lightfoot, 1997). Imagery is particularly helpful in getting a child through a medical procedure with a safe and effective level of sedation or analgesia and as little movement as possible. Suggestions to breathe deeply and to relax or be comfortable are combined with vivid images of a favorite place. It is best to introduce the child to breathing techniques and explore favorite places prior to the procedure. In critical or emergency situations, however, imagery has been successfully employed without these preliminaries (Kohen, 2000).

Distraction imagery is most useful for severe pain that is exhausting and for dealing with painful procedures. Suggestions for drawing attention completely from the physical pain include floating or other pleasant sensations, recalling a pleasant past experience or feeling, or distracting oneself from the pain source by rubbing the fingers together or squeezing and releasing the hands.

Several studies document the effectiveness of imagery to reduce acute procedural pain in children. Broome, Rehwaldt, and Fogg (1998) taught relaxation, distraction, and imagery to 28 children and adolescents undergoing lumbar puncture (LP) for cancer treatment. Although little change in pain behaviors was observed by staff during the LP, the children reported a significant improvement in their pain (there was no control group, however). Similarly, 30 children undergoing bone marrow biopsy who received either clinical hypnosis (relaxation and visual imagery followed by hypnotic suggestions to induce the feeling of anesthesia) or cognitive restructuring techniques with relaxation reported less pain and anxiety than a standard control group (Liossi & Hatira, 1999). In 26 children undergoing elective surgical procedures, preoperative imagery reduced postoperative pain scores and length of stay in comparison to standard preoperative education where the amount of pain medication used was the same (Lambert, 1996). Two other studies measuring the effectiveness of imagery in reducing procedural pain in children found no differences in distress behaviors and pain with cardiac catheterization in comparison to a control group (Pederson, 1995) and during burn dressing changes (Foertsch, O'Hara, Stoddard, & Kealy, 1998).

The focus with moderate pain is to alter the interpretation or perception of pain. Metaphors for pain can be used to dissociate from the pain and gain control (initially over the metaphor itself), thereby reducing the intensity of the pain. Another alternative is to identify pleasant sensations with the metaphor. Associations with hot or cold temperature also can be used, with the individual concentrating on raising and lowering the intensity or level and associating pleasant sensations with different temperatures.

Focusing and transferring analgesia is most effective for mild pain. Several techniques can be used, such as imagining the area being injected with anesthetic, being wooden, or being painted a color that numbs the area. It is helpful to numb an unaffected area first, such as a "hand in glove" anesthesia, and then transfer that numbness to the painful area (Levitan, 1992). Although elements of relaxation, vividness, and distraction were important to pain reduction, Zachariae and Bjerring (1994) found that focused analgesia was the most effective in reducing acute pain, particularly in subjects with high hypnotizable ratings.

Cancer Pain

Pain specific to cancer and its treatment can be acute or chronic. In a randomized pretest-posttest study of 67 hospitalized patients with cancer pain, imagery combined with progressive muscle relaxation reduced pain sensation, intensity, and severity and lowered non-opioid breakthrough analgesia use (Sloman, 1995). Similarly, in two clinical trials of bone marrow transplant patients, Syrjala and colleagues measured reduced levels of mucositis-related pain in the imagery/hypnosis group (Syrjala, Cummings, & Donaldson, 1992; Syrjala, Donaldson, Davis, Kippes, & Carr, 1995). Twice weekly imagery sessions included progressive muscle relaxation, deep relaxation, transference of sensations, and individualized imagery.

Despite its use in cancer, there are few randomized controlled studies documenting the effectiveness of imagery for cancer-related pain (Wallace, 1997). However, a National Institutes of Health technology assessment panel concluded that behavioral therapies for chronic cancer pain be accepted as standard treatment and reimbursed similar to medical treatments (Eastman, 1995). Kwekkeboom (1999) proposed a model to help predict the the effectiveness of cognitive-behavioral cancer pain management strategies. Factors influencing the effectiveness of use include prior use, perceived credibility of the strategy, and fit with the patient's preferred coping style. Documentation is needed on specific interventions used, outcomes affected by imagery, and factors influencing effectiveness.

Cancer Outcomes

Although several prospective randomized studies found that imagery increased survival in patients with cancer (Fawzy et al., 1993; Walker, 1998), many other factors also influence cancer outcomes. Psychosocial factors such as depression (Walker, 1998) and diagnostic factors such as stage of disease (Ratcliffe, Dawson, & Walker, 1995) are consistent covariates in explaining survival outcomes.

A common explanation for how imagery may improve cancer outcomes is postulated through increasing cellular immune function. Some studies have demonstrated increases in natural killer cytotoxicity (Fawzy et al., 1990, 1993; Gruber et al., 1993; Walker et al., 1996) and T-cell responses (Gruber et al., 1993), while others have found no differences (Post-White et al., 1996; Richardson et al., 1997) or decreases (Zachariae et al., 1994) in natural killer cell numbers and cytotoxicity. Despite inconclusive effects on cancer outcome, imagery interventions have consistently improved coping responses and psychological states in patients with cancer, suggesting that imagery may mediate psychoneuroimmune outcomes in breast cancer. Further study is needed to determine the clinical significance of immunological effects.

FUTURE RESEARCH

Despite documented relationships between the mind and the body, many of the intervention trials that test the effectiveness of guided imagery and other mind-body interventions lack the scientific rigor of randomized controlled clinical trials. Key questions that remain to be answered are whether psychoneuroimmune responses to imagery influence clinical outcomes and quality of life and how they work to mediate psychosocial and clinical outcomes. Determining personal preferences for the use of imagery and specific types of imagery is important to demonstrating significant clinical effects. Measuring clinical outcomes relevant to quality of life and health/illness states is critical to demonstrating cost-effectiveness and efficacy of imagery as an intervention that is useful in practice. The following questions should be explored:

1. Is imagery more effective than relaxation alone in producing stress-reducing outcomes?

2. Does the type of imagery (outcome or process) produce different outcomes? Does imaging the immune system in cancer actually influence immune response?

3. Are there certain characteristics of individuals that determine their ability to respond to imagery and produce desired outcomes? Are there certain individuals or conditions for whom imagery should not be recommended?

4. What are the long-term effects of imagery? Can imagery reduce stress, improve coping, enhance well-being, create healthier lifestyles, and reduce illness in individuals over time?

REFERENCES

Achterberg, J. (1985). *Imagery in healing: Shamanism and modern medicine.* Boston: Shambhala.

Achterberg, J., & Lawlis, G. F. (1984). *Imagery and disease: Diagnostic tools?* Champaign, IL: Institute for Personality and Ability Testing.

Ader, R., Felten, D. L., & Cohen, N. (1991). *Psychoneuroimmunology* (2nd ed.). San Diego, CA: Academic Press.

Ashton, C., Whitworth, G. C., Seldomridge, J. A., Shapiro, P. A., Weinberg, A. D., Smith, C. R., Rose, A., Fisher, S., & Oz, M. C. (1997). Self-hypnosis reduces anxiety following coronary artery bypass surgery: A prospective, randomized trial. *Journal of Cardiovascular Surgery, 38,* 69–75.

Baider, L., Uziely, B., & De-Nour, A. K. (1994). Progressive muscle relaxation and guided imagery in cancer patients. *General Hospital Psychiatry, 16*(5), 340–347.

Benson, H. (1993). The relaxation response. In D. Goleman & J. Gurin (Eds.), *Mind/body medicine* (pp. 233-258). Yonkers, NY: Consumers Union of United States, Inc.

Black, P. H. (1995). Psychoneuroimmunology: Brain and immunity. *Scientific American Science and Medicine, 2*(6), 16–25.

Bonneau, R. H., Mormede, P., Vogler, G. P., McClearn, G. E., & Jones, B. C. (1998). A genetic basis for neuroendocrine-immune interactions. *Brain, Behavior, and Immunity, 12,* 83–89.

Broome, M. E., Rehwaldt, M., & Fogg, L. (1998). Relationships between cognitive behavioral techniques, temperament, observed distress, and pain reports in children and adolescents during lumbar puncture. *Journal of Pediatric Nursing, 13*(1), 48–51.

Cacioppo, J. T., Berntson, G. G., Malarkey, W. B., Kiecolt-Glaser, J. K., Sheridan, J. F., Poehlmann, K. M., Burleson, M. H., Ernst, J. M., Hawkley, L. C., & Glaser, R. (1998). Autonomic, neuroendocrine, and immune responses to psychological stress: The reactivity hypothesis. *Annals of the New York Academy of Sciences, 1*(840), 664–673.

Decker, T. W., & Cline-Elsen, J. (1992). Relaxation therapy as an adjunct in radiation oncology. *Journal of Clinical Psychology, 48*(3), 388–393.

Dossey, B. (1995). Complementary modalities Part 3: Using imagery to help your patient heal. *American Journal of Nursing, 96*(6), 41–47.

Eastman, P. (1995). Panel endorses behavioral therapy for cancer pain (news). *Journal of the National Cancer Institute, 87*(22), 1666–1667.

Fawzy, F. I., Fawzy, N., Hyun, L. S., Elashoff, R., Guthrie, D., Fahy, J. L., & Morton, D. L. (1993). Malignant melanoma: Effects of an early structured psychiatric intervention, coping and affective state on recurrence and survival 6 years later. *Archives of General Psychiatry, 50,* 681–689.

Fawzy, F. I., Kemeny, M. E., Fawzy, N. W., Elashoff, M. D., Cousins, N., & Fahey, J. L. (1990). A structured psychiatric intervention for cancer patients II. Changes over time in immunological measures. *Archives of General Psychiatry, 47,* 729–735.

Foertsch, C. E, O'Hara, M. W., Stoddard, F. J., & Kealey, G. P. (1998) Treatment-resistant pain and distess during pediatric burn-dressing changes. *Journal of Burn Care and Rehabilitation, 19,* 219–224.

Goleman, D., & Gurin, J. (1993) (Eds.). *Mind/body medicine.* Yonkers, NY: Consumer Reports Books.

Gruber, B. L., Hersh, S. P., Hall, N. R., Waletzky, L. R., Kunz, J. F., Carpenter, J. K., Kverno, K. S., & Weiss, S. M. (1993). Immunological responses of breast cancer patients to behavioral interventions. *Biofeedback and Self Regulation, 18*(1), 1–22.

Keller, V. (1995). Management of nausea and vomiting in children. *Journal of Pediatric Nursing, 10*(5), 280–286.

Kohen, D. (2000, June). *Integrating hypnosis into practice.* Introductory Workshop in Clinical Hypnosis. University of Minnesota at St. Paul and the Minnesota Society of Clinical Hypnosis.

Kolcaba, K., & Fox, C. (1999). The effects of guided imagery on comfort of women with early stage breast cancer undergoing radiation therapy. *Oncology Nursing Forum, 26*(1), 67–72.

Kwekkeboom, K. (1999). A model for cognitive-behavioral interventions in cancer pain management. *Image: Journal of Nursing Scholarship, 31,* 151–156.

Kwekkeboom, K., Huseby-Moore, K., & Ward, S. (1998). Imaging ability and effective use of guided imagery. *Research in Nursing and Health, 21,* 189–198.

Lambert, S. (1996). The effects of hypnosis/guided imagery on the postoperative course of children. *Developmental and Behavioral Pediatrics, 17*(5), 307–310.

Lambert, S. (1999). Distraction, imagery, and hypnosis: Techniques for management of children's pain. *Journal of Child and Family Nursing, 2*(1), 5–15.

Levitan, A. A. (1992). The use of hypnosis with cancer patients. *Psychiatric Medicine, 10*(1), 119-131.

Liossi, C., & Hatira, P. (1999). Clinical hypnosis versus cognitive behavioral training for pain management with pediatric cancer patients undergoing bone marrow aspirations. *The International Journal of Clinical Hypnosis, 47*(2), 104–116.

Olness, K., & Kohen, D. (1996). *Hypnosis and hypnotherapy with children* (3rd ed.) New York: Guilford Press.

Pederson, C. (1995). Effect of imagery on children's pain and anxiety during cardiac catheterization. *Journal of Pediatric Nursing, 10*(6), 365–374.

Pert, C. B., Dreher, H. E., & Ruff, M. R. (1998). The psychosomatic network: Foundations of mind-body medicine. *Alternative Therapies, 4*(4), 30–41.

Post-White, J., & Johnson, M. (1991). Complementary nursing therapies in clinical oncology practice: Relaxation and imagery. *Dimensions in Oncology Nursing, 5*(2), 15–20.

Post-White, J., Schroeder, L., Hannahan, A., Johnston, M. K., Salscheider, N., & Grandt, N. (1996). Response to imagery/support in breast cancer survivors. *Oncology Nursing Forum*, 23(2), 355.

Ratcliffe, M. A., Dawson, A. A., & Walker, L. G. (1995). Personality inventory L-scores in patients with Hodgkin's disease and non-Hodgkin's lymphoma. *Psycho-Oncology*, 4, 39–45.

Rees, B. L. (1995). Effect of relaxation with guided imagery on anxiety, depression, and self-esteem in primaparas. *Journal of Holistic Nursing*, 13(3), 255–267.

Richardson, M. A., Post-White, J., Grimm, E. A., Moye, L. A., Singletary, S. E., & Justice, B. (1997). Coping, life attitudes, and immune responses to imagery and group support after breast cancer. *Alternative Therapies in Health and Medicine*, 3(5), 62–70.

Rusy, L. M., & Weisman, S. J. (2000). Complementary therapies for acute pediatric pain management. *Pediatric Clinics of North America*, 47(3), 589–599.

Sloman, R. (1995). Relaxation and the relief of cancer pain. *Nursing Clinics of North America*, 30(4), 697–709.

Spira, J. L., & Spiegel, D. (1992). Hypnosis and related techniques in pain management. *Hospice Journal*, 8(1,2), 89–119.

Steggles, S., Damore-Petingola, S., Maxwell, J., & Lightfoot, N. (1997). Hypnosis for children and adolescents with cancer: An annotated bibliography 1985-1995. *Journal of Pediatric Oncology Nursing*, 14(1), 27–32.

Stevens, M. M., Pozza, L. D., Cavelletto, B., Cooper, M. G., & Kilham, H. A. (1994). Pain and symptom control in paediatric palliative care. *Cancer Surveys*, 21, 211–231.

Syrjala, K. L., Cummings, C., & Donaldson, G. W. (1992). Hypnosis or cognitive behavioral training for the reduction of pain and nausea during cancer treatment: A controlled clinical trial. *Pain*, 48, 137–146.

Syrjala, K. L., Donaldson, G. W., Davis, M. W., Kippes, M. E., & Carr, J. E. (1995). Relaxation and imagery and cognitive-behavioral training reduce pain during cancer treatment: A controlled clinical trial. *Pain*, 63, 189–198.

Tellegen, A. (1993). *Multidimensional Personality Questionnaire manual*. Minneapolis: University of Minnesota Press.

Thompson, M. B., & Coppens, N. M. (1994). The effects of guided imagery on anxiety levels and movement of clients undergoing magnetic resonance imaging. *Holistic Nursing Practice*, 8(2), 59–69.

Troesch, L. M., Rodehaver, C. B., Delaney, E. A., & Yanes, B. (1993). The influence of guided imagery on chemotherapy-related nausea and vomiting. *Oncology Nursing Forum*, 20(8), 1179–1185.

Walker, L. G. (1998). Hypnosis and cancer: Host defences, quality of life and survival. *Contemporary Hypnosis*, 15(1), 34–38.

Walker, L. G., Miller, I., Walker, M. B., Simpson, E., Ogston, K., Segar, A., Heys, S. D., Ah-See, A. K., Hutcheon, A. W, Sarkar, T. K., & Eremin, O. (1996). Immunological effects of relaxation training and guided imagery in women with locally advanced breast cancer. *Psycho-Oncology*, 5(3) (Suppl. 16).

Wallace, K. (1997). Analysis of recent literature concerning relaxation and imagery interventions for cancer pain. *Cancer Nursing, 20*(2), 79–87.

Zachariae, R., & Bjerring, P. (1994). Laser-induced pain-related brain potentials and sensory pain ratings in high and low hypnotizable subjects during hypnotic suggestions of relaxation, dissociated imaging, focused analgesia, and placebo. *International Journal of Clinical and Experimental Hypnosis, 42,* 56–80.

Zachariae, R., Hanson, J. B., Andersen, M., Jinquan, T., Peterson, K. S., Simonson, C., Zachariae, C., & Thestrup-Pederson, K. (1994). Changes in cellular immune function after specific guided imaging and relaxation in high and low hypnotizable healthy subjects. *Psychotherapy and Psychosomatics, 61,* 74–92.

Zachariae, R., Oster, H., Bjerring, P., & Kragballe, K. (1996). Effects of psychologic intervention on psoriasis: a preliminary report. *Journal of American Academy of Dermatology, 34*(6), 1008–1015.

6

Music Intervention

Linda Chlan

Music has been used throughout history as a treatment modality. From the time of the ancient Egyptians, the power of music to affect health has been noted. Nursing's pioneering leader Florence Nightingale recognized the healing power of music (1860/1969). Today nurses can implement music in a variety of settings to benefit patients and clients.

DEFINITIONS

Merriam-Webster's collegiate dictionary defines music as "the science or art of ordering tones or sounds in succession, in combination, and in temporal relationships to produce a composition having unity and continuity" (Woolf, 1979). Alvin (1975) delineated five main elements of music. The character of a piece of music and its effects depend on the qualities of these elements and their relationships to one another.

- *Frequency or pitch* is produced by the number of vibrations of a sound; the highness or lowness of a musical tone noted by the letters A, B, C, D, E, F, G. Rapid vibrations tend to act as a stimulant, whereas slow vibrations bring about relaxation.
- *Intensity* creates the volume of the sound, related to the amplitude of the vibrations. A person's like or dislike of certain music depends on intensity, which can be used to produce intimacy (soft music) or power (loud music).
- *Tone color* or *timbre* is a nonrhythmical, subjective property that results from harmony. Psychological significance results from the timbre of music because of associations with past events or feelings.

- *Interval* is the distance between two notes related to pitch, which creates melody and harmony. Melody results from how musical pitches are sequenced and the interval between them. Harmony results in the way pitches are sounded together, described by the listener as consonant (conveying the feeling of restfulness) or dissonant (conveying the feeling of tension). Cultural norms determine what is deemed enjoyable and pleasant by a listener.
- Duration creates *rhythm* and *tempo*. Duration refers to the length of sounds, and rhythm is a time pattern fitted into a certain speed. Rhythm is what influences one to move with music in a certain manner and can convey peace and security, while repetitive rhythms can elicit feelings of depression. Continuous sounds that are repeated at a slow pace and become gradually slower produce decreased levels of responsiveness. Strong rhythms can awaken feelings of power and control.

From a nursing perspective, music intervention is the use of music for therapeutic purposes to promote patient/client health and well-being. Music therapists are employed in many health care facilities, and countless situations exist in which nurses can implement music into a patient's plan of care. In order not to confuse the practice of music therapy with the use of music from a nursing perspective, the term music intervention will be used in this chapter.

SCIENTIFIC BASIS

Music is complex and affects the physiological, psychological, and spiritual aspects of human beings. Individual responses to music can be influenced by personal preferences, the environment, education, and cultural factors.

Entrainment, a physics principle, is a process whereby two objects vibrating at similar frequencies will tend to cause mutual sympathetic resonance, resulting in their vibrating at the same frequency (Maranto, 1993). Musical tempos may be used to synchronize or entrain the physiological state; changes in body rhythms (e.g., heart rate or breathing pattern) are caused by musical variations (Bonny, 1986). Music has the potential to entrain heart rate via its pulse or tempo, or to entrain breathing through its rhythm (Maranto, 1993). Bonny noted that entrainment can utilize not only the tempo of a musical selection, but also the mood of the music to effect changes in mood state and body rhythms.

Likewise, music can serve as a powerful distraction technique. Music intervention provides a patient/client with a familiar, comforting stimulus that can evoke pleasurable sensations while refocusing one's attention onto the music instead of on stressful thoughts or other environmental stimuli.

INTERVENTION

Determination of a person's musical preferences through assessment is essential; among the tools developed for use by nurses is one by Chlan and Tracy (1999). The assessment instrument elicits information on how frequently music is listened to, the type of preferred musical selections, and the purpose for which a person listens to music. For some people the purpose of listening to music may be to relax while others may prefer music stimulates and invigorates them. After assessment data have been gathered, appropriate techniques with specific music can then be implemented.

TECHNIQUES

The use of music can take many forms, from listening to selected tapes to singing or playing an instrument. A number of factors should be kept in mind when considering the specific technique: the type of music and personal preferences, active versus passive involvement, use in a group or on an individual basis, length of time to use music, and the desired outcomes. Two of the more commonly used music techniques by nurses will be discussed here: listening and group work.

Listening

Providing the means for patients to listen to musical selections is the technique most frequently implemented by nurses, and cassette tapes and compact discs make it easy to provide music for patients in all types of settings. Tapes have many advantages. Tape players are relatively inexpensive; they are small and can be used even in the most crowded confines such as critical care units. Auto-reverse capabilities allow the patient to listen to music for any length of time without having to be interrupted to turn the tape over. Although more expensive than tapes, CDs have superior sound clarity and track-seeking that allows immediate selection of a desired piece. Comfortable headphones allow patients private listening that does not disturb others.

For a very modest outlay of money, a nursing unit can establish a tape library containing a wide variety of selections to meet various musical preferences. It is also easy to individualize tapes to meet the preferences of each patient. (Attention to copyright laws is necessary when reproducing tapes.)

While various musical genres are available on the radio, commercial messages and talking are deterrents to using them for music intervention. Likewise, one cannot control the quality of the radio signal reception nor the specific music selections.

Individual Versus Group

Music can be used for patient groups as a powerful integrating force. Music creates interrelationships among the members, and between the listener and the music. Canadian nurses implemented karaoke for groups of residents with chronic conditions to enhance their quality of life by connecting with others on the unit and with people from the past (Mavely & Mitchell, 1994). However, diversity in the preference of individuals in a group or securing an appropriate site for a group session may necessitate implementing music on an individual basis; groups also require more planning than do individual sessions.

TYPES OF MUSIC FOR INTERVENTION

Careful attention to the selection of the music contributes to its therapeutic effects. For example, music to induce relaxation has a regular rhythm, no extreme pitch or dynamics, and a melodic sound that is smooth and flowing (Bonny, 1986). Past experiences can influence one's response to music as well. Specific selections may be associated with happy or sad occasions and events, and cultural influences will also impact one's musical preferences.

Older persons may prefer patriotic and popular songs from an earlier era or hymns with slower tempos played with familiar instruments (Moore, Staum, & Brotons, 1992). Religious music may be welcomed by many when this type of music is not readily available on the radio, and providing religious music tapes will fill a void for many who are unable to attend religious services.

Classical music is thought to evoke greater enjoyment and interest with repeated listening, while popular music declines in effectiveness with repetition (Bonny, 1986). Bonny feels that patients in a weakened state respond less to popular music and are more receptive to the meaningful stimulus of classical music that has endured over time. In any event, providing a choice and consideration for a person's musical preferences are imperative.

New Age, synthesized, or nontraditional music has become very popular. This type of music differs from traditional music, which is characterized by tension and release (Guzzetta, 1995). However, some experts feel that this type of synthesized music is not appropriate for relaxation due to the novelty of the stimulus and the absence of the usual form found in more traditional and American music (Bonny, 1986; Hanser, 1988).

GUIDELINES

Music intervention for the purposes of relaxation utilizes music as a pleasant stimulus to block out sensations of anxiety, fear, and tension and to divert attention from unpleasant thoughts (Thaut, 1990). A minimum of 20 minutes is necessary to induce relaxation along with some form of relaxation exercise, such as deep breathing, prior to initiating music intervention (Guzzetta, 1995).

While the definition of relaxing music may vary by individual, factors affecting the response to music include musical preferences and familiar selections. Music of a relaxing nature should have a tempo at or below a resting heart rate (72 beats or less); predictable dynamics; fluid melodic movement; pleasing harmonies; regular rhythm without sudden changes; and tonal qualities that include strings, flute, piano, or specially synthesized music (Robb, Nichols, Rutan, Bishop, & Parker, 1995). One of the most widely used classical music selections for relaxation is Pachelbel's Canon in D Major, which is frequently included in commercially available relaxation tapes. Table 6.1 outlines the basic steps for implementing music intervention for promoting relaxation.

MEASUREMENT OF OUTCOMES

The outcome indices for evaluating the effectiveness of music vary, depending on the purpose for which music is implemented. Outcomes may be physiological or psychological alterations and include a decrease in anxiety or stress arousal, promotion of relaxation, an increase in social interaction, and an increase in overall well-being. Table 6.2 provides measurement indices that have been used with specific populations. In addition to those listed in the table, heart rate variability (White, 1999) and respiratory muscle strength (Wiens, Reimer, & Guyn, 1999) also have been examined in response to music.

PRECAUTIONS

Adaptation occurs if the auditory system is continually exposed to the same type of stimulus (Farber, 1982). Neural adaptation can occur after 3 minutes of continuous exposure, resulting in the music's no longer being the stimulant or calming influence intended. Use of stimulation such as music in phase I following head injury may increase intracranial pressure. Music of a stimulating quality should be delayed until the autonomic nervous system has stabilized. Quiet music may be used to induce relaxation and block the

TABLE 6.1 Guidelines for Music Intervention for Relaxation

1. Ascertain that patient has adequate hearing.
2. Ascertain patient's like/dislike for music.
3. Assess music preferences and previous experience with music for relaxation; assist with tape/CD selections as needed.
4. Determine agreed-upon goals for music intervention with patient.
5. Complete all nursing cares prior to intervention; allow at least 20 minutes of uninterrupted listening time.
6. Gather equipment (CD or cassette tape-player, cassettes/CDs, headphones, batteries) and ensure all are in good working order. Provide the patient a choice of "relaxing" selections.
7. Assist patient to a comfortable position, as needed; ensure call-light is within easy reach.
8. Assist patient with equipment as needed.
9. Enhance environment as needed (draw blinds, close door, turn off overhead lights, etc.).
10. Post a Do Not Disturb sign to minimize unnecessary interruptions.
11. Encourage and provide patient with opportunities to "practice" relaxation with music.
12. Document goal attainment. Revise intervention as needed.

irritating sounds from the environment; however, the patient's individual response to music should be monitored.

Careful control of volume is essential. Permanent ear damage results from exposure to high frequencies and volumes. Decibels higher than 90 dBSL cause discomfort (Idzoriek, 1982), and fatigue occurs more frequently when stimulation is at higher frequencies (Farber, 1982).

Initiating music intervention without first assessing a person's likes and dislikes may produce deleterious effects. Because of music's effect on the limbic system, it can bring about intense emotional responses.

USES

Music has been tested as a therapeutic intervention with many different patient populations, with a majority of the nursing literature focusing on individualized music listening. Table 6.2 shows those patient populations and purposes for which music has been implemented. Two frequent uses will be highlighted here.

TABLE 6.2   Uses of Music Intervention

Orientation/minimizing disruptive behaviors
    Older adults (Clark, Lipe, & Bilbrey, 1998; Gerdner & Swanson, 1993;
        Gerdner, 1997; Janelli, Kanski, Jones, & Kennedy, 1995; Sambandham &
        Schirm, 1995; Snyder & Olson, 1996)
    Restrained patients (Janelli & Kanski, 1998)

Decreasing anxiety
    Pediatrics (Klein & Winkelstein, 1996)
    Surgical (Augustin & Hains, 1996; Kaempf & Amodei, 1989; Steelman, 1990;
        Stevens, 1990)
    Coronary care unit (Bolwerk, 1990; White, 1992, 1999)

Pain management
    Acute pain (Good, 1995; Good et al., 1999)
    Chronic pain (Schorr, 1993)
    Cancer-related pain (Beck, 1991)
    Invasive procedures/pediatrics (Berlin, 1998)

Stress reduction and relaxation
    NICU patients (Burke et al., 1995; Collins & Kuck, 1991)
    Ventilator-dependent ICU patients (Chlan, 1995, 1998)
    Adult ICU patients (Updike, 1990)
    Coronary care patients/post-myocardial infarction (Guzzetta, 1989; White, 1999)

Stimulation
    Depression in older adults (Hanser & Thompson, 1994)
    Sleep disturbances in older adults (Mornhinweg & Voignier, 1995)
    Head injury (Jones, Hux, Morton-Anderson, & Knepper, 1994)

Distraction/diversion
    High-dose chemotherapy (Ezzone, Baker, Rosselet, & Terepka, 1998)
    Intravenous catheter insertion (Jacobsen, 1999)
    Children's immunizations (Megel, Houser, & Gleaves, 1998)

Decreasing Anxiety

One of the strongest effects of music is anxiety reduction (Standley, 1986).
Music can enhance the immediate environment, provide a diversion, and
lessen the impact of potentially disturbing sounds for pediatric patients
(Klein & Winkelstein, 1996); for patients experiencing a variety of surgical
procedures (Augustin & Hains, 1996; Steelman, 1990; Stevens, 1990); coronary care unit patients (Bolwerk, 1990; White, 1992, 1999); and ventilator-
dependent ICU patients (Chlan, 1998).

Distraction

Music is an effective intervention for distraction, particularly for procedures that induce untoward symptoms and distress. Music has been found to be an effective diversional adjunct in the management of nausea and vomiting induced by chemotherapy (Ezzone, Baker, Rosselet, & Terepka, 1998); for distress in children undergoing immunizations (Megel, Houser, & Gleaves, 1998); or for adults during intravenous catheter insertion (Jacobsen, 1999).

FUTURE RESEARCH

While the number of publications examining various patient responses to music has been increasing (Snyder & Chlan, 1999), the following are areas in which research is needed in order to build the scientific base of music intervention:

1. Stress is a major response to illness that can adversely affect immune status. What are the effects of various types of music listening for patients on their immune functions (e.g., salivary cortisol)?
2. Little direction is available for prescribing music for intervention. What is the most efficacious music prescription? When, how much, how often?
3. A majority of nursing research studies testing the effects of music have employed designs restricted to immediate or short-term effects of the intervention. Therefore, longitudinal studies are needed to determine what, if any, are the long-term effects or benefits of music intervention?

While intervention research itself is labor-intensive, there is a need for larger studies on music intervention, such as multicenter clinical trials with measurement of salient outcome variables. The knowledge base of music intervention to promote patient/client health and well-being can be expanded through high-quality research and by dissemination of those findings.

REFERENCES

Alvin, J. (1975). *Music therapy.* New York: Basic Books.

Augustin, P., & Hains, A. (1996). Effect of music on ambulatory surgery patients' preoperative anxiety. *AORN Journal, 63*(4), 750–758.

Beck, S. (1991). The therapeutic use of music for cancer-related pain. *Oncology Nursing Forum, 18*(8), 1327–1337.

Berlin, B. (1998). Music therapy with children during invasive procedures: Our emergency department's experience. *Journal of Emergency Nursing, 24*(6), 607–608.

Bolwerk, C. (1990). Effects of relaxing music on state anxiety in myocardial infarction patients. *Critical Care Nursing Quarterly, 13*(2), 63–72.

Bonny, H. (1986). Music and healing. *Music Therapy, 6*(1), 3–12.

Burke, M., Walsh, J., Oehler, J., & Gingras, J. (1995). Music therapy following suctioning. *Neonatal Network, 14*(7), 41–49.

Chlan, L. (1995). Psychophysiologic responses of mechanically ventilated patients to music: A pilot study. *American Journal of Critical Care, 4*(3), 233–238.

Chlan, L. (1998). Effectiveness of a music therapy intervention on relaxation and anxiety for patients receiving ventilatory assistance. *Heart and Lung, 27*(3), 169–176.

Chlan, L., & Tracy, M. (1999). Music therapy in critical care: Indications and guidelines for intervention. *Critical Care Nurse, 19*(3), 35–41.

Clark, M., Lipe, A., & Bilbrey, M. (1998). Use of music to decrease aggressive behavior in people with dementia. *Journal of Gerontological Nursing, 24*(7), 10–17.

Collins, S., & Kuck, K. (1991). Music therapy in the neonatal intensive care unit. *Neonatal Network, 9*(6), 23–26.

Ezzone, S., Baker, C., Rosselet, R., & Terepka, E. (1998). Music as an adjunct to antiemetic therapy. *Oncology Nursing Forum, 25*(9), 1551–1556.

Farber, S. (1982). *Neurorehabilitation.* Philadelphia: W.B. Saunders.

Gerdner, L. (1997). An individualized music intervention for agitation. *Journal of the American Psychiatric Nurses Association, 3*(6), 177–184.

Gerdner, L., & Swanson, E. (1993). Effects of individualized music on confused and agitated elderly patients. *Archives of Psychiatric Nursing, 7*(5), 284–291.

Good, M. (1995). A comparison of the effects of jaw relaxation and music on postoperative pain. *Nursing Research, 44*(1), 52–57.

Good, M., Stanton-Hicks, M., Grass, J., Anderson, G., Choi, C., Schoolmeesters, L., & Salman, A. (1999). Relief of postoperative pain with jaw relaxation, music and their combination. *Pain, 81*(1, 2), 163–172.

Guzzetta, C. E. (1989). Effects of relaxation and music therapy on patients in a coronary care unit with presumptive acute myocardial infarction. *Heart & Lung, 18*(6), 609–616.

Guzzetta, C. (1995). Music therapy: Hearing the melody of the soul. In B. Dossey, L. Keegan, C. Guzzetta, & L. Kolkmeier (Eds.), *Holistic nursing* (pp. 670–698). Gaithersburg, MD: Aspen.

Hanser, S. (1988). Controversy in music listening/stress reduction research. *The Arts in Psychotherapy, 15*(2), 211–217.

Hanser, S., & Thompson, L. (1994). Effects of a music therapy strategy on depressed older adults. *Journal of Gerontology, 49*(6), 265–269.

Idzoriek, P. (1982). *Comparison of auditory and strong tactile stimuli on responsiveness.* Unpublished Plan B Project. University of Minnesota, School of Nursing, Minneapolis.

Jacobsen, A. (1999). Intradermal normal saline solution, self-selected music, and insertion difficulty effects on intravenous insertion pain. *Heart & Lung, 28*(2), 114–122.

Janelli, L., & Kanski, G. (1998). Music for untying restrained patients. *Journal of the New York State Nurses Association, 29*(1), 13–15.

Janelli, L., Kanski, G., Jones, H., & Kennedy, M. (1995). Exploring music intervention with restrained patients. *Nursing Forum, 30*(4), 12–18.

Jones, R., Hux, C., Morton-Anderson, A., & Knepper, L. (1994). Auditory stimulation effect on a comatose survivor of traumatic brain injury. *Archives of Physical Medicine and Rehabilitation, 75*(1), 164–171.

Kaempf, G., & Amodei, M. (1989). The effect of music on anxiety. *AORN Journal, 50*(1), 112–118.

Klein, S., & Winkelstein, M. (1996). Enhancing pediatric health care with music. *Pediatric Health Care, 10*(1), 74–81.

Maranto, C. (1993). Applications of music in medicine. In M. Heal & T. Wigram (Eds.), *Music therapy in health and education* (pp. 153–174). London: Jessica Kingsley.

Mavely, R., & Mitchell, G. (1994). Consider karaoke. *Canadian Nurse, 90*(1), 22–24.

Megel, M., Houser, C., & Gleaves, L. (1998). Children's responses to immunization: Lullabies as a distraction. *Issues in Comprehensive Pediatric Nursing, 21*(3), 129–145.

Moore, R., Staum, M., & Brotons, M. (1992). Music preferences of the elderly: Repertoire, vocal ranges, tempos, and accompaniments for singing. *Journal of Music Therapy, 29*(4), 236–252.

Mornhinweg, G., & Voignier, R. (1995). Music for sleep disturbance in the elderly. *Journal of Holistic Nursing, 13*(3), 248–254.

Nightingale, F. (1860/1969). *Notes on nursing.* New York: Dover.

Robb, S., Nichols, R., Rutan, R., Bishop, B., & Parker, J. (1995). The effects of music-assisted relaxation on preoperative anxiety. *Journal of Music Therapy, 32*(1), 3–12.

Sambandham, M., & Schirm, V. (1995). Music as a nursing intervention for residents with Alzheimer's disease in long-term care. *Geriatric Nursing, 16*(2), 79–83.

Schorr, J. (1993). Music and pattern change in chronic pain. *Advances in Nursing Science, 15*(4), 27–36.

Snyder, M., & Chlan, L. (1999). Music therapy. In J. Fitzpatrick (Ed.), *Annual review of nursing research, 17,* 3–25. New York: Springer.

Snyder, M., & Olson, J. (1996). Music and hand massage interventions to produce relaxation and reduce aggressive behaviors in cognitively impaired elders: A pilot study. *Clinical Gerontologist, 17*(1), 64–69.

Standley, J. (1986). Music research in medical/dental treatment: Meta-analysis and clinical applications. *Journal of Music Therapy, 23*(2), 56–122.

Steelman, V. (1990). Intraoperative music therapy. *AORN Journal, 52*(5), 1026–1034.

Stevens, K. (1990). Patients' perceptions of music during surgery. *Journal of Advanced Nursing, 15*(6), 1045–1051.

Thaut, M. (1990). Physiological and motor responses to music stimuli. In R. Unkefer (Ed.), *Music therapy in the treatment of adults with mental disorders: Theoretical bases and clinical interventions* (pp. 33–49). New York: Schirmer Books.

Updike, P. (1990). Music therapy results for ICU patients. *Dimensions of Critical Care Nursing*, 9(1), 39–45.

White, J. (1992). Music therapy: An intervention to reduce anxiety in the myocardial infarction patient. *Clinical Nurse Specialist*, 6(2), 58–63.

White, J. (1999). Effects of relaxing music on cardiac autonomic balance and anxiety after acute myocardial infarction. *American Journal of Critical Care*, 8(4), 220–230.

Wiens, M., Reimer, M., & Guyn, H. (1999). Music therapy as a treatment method for improving respiratory muscle strength in patients with advanced multiple sclerosis: A pilot study. *Rehabilitation Nursing*, 24(2), 74–80.

Woolf, H. (Ed.) (1979). *Merriam-Webster's collegiate dictionary* (9th ed.). Springfield, MA: Merriam-Webster.

7

Humor

Kevin Smith

A merry heart doeth good like a medicine, but a broken spirit drieth the bones.
— Proverbs 17:22

Throughout history, many have accorded a beneficial effect to joy and mirth. Greek philosophers including Plato and Aristotle wrote treatises on humor (McGhee, 1979). The German philosopher Immanuel Kant, in 1790, set forth similar physical effects of humor and defined humor as a talent that enabled one to look at things from a different perspective (Haig, 1988). In medieval physiology, the definition of humor was "moisture" or "vapor." *Humor* referred to the four principal fluids of the body: blood, phlegm, choler (yellow bile), and melancholy (black bile). A proper balance of the four was called good humor, and a preponderance of any one constituted ill humor (Robinson, 1991).

That humor and laughter can improve our ability to cope with difficulties and to stay healthy is a popular notion. Interest in this area has increased since Norman Cousins' account of the role of laughter in his recovery from a painful collagen disorder (1979). The belief that humor and laughter positively influence health and the scientific evidence will be reviewed to provide a basis for the use of humor by nurses and others providing health care.

Nursing journal articles continue to address many facets of humor, such as laughter and stress management (Paquet, 1993; Woodhouse, 1993); humor as a nursing intervention (Hunt, 1993; Mornhinweg & Voignier, 1995); humor and the older adult (Herth, 1993); humor and healing (Macaluso, 1993); and the positive physiologic effects of humor (Lambert & Lambert, 1995). Humor organizations and publications are increasing, humor workshops are being offered to nurses and other health care providers, and many continuing education offerings are incorporating humorous presentations or activities.

Humor can be used as a specific therapy or can be used with other therapies. In conjunction with other therapies it can be considered a parallel intervention. The goals in using humor as an intervention are to enhance the well-being of the client, to enhance the therapeutic relationship between the nurse and the client, and to bring hope and joy to the situation. Humor creates an outlet for stress for both the client and nurse. It can be used to foster trust and a comfortable environment for the client. Virtually anyone can develop the requisite skills needed to use humor as an intervention.

DEFINITION

Humor is the good-natured side of truth.

—Mark Twain

The American Association for Therapeutic Humor (2000) defines therapeutic humor as follows:

> Any intervention that promotes health and wellness by stimulating a playful discovery, expression of appreciation of the absurdity or incongruity of life's situations. This intervention may enhance health or be used as a complementary treatment of illness to facilitate healing or coping, whether physical, emotional, cognitive, social or spiritual. (p. 3)

Nurse and humor expert Vera Robinson (1978) described the phenomenon of humor as "any communication which is perceived by any of the interacting parties as humorous and leads to laughing, smiling or a feeling of amusement" (p. 193). The dictionary defines it as "the quality of being laughable or comical," and "the ability to perceive, enjoy, or express what is comical or funny." Humor can be the process of either producing or perceiving the comical. What is personally defined or perceived as funny and its physical manifestations varies among individuals. However, there are predictable stimuli for laughter and usual responses.

WHY DO WE LAUGH?

There are many different reasons. Sometimes the response is simply for the fun of it; sometimes it is for more important reasons. Here we will discuss four basic theories for the laughter response: surprise, superiority, incongruity, and release.

1. *Surprise.* Good humor or a good joke may catch one off guard. The surprise in itself causes a person to laugh. Another type of surprise humor is shock humor. This could be a startling or loud punch line or even something taboo or vulgar. Shock humor has caused many a mother to say, "Please do not encourage her." Shock humor is not recommended in clinical or therapeutic settings.

2. *Superiority.* The theory of superiority laughter (Robinson, 1991) involves situations in which laughter occurs when one feels superior to an individual or a group. One's laughter is in response to the inferiority, stupidity, or the misfortunes of others. In its most simple form this would be slapstick humor; a more sophisticated form would be political satire. It has been suggested that the essential effect of humor is derived from a sense of mastery or ego strength (Lefcourt & Martin, 1986).

3. *Incongruity.* Schafner (1981) concisely describes this theory as laughter occurring because of "a perception of an incongruity in a ludicrous context." For example, a man walks in to a psychiatrist's office with a duck on his head. The duck says, "Doc, you got to help me get this guy off my tail." Two ideas are juxtaposed in an impossible or absurd situation. The incongruity theory advanced by Kant and other philosophers like Schopenhauer and Spencer emphasized the importance of a sudden surprise, shock, conflict of ideas, or incongruity as a trigger for laughter (Liechty, 1987). Asimov (1992) argues that incongruities put the listener, for a brief moment, in a fantasy world. This suspension of reality readies the listener for the crowning bit of fantasy or the punch line that results in laughter.

4. *Release.* The basic premise of the release theory, as a laughter stimulus, is that humor and laughter help to release tensions and anxieties. Freud (1905/1960) viewed humor as a coping tool that allows individuals to reduce tension by expressing hostile or obscene impulses in a socially acceptable manner. Morreal (1983) called this the relief theory and notes that humor which produces laughter is a method for venting nervous energy. This release type of laughter is often enhanced in group situations where many share the same anxiety.

HUMOR STYLES

Most of the humor that is employed on a daily basis with staff and patients is of the spontaneous type: situational humor that arises out of the normal absurdities of today's activities. This type of humor is also a very effective communication tool when used to break the ice with patients or co-workers. An attempt is made to lighten up the situation; this is a sign of caring and allows for a free exchange of thoughts, feelings and emotions. Formal humor, or premeditated acts of humor (Smith, 1995), include the sharing of jokes, cartoons, humorous articles or stories, novelty toys or gag gifts, and practical jokes. Formal humor, like most forms of humor, is usually only effective when it is relevant to the situation in which it is presented. Other more specific humor styles include self-deprecating humor, puns and plays on words, ethnic humor, sarcastic humor, and gallows humor.

Self-deprecating humor may be the most effective and powerful humor tool that nurses can develop and use. To show that one is able to laugh at oneself demonstrates that one is a normal human being with weaknesses while at the same time displaying a level confidence, self-awareness, and self-esteem. Ronald Reagan used this type of humor effectively when he was being taken to the operating room after an assassination attempt. He quipped, "I hope my surgeon is a Republican" (Klein, 1989). Paulsen (1989) stated that gently poking fun at oneself acts as a social lubricant. It shows that a person is at ease with the situation. People are often suspicious or afraid of those without any sense of humor.

Puns and plays on words are simple and straightforward humor styles. Some consider puns to be the lowest form of humor, but pun enthusiasts include Asimov and Freud. Puns typically produce groans rather than laughter. For example, "With friends like you, who needs enemas?"

Ethnic humor is often regional. Using one's own ethnicity or profession as the target of the joke is the most acceptable approach. Sarcastic humor is somewhat risky; overheard sarcasm can make a patient or others think they are the target of the sarcastic comments. Freud (1960) developed a theory about why people laugh at tragedy and death, which he called gallows humor. Such grim humor is typically seen when people are faced with considerable stress. He theorized that jokes allow people to express unconscious aggressive or sexual impulses. Obrdlik (1942) asserted that the phenomenon of gallows humor has a definite social purpose. It provides a psychological escape and strengthens the morale of the group and in some situations undermines the morale of the oppressors. Gallows humor is frequently used in situations where individuals are under significant stress, such as emergency rooms, intensive care units, operating rooms, and morgues.

SCIENTIFIC BASIS

Many of the positive physiological effects of humor and laughter have been studied. Humor is considered the stimulus and laughter the response. Laughter creates a cascade of physiological changes in the body. Fry (1971) studied the effects of mirthful laughter on heart rate and on the oxygen saturation level of peripheral blood and respiratory phenomena. He found that both the arousal and cathartic effects are paralleled in the physiological. In contrast to other emotions, laughter involves extensive physical activity. It increases respiratory activity and oxygen exchange, increases muscular activity and heart rate, and stimulates the cardiovascular system, the sympathetic nervous system, and the production of catecholamines. The arousal state is followed by the relaxation state in which respiration rate, heart rate, and muscle tension return to normal. Although the oxygen saturation of peripheral blood is not affected during this relaxation state, blood pressure is reduced and a state exists similar to the impact of hearty exercise. Fry and Savin (1982) investigated the effects of humor on arterial blood pressure using direct arterial cannulization. Findings showed increases in systolic and diastolic blood pressure that were directly related to the intensity and length of laughter. Blood pressure decreased immediately after the laughter to below the pre-laughter baseline.

Many studies have found that humor and laughter increase levels of salivary immunoglobulin A (S-IgA), a vital immune system protein that is the body's first line of defense against respiratory illnesses. In a controlled study, Dillon, Minchoff, and Baker (1985) demonstrated increased levels of S-IgA in college students who were exposed to a humorous intervention, viewing a humorous video. Martin and Dobbin (1988) measured subjects' sense of humor, stress levels, and S-IgA levels and demonstrated that subjects with low scores on the humor scales showed a greater negative relationship between stress and S-IgA than did subjects with high humor scores. Stone, Valdimarsdottir, Jandorf, Cox, and Neale (1987) found that the S-IgA response level was lower on days of negative mood and higher on days of positive mood. Lambert and Lambert (1995) produced similar findings with S-IgA levels in well fifth-grade students.

Berk and colleagues studied the effects of laughter on the neuroendocrine, stress hormones (Berk, Tan, & Fry, 1989), and immune parameters (Berk, Tan, Napier, & Erby, 1989). They found a complex autonomic response with each catecholamine, suggesting that laughter may be an antagonist to the classical stress response. They demonstrated that laughter lowered serum cortisol levels, increased the amount of activated T-lymphocytes, and increased the number and activity of natural killer cells. Laughter stimulated the immune system, counteracting the immunosuppressive effects of stress.

Friedman and Ulmer (1984) assigned hundreds of heart-attack survivors to one of two groups. The control group received standard advice regarding medications, diet, and exercise. The treatment group received additional counseling on relaxation, smiling, laughing at themselves, admitting mistakes, taking time to enjoy life, and renewing their religious faith. Over 3 years, the treatment group experienced half as many repeat heart attacks as the control group.

PSYCHOLOGICAL PERSPECTIVES

Humor has been considered an adaptive coping mechanism. Freud (1905/1960) regarded humor and laughter as one of the few socially acceptable means for releasing pent-up frustrations and anger, a cathartic mechanism for preserving psychic or emotional energy. Humor and laughter alter our perspective in various situations. Laughter can counteract negative emotions; it allows people to transcend predicaments, conquer painful circumstances, and cope with difficulties. By focusing energy elsewhere, humor can diffuse the stress of difficult events (Klein, 1989). The use of humor has been shown to reduce threat-induced anxiety (Yovetich, Dale, & Hudak, 1990).

INTERVENTION

There are many approaches, techniques, and tools that can be used for utilizing humor as an intervention. A first step in deciding how and when to use humor is to complete a humor assessment, first of yourself, then of your patient.

ASSESSMENT

A humor interview guide was developed to explore older adults' perceptions of humor (Herth, 1993; see Table 7.1). This assessment could be adapted for use in clinical setting or used in research. The assessment is completed by the provider, then by the client.

When completing a self-assessment of one's own sense of humor, one should consider what type of humor seems most natural. Consider preferences for spontaneity versus formal humor. The comfort levels of the provider and client should also be considered. Like all skills, you can always work on improving your sense of humor. Strickland (1993) says that the first and biggest barrier to using humor is the fear of appearing foolish or of losing control over one's self-image.

Part of a humor assessment of a patient is determining what type of humor is appropriate to use for the client and the particular situation. Humor that is divisive in any way should be avoided. Find out the patient's and family's prior use of humor and whether they currently appreciate and value humor and laughter (Davidhizar & Bowen 1992). Spontaneous comments on a neutral topic such as the weather, equipment, or yourself can help you to see if the individual is open to humor, though readiness for humor may or may not be apparent.

TABLE 7.1   Humor Assessment Interview Guide

1. When you think of humor, what kinds of images or thoughts come to mind?
2. Was humor a part of your life when you were younger?
3. Is humor still a part of your life?
4. How has humor been helpful or not helpful at this time in your life?
5. If humor is helpful, what do you do to maintain humor in your life?
6. Are there certain times when you appreciate humor more than other times?
7. When has humor been a negative experience?
8. What types of activities do you find amusing or enjoyable?

Note: From "Humor and the Older Adult," by K. A. Herth, 1993, *Applied Nursing Research*, 64, pp. 146–153. Copyright 1993, Philadelphia, PA: W. B. Saunders Company. Used with permission.

TECHNIQUES

Table 7.2 shows a variety of approaches to intervention. Ackerman, Henry, Graham, and Coffey (1994) developed a model for incorporating humor into the health care setting and described the steps to create a humor program. Humorous materials were made available to patients through a "chuckle wagon" cart that was taken to patients' rooms. A humor-resource center was developed to assist nurses in incorporating humor into their patient care, and a patient satisfaction evaluation tool was developed to assess the patients' response to the humor cart. Table 7.3 provides several humor Web sites that contain material for humor interventions.

MEASUREMENT OF EFFECTIVENESS

Although physical laughter is not an essential outcome of humor, physical responses to a humor intervention are obvious indicators of effectiveness. According to Black (1984), the multiple physical manifestations of the laughter response cover a range from smiling to belly laughing. Other positive responses may be the relief of symptoms, facial expression, degree of involvement in activities, and strengthening of the relationship between caregiver and client.

Lefcourt and Martin (1986) developed the Situational Humor Response Questionnaire (SHRQ) for determining an individual's response to particular types of humor. It has been used in numerous studies and has been validated as effectively measuring humor. Diverse factors, such as developmental or cultural factors, may also influence an individual's response to humor. It is important to be alert to the variations and subtleties of a patient's response.

TABLE 7.2   Selected Techniques and Activities to Provide and
             Support Humor Interventions

1. Assemble/collect humor resources (create humor rooms, humor carts, humorous videos).
2. Invite guest performers (comedians, magicians, clowns).
3. Wear a humorous item, silly button, necktie, etc.
4. Display humorous photos of staff.
5. Have a cartoon bulletin board with favorites from staff and patients displayed each week.
6. Play music that encourages playful movement.
7. Support and applaud the efforts of staff and patients to use humor.

USES

Humor can be used in many situations. It may be effectively used in highly stressful situations to overcome tensions and to facilitate patient catharsis or expression of fear and anxiety. Ziv (1984) described the use of humor as a defense mechanism for dealing with anxieties. As a provider of patient care, one must be sensitive to the fact that the use of humor could be the patient's attempt to avoid facing more serious issues or feelings. Humorous distraction may be used to reduce preoperative anxiety (Gaberson, 1991). Humor has also been used as an adjunct for enhancing postoperative recall of the exercise routines that were taught preoperatively (Parfitt, 1990). It may be used effectively for problems associated with communication, anxiety, grieving, powerlessness, or social isolation (Hunt, 1993). The psychological impact of humor and laughter has been studied as an adjunct in the management of psychiatric patients (Saper, 1988, 1990) and may be an effective intervention as part of psychotherapy (Rosenheim & Golan, 1986). Moody (1978) studied and has incorporated the use of positive emotions and humor in dealing with the fear, anxiety, and pain that go along with cancer and other chronic conditions. Humor also has been advocated as an intervention for elderly clients (Hulse, 1994).

Humor may be used to increase comfort or raise the pain threshold. Cogan, Cogan, Waltz, and McCue (1987) studied the effects of laughter and relaxation on discomfort thresholds. In a group of volunteers, tolerance levels of physical discomfort were measured after members of the group either listened to a laughter-inducing narrative, an uninteresting narrative tape, or had no intervention. Patient discomfort thresholds increased (patients could handle more pain) in the laughter-inducing scenario.

TABLE 7.3   Selected On-line Humor Resources

1. *American Association for Therapeutic Humor:* www.aath.org
2. *Humor and Health Institute:* www.intop.net~jrdunn/
3. *The Joyful Noiseletter:* www.joyfulnoiseletter.com
4. *The Humor Project:* www.humorproject.com

Situations involving short-term pain such as some nursing treatments (e.g., injections) and recovery from procedures or surgery are particularly appropriate for the use of humor.

PRECAUTIONS

There are a variety of factors that practitioners should consider when using humor. The timing of the use of humor in the clinical setting is crucial to its success. Leiber (1986) cautioned that one must assess the patient's receptiveness to humor. Crane (1987) states that there are times when humor is contraindicated. What may be funny to a patient when they are feeling well may not seem funny during an illness episode. Humor and laughter have no place at the height of a crisis, although they can be useful to allay tension as the crisis subsides. Inside jokes among health care professionals can seem offensive or callous to outsiders who may overhear them. Laughing *at* others negates confidence and destroys teamwork, whereas laughing *with* others builds confidence, brings people together, and pokes fun at our common dilemmas (Goodman, 1992). Patients may use inappropriate or sexually aggressive remarks under the pretext of joking, in which case further assessment may be indicated to determine the underlying reason for the aggressive verbal behavior.

FUTURE RESEARCH

The therapeutic use of humor by nurses has been and will continue to be an important aspect of providing patient care. Awareness of the importance of humor is increasing as demonstrated by the plethora of articles published in support of humor as an intervention, numerous scientific studies regarding its use, and an increase in the number of educational offerings. An understanding is needed of how humor, laughter, and positive emotions benefit the physiology and potential healing capacity of individuals. Nurses can use this same information to incorporate humor into their lives to make their work and personal lives more enjoyable and to become more effective providers of care. Research questions to be addressed include:

1. What are the physiological effects of humor on patients who are critically ill?
2. How can the use of humor be taught and the effectiveness of its use be measured?
3. Can the systematic use of humor speed healing or enhance outcomes of acute illness?
4. Can humor be utilized in care environments to reduce stress and enhance nurse satisfaction and retention?

REFERENCES

Ackerman, M., Henry, M., Graham, K., & Coffey, N. (1994). Humor won, humor too: A model to incorporate humor into the health care setting (revised). *Nursing Forum, 29*(2), 15–21.

American Association for Therapeutic Humor. (2000). [on-line] www.aath.org

Asimov, A. (1992). *Asimov laughs again.* New York: HarperCollins.

Berk, L., Tan, S., & Fry, W. (1989). Neuroendocrine and stress hormone changes during mirthful laughter. *American Journal of Medical Sciences, 298*(6), 390–396.

Berk, L., Tan, S., Napier, B., & Eby, W. (1989). Eustress of mirthful laughter modifies natural killer cell activity. *Clinical Research, 37*(1), 115A.

Black, D. (1984). Laughter. *Journal of the American Medical Association, 25*(21), 2995–2998.

Cogan, R., Cogan, D., Waltz, W., & McCue, M. (1987). Effects of laughter and relaxation on discomfort thresholds. *Journal of Behavioral Medicine, 10*, 139–144.

Cousins, N. (1979). *Anatomy of an illness.* New York: W.W. Norton.

Crane, A. L. (1987). Why sickness can be a laughing matter. *RN, 50*, 41–42.

Davidhizar, R., & Bowen, M. (1992). The dynamics of laughter. *Archives of Psychiatric Nursing, 6*(2), 132–137.

Dillon, K., Minchoff, B., & Baker, K. (1985). Positive emotional states and enhancement of the immune system. *International Journal of Psychiatry in Medicine, 15*(1), 3–17.

Freud, S. (1960). *Jokes and their relation to the unconscious.* New York: W.W. Norton. (Originally: *DerWitz und seine Beziehung zum Unbewussten.* Leizig and Vienna: Durtricke, 1905).

Friedman, M., & Ulmer, D. (1984). *Treating type A behavior—and your heart.* New York: Knopf.

Fry, W. (1971). Mirth and oxygen saturation of peripheral blood. *Psychotherapy and Psychosomatics, 19*, 76–84.

Fry, W. F., & Savin, M. (1988). Mirthful laughter and blood pressure. *Humor, 1,* 49–62.

Gaberson, K. (1991). The effect of humorous distraction on preoperative anxiety. *AORN Journal, 54*(6), 1258–1264.

Goodman, J. (1992). Laughing matters: Taking your job seriously and yourself lightly. *Journal of the American Medical Association, 267*(13),1858.

Haig, R. A. (1988). *The anatomy of humor: Biopsychosocial and therapeutic perspectives.* Springfield, IL: Charles C. Thomas.

Herth, K. A. (1993). Humor and the older adult. *Applied Nursing Research, 6*(4), 146–153.

Hulse, J. (1994). Humor: A nursing intervention for the elderly. *Geriatric Nursing, 15*(2), 88–90.

Hunt, A. H. (1993). Humor as a nursing intervention. *Cancer Nursing, 16*(1), 34–39.

Klein, A. (1989). *The healing power of humor.* Los Angeles: Jeremy P. Tarcher.

Lambert, R., & Lambert, N. K. (1995). The effects of humor on secretory immunoglobulin-A levels in school-aged children. *Pediatric Nursing, 21*(1), 16–19.

Lefcourt, H. M., & Martin, R. A. (1986). *Humor and life stress: Antidote to adversity.* New York: Springer-Verlag.

Leiber, D. B. (1986). Laughter and humor in critical care. *Dimensions in Critical Care Nursing, 5*(3), 162–170.

Liechty, R. D. (1987). Humor and the surgeon. *Archives of Surgery, 122,* 519–522.

Macaluso, M. C. (1993). Humor, health and healing. *American Nephrology Nurses Association Journal, 20*(1), 14–16.

Martin, R., & Dobbin, J. (1988). Sense of humor, hassles, and immunoglobulin evidence for a stress-moderating effect of humor. *International Journal of Psychiatry in Medicine, 18*(2), 93–105.

McGhee, P. (1979). *Humor: Its orgin and development.* San Francisco: W.H. Freeman.

Moody, R. A. (1978). *Laugh after laugh.* Jacksonville, FL: Headwaters Press.

Mornhinweg, G., & Voignier, R. (1995). Holistic nursing interventions. *Orthopedic Nursing, 14*(4), 20–24.

Morreal, J. (1983). *Taking laughter seriously.* Albany: State University of New York Press.

Obrldik, A. (1942). Gallows humor: A sociological phenomenon. *American Journal of Sociology, 47,* 709–716.

Paquet, J. (1993, November/December). Laughter and stress management. *Today's OR Nurse,* 13–17.

Parfitt, J. M. (1990). Humorous preoperative teaching: Effect of recall of postoperative exercise routines. *AORN Journal, 52*(1), 114–120.

Paulsen, T. (1989). *Making humor work: Take your job seriously and yourself lightly.* Los Altos, CA: Crisp.

Robinson, V. (1978). Humor in nursing. In C. Carlson & B. Blackwell, (Eds.), *Behavioral concepts and nursing interventions.* Philadelphia: J.B. Lippincott.

Robinson, V. M. (1991). *Humor and the health professions* (2nd ed.). Thorofare, NJ: Slack.

Rosenheim, E., & Golan, G. (1986). Patients' reactions to humorous interventions in psychotherapy. *American Journal of Psychotherapy, 40*(1), 110–124.

Saper, B. (1990). The therapeutic use of humor for psychiatric disturbances in adolescents and adults. *Psychiatric Quarterly, 61*(4), 261–272.

Saper, B. (1988). Humor in psychiatric healing. *Psychiatric Quarterly, 59*(4), 306–319.

Schaefner, N. (1981). *The art of laughter.* New York: Columbia University Press.

Simon, J. M. (1989) Humor techniques for oncology nurses. *Oncology Nursing Forum, 16*(5), 667–670.

Smith, K. L. (1995). *Medicinal mirth: The art and science of therapuetic humor.* Presentation to North Memorial Hospice and Home Care, Minneapolis.

Stone, A., Valdimarsdottir, H., Jandorf, L., Cox, D., & Neale, J. (1987). Evidence that IgA antibody is associated with daily mood. *Journal of Personality and Social Psychology, 52,* 988–993.

Strickland, D. (1993, November/December). Seriously, laughter matters. *Today's OR Nurse,* 19–24.

Woodhouse, D. K. (1993). The aspects of humor in dealing with stress. *Nursing Administration Quarterly, 18*(1), 80–89.

Yovetich, N. A., Dale, A., & Hudak, M. (1990). Benefits of humor in reduction of threat induced anxiety. *Psychological Reports, 66,* 51–58.

Ziv, A. (1984). *Personality and sense of humor.* New York: Springer-Verlag.

8

Yoga

Miriam E. Cameron

Regardless of age, health, religion, or education, anyone can benefit from doing yoga. The practice of yoga heals and strengthens the body, sharpens the mind, and calms the spirit. As the body, mind, and spirit come into harmony with one another and with the infinite, the person experiences compassion, well-being, and inner peace. Yoga does not require drugs, expensive equipment, or surgery. Because of the efficacy, cost-effectiveness, and lack of side effects, yoga is an effective aid in health and healing (Mehta, Mehta, & Mehta, 1999). Nurses do yoga themselves, and they use yoga as a complementary, alternative, and primary therapy in nursing practice. This chapter focuses on yoga postures and breathing as a nursing intervention.

DEFINITION

Yoga, an ancient Indian science, means union or joining together of the individual and universal spirit. More than 2,000 years ago, Patanjali systemized yoga into a treatise, *Yoga Sutra*, which continues to be the authoritative text. With its unique blend of theoretical knowledge and practical application, yoga has eight interconnected limbs, or aspects of the whole, that lead progressively to higher stages of health, awareness, and spirituality. The first five limbs still the mind in order to attain the last three. The eight limbs and Sanskrit names are as follows:

1. Universal ethical principles (*yama*): nonviolence, truthfulness, non-stealing, chastity, and noncovetousness. The individual avoids harming any living being and becomes gentle, loving, free from anger, and helpful to other people.

81

2. Personal conduct (*niyma*): purity, commitment, contentment, self-study, and surrender to the infinite. The person eats small amounts of high-quality food that provide *prana* or life force and lets go of egoism, which underlies unhappiness, pain, and most diseases.

3. Yoga postures (*asanas*): carefully designed movements to methodically stretch, condition, and massage the body. These postures are performed deliberately without strain.

4. Yoga breathing (*pranayama*): regulation and refinement of the inhalation, exhalation, and retention of breath. The person learns that the breath, consisting of air and *prana*, affects well-being and determines to a great extent the length and quality of life.

5. Control of the senses (*pratyahara*): temporary withdrawal of the senses from the external to the inner world. External disturbances are unable to cross the threshold of the inner world.

6. Concentration of the mind (*dharana*): the mind focuses steadily and without interruption on a particular point or object. Examples of such objects are the breath and a lit candle.

7. Meditation (*dhyana*): a profound state of quiet and relaxation. The person temporarily withdraws from the external world and develops awareness of the inner self and the infinite.

8. Absorption into the infinite (*samadhi*): a transcendent state of truth and wisdom that is beyond meditation. The individual experiences true joy and inner peace (Mehta, Mehta, & Mehta, 1999).

SCIENTIFIC BASIS

For centuries, yogis in India have made health claims about yoga. Recently, researchers have found that regular practice of yoga postures and breathing produces significant health benefits. For example, yoga improved perceptual motor skills (Manjunath & Telles, 1999; Raghuraj & Telles, 1997), increased work output, and reduced ventilation and level of oxygen consumption (Raju, Prasad, Venkata, Murthy, & Reddy, 1997). Moreover, yoga decreased stress (Anand, 1999) and anxiety (Khasky & Smith, 1999). Medical students who did yoga were less likely to fail exams and feel irritable; they had a relaxed feeling of well-being, optimism, and self-confidence; and they improved their efficiency, interpersonal relationships, concentration, and attentiveness (Malathi & Damodaran, 1999).

Research indicates that yoga postures and breathing produce effects different from other exercise programs. Yoga both treats symptoms and prevents recurrences or the onset of symptoms. For example, poor body alignment and breathing are major factors in health problems. Yoga improves body alignment and breathing, as well as circulation, use of the extremities, and mindfulness. Consequently, the vital organs and endocrine glands become rehabilitated so they consume little energy and produce optimal efficiency. The person experiences self-regulation, healing, and well-being (Farrell, Ross, & Sehgal, 1999; Sequeira, 1999).

INTERVENTION

Various Postures and Breathing Techniques

Because yoga is an experiential therapy, the best way to learn yoga is to do it. Numerous books, classes, and videos are available for students from beginning to advanced levels. Table 8.1 describes *savasana*, a posture for calming the body and mind. Table 8.2 explains *bharadvajasana*, which relaxes and tones the spine and internal organs. Thousands of other yoga postures and breathing techniques condition all parts of the body (Mehta, Mehta, & Mehta, 1999).

Measurement of Outcomes

Nurses can measure outcomes by asking individuals how they feel after doing yoga. Most health problems develop over time, and yoga may not alleviate them right away. Minor difficulties often respond quickly, but serious problems require sustained, patient practice. Yoga philosophy advocates gradual change. Optimal benefits occur from regular practice. Short-term outcomes are notable, however, for they include a more relaxed attitude, decreased anxiety, improved balance, and increased musculoskeletal flexibility. Faithful practitioners experience long-term outcomes of better physical, spiritual, and mental health, including weight regulation and mental clarity.

Precautions

Complications may result from performing yoga postures and breathing in a harmful manner, such as straining to do yoga postures. Because yoga was designed to develop human potential, yoga philosophy does not encourage anything unnatural or hurtful. Adverse effects can be avoided by doing yoga gently and in moderation and by developing an attitude of noncompetition and nonmaleficence. Although yoga teachers and other aids can be helpful in providing guidance, individuals must seek their own inner wisdom (Mehta, Mehta, & Mehta, 1999).

TABLE 8.1   *Savasana* (Corpse Posture)

1. Lie down on a flat surface, such as a bed or a mat on the floor, making sure to keep your trunk and legs in line. If you wish, place a small pillow under your head and neck.

2. Settle your back and extend your trunk, arms, and legs so you are comfortable and can relax. If this position hurts your lower back, bend your knees and put your feet flat on the bed or mat.

3. Turn your upper arms out, with your palms up and your fingers curling naturally.

4. Close your eyes; keep your eyes still and your face relaxed.

5. Breathe slowly, evenly, and quietly through your nose and from your abdomen.

6. Do not let your mind wander, but focus on your body and breath.

7. Allow your body to sink into the bed or mat.

8. Stay quietly for 5 to 10 minutes or more.

9. Slowly open your eyes and bend your knees.

10. Turn to one side, and stay for a moment; then turn to the other side before getting up.

Savasana encourages your body to become as still as a corpse and your mind to be at peace. With practice, you will be able to call on this quietness at will.

Note: Adapted from *Yoga the Iyengar Way,* by S. Mehta, M. Mehta, and S. Mehta, 1999, New York: Alfred A. Knopf.

USES

Nurses report using yoga postures and breathing techniques in their work involving long-term care, HIV/AIDS, labor and delivery, mental health, substance abuse, pain management, respiratory problems, health promotion, surgery, postoperative care, rehabilitation, and other areas. Yoga classes at work help nurses to reduce their own job-related health problems, such as carpal tunnel syndrome and neck, shoulder, and back pain (Collins, 1998; Gimbel, 1998; Luskin et al., 2000). Case studies have been published about the advantages of yoga for individuals who have diabetes, arthritis, cold and flu symptoms, cancer, injuries, problems with the endocrine and nervous systems, spinal difficulties, insomnia, Crohn's disease, and other conditions (Dunn, 2000; Pirisi, 2000; Staff Editors, 2000). Doing yoga reduced the stress of children in a community home (Telles, Narendran, Raghuraj, Nagarathna, & Nagendra, 1997) and inner city, bilingual adults (Roth & Creaser, 1997).

TABLE 8.2 *Bharadvajasana I* (Seated Spinal Twist)

1. Sit straight and tall on the floor or in a chair or wheelchair with your shoulders back.
2. Face forward and balance your head over your spine so your neck muscles are soft.
3. To twist to the right, place your right hand on the floor, seat or arm of the chair in which you are sitting.
4. Place the back of your left hand on your outer right knee or thigh. If you are sitting on the floor, bend your legs to the left.
5. Without hurrying, begin with every exhalation to rotate your body to the right.
6. Slowly turn your head to the right, making sure to balance your head directly on top of your spine.
7. Look as far to the right as you can, and hold the posture until your muscles relax.
8. Continue to breathe slowly, deeply, and evenly through your nose and from your abdomen.
9. After completing the twist to the right, twist to the left by following the same steps in the opposite direction.

Bharadvajasana releases tension and strengthens the spine, neck, and shoulders; tones and cleanses the internal organs; and quiets the nervous system.

Note: Adapted from "Bharadvajasana I," by D. Benitez, 2000, *Yoga Journal, 147,* pp. 22–23.

Table 8.3 lists research findings about the benefits of using yoga for specific health problems.

FUTURE RESEARCH

Additional research is needed to understand more completely how yoga postures and breathing aid health and healing. Longitudinal studies are lacking about the long-term results of doing yoga. To study yoga effectively, researchers may need to develop new, holistic research methodologies. Some research questions are

1. What yoga postures and breathing techniques are therapeutic for particular health problems?
2. What yoga postures and breathing techniques are beneficial to use as part of nursing care?

TABLE 8.3   Research Findings: The Benefits of Yoga for Specific Health Problems

- Reduced pain (Hudson, 1998; Kabat-Zinn, 1993; Jain, Nagarathna, Nagendra, & Telles, 1999).
- Improved musculoskeletal strength (Garfinkel & Schumacher, 2000).
- Relieved carpal tunnel syndrome (Garfinkel et al., 1998; Sequeira, 1999).
- Lowered blood pressure (Anand, 1999; Selvamurthy et al., 1998).
- Reduced risks for and managed heart disease (Mahajan, Reddy, & Sachdeva, 1999; Ornish, 1993; Pandya, Vyas, & Vyas, 1999; Schmidt, Wijga, Muhlen, Brabant, & Wagner, 1997).
- Improved mental ability, motor coordination, and social skills of mentally disabled persons; restored some functional ability for physically disabled persons; decreased abnormal anxiety levels of visually impaired children; improved sleep, appetite, and general well-being of socially disadvantaged adults and children; decreased substance abuse (Telles & Naveen, 1997).
- Exerted antidepressant effects (Naga, Janakiramaiah, Gangadhar, & Subbakrishna, 1998).
- Increased relaxation, positive attitude, and exercise tolerance and led to less use of beta-adrenergic inhalers for individuals with asthma (Vedanthan, et al., Nagarathna, 1998).

3. What characterizes individuals who practice yoga regularly, compared with persons who do not use yoga at all or who stop doing yoga?
4. What are effective strategies for encouraging individuals to do yoga regularly?
5. What are effective strategies for teaching nurses to use yoga as a nursing intervention?

REFERENCES

Anand, M. P. (1999). Non-pharmacological management of essential hypertension. *Journal of the Indian Medical Association, 97*, 220–225.

Benitez, D. (2000, July/August). Bharadvajasana I. *Yoga Journal, 147*, 22–23.

Collins, C. (1998). Yoga: Intuition, preventive medicine, and treatment. *Journal of Obstetric, Gynecologic, and Neonatal Nursing, 27*, 563–568.

Dunn, S. (2000, July/August). How yoga saved my life. *Yoga Journal, 154*, 79–83, 160–163.

Farrell, S. J., Ross, A. D. M., & Sehgal, K. V. (1999). Eastern movement therapies. *Physical Medicine and Rehabilitation Clinics of North America, 10*, 617–629.

Garfinkel, M., & Schumacher, H. R., Jr. (2000). Yoga. *Rheumatic Diseases Clinics of North America, 26*(1), 125–132.

Gimbel, M. A. (1998). Yoga, meditation, and imagery: Clinical applications. *Nurse Practitioner Forum, 9,* 243–255.

Hudson, S. (1998). Yoga aids in back pain. *Australian Nursing Journal, 5*(9), 27.

Jain, A., Nagarathna, R., Nagendra, H. R., & Telles, S. (1999). Effect of "pranic" healing in chronic musculoskeletal pain—A single blind control study. *International Journal of Complementary Medicine, 17*(8), 14–17.

Kabat-Zinn, J. (1993). Meditation. In B. Moyers (Ed.), *Healing and the mind* (pp. 115–143). New York: Doubleday.

Khasky, A. D., & Smith, J. C. (1999). Stress, relaxation states, and creativity. *Perceptual and Motor Skills, 88,* 409–416.

Luskin, F. M., Newell, K. A., Griffith, M., Holmes, M., Telles, S., DiNucci, E., Marvasti, F. F., Hill, M., Pelletier, K. R., & Haskell, W. L. (2000). A review of mind/body therapies in the treatment of musculoskeletal disorders with implications for the elderly. *Alternative Therapies in Health and Medicine, 6*(2), 46–56.

Mahajan, A. S., Reddy, K. S., & Sachdeva, U. (1999). Lipid profile of coronary risk subjects following yogic lifestyle intervention. *Indian Heart Journal, 51*(1), 37–40.

Malathi, A., & Damodaran, A. (1999). Stress due to exams in medical students—Role of yoga. *Indian Journal of Physiology and Pharmacology, 43,* 218–224.

Manjunath, N. K., & Telles, S. (1999). Factors influencing changes in tweezer dexterity scores following yoga training. *Indian Journal of Physiology and Pharmacology, 43,* 225–229.

Mehta, S., Mehta, M., & Mehta, S. (1999). *Yoga the Iyengar way.* New York: Alfred A. Knopf.

Naga, V. M. P. J., Janakiramaiah, N., Gangadhar, B. N., & Subbakrishna, D. K. (1998). P300 amplitude and antidepressant response to Sudarshan Kriya Yoga (SKY). *Journal of Affective Disorders, 50*(1), 45–48.

Ornish, D. (1993). Changing life habits. In B. Moyers (Ed.), *Healing and the mind* (pp. 87–113). New York: Doubleday.

Pandya, D. P., Vyas, V. H., & Vyas, S. H. (1999). Mind-body therapy in the management and prevention of coronary disease. *Comprehensive Therapy, 25,* 283–293.

Pirisi, A. (2000, February). Seven poses to relieve cold and flu symptoms. *Yoga Journal, 151,* 102–112.

Raghuraj, P., & Telles, S. (1997). Muscle power, dexterity skill, and visual perception in community home girls trained in yoga or sports and in regular schoolgirls. *Indian Journal of Physiology and Pharmacology, 41,* 409–415.

Raju, P. S., Prasad, K. V., Venkata, R. Y., Murthy, K. J., & Reddy, M. V. (1997). Influence of intensive yoga training on physiological changes in 6 adult women: A case report. *Journal of Alternative and Complementary Medicine, 3,* 291–295.

Roth, B., & Creaser, T. (1997). Mindfulness meditation-based stress reduction: Experience with a bilingual inner-city program. *Nurse Practitioner, 22,* 150–152, 154, 157.

Schmidt, T., Wijga, A., Von Zur Muhlen, A., Brabant, G., & Wagner, T. O. (1997). Changes in cardiovascular risk factors and hormones during a comprehensive residential three month kriya yoga training and vegetarian nutrition. *Acta Physiologica Scandinavica. Supplementum. 640,* 158–162.

Selvamurthy, W., Sridharan, K., Ray, U. S., Tiwary, R. S., Hegde, K. S., Radhakrishan, U., & Sinha, K. C. (1998). A new physiological approach to control essential hypertension. *Indian Journal of Physiology and Pharmacology, 42,* 205–213.

Sequeira, W. (1999). Yoga in treatment of carpal-tunnel syndrome. *The Lancet, 353,* 689–690.

Staff Editors. (2000, October). Ask us. *Yoga Journal, 155,* 60–62.

Telles, S., Narendran, S., Raghuraj, P., Nagarathna, R., & Nagendra, H. R. (1997). Comparison of changes in autonomic and respiratory parameters of girls after yoga and games at a community home. *Perceptual and Motor Skills, 84,* 251–257.

Telles, S., & Naveen, K. V. (1997). Yoga for rehabilitation: An overview. *Indian Journal of Medical Sciences, 51,* 123–127.

Vedanthan, P. K., Kesavalu, L. N., Murthy, K. C., Duvall, K., Hall, M. J., Baker, S., & Nagarathna, S. (1998). Clinical study of yoga techniques in university students with asthma: A controlled study. *Allergy and Asthma Proceedings, 19*(1), 3–9.

9

Biofeedback

Marion Good

DEFINITION

Biofeedback, an intervention of relatively recent origin, is based on a holistic perspective in which psyche and soma are not separated. The goal of biofeedback is increased control over one's functioning. Biofeedback is defined by Williams, Nigl, and Savine (1981) as

> The technique of using equipment (usually electronic) to reveal to human beings some of their internal physiological events, normal and abnormal, in the form of visual and auditory signals in order to teach them to manipulate these otherwise involuntary or unfelt events by manipulating the displayed signals. This technique inserts a person's volition into the gap of an open feedback loop, hence the artificial name of biofeedback. (p. 22)

The holistic philosophy behind biofeedback and its focus on helping persons gain more control over their functioning makes the intervention an appropriate one for nurses to use.

Biofeedback has been used to control functions related to all areas of the nervous system: brain activity and somatic and autonomic nervous system (ANS) responses. These responses are monitored and feedback is provided to the patient concerning the degree of control achieved so that the person can eventually control the response without feedback.

SCIENTIFIC BASIS

Biofeedback originated from research in the fields of psychophysiology, learning theory, and behavioral theory. For centuries it was believed that responses such as heart rate and respiration were beyond the individual's control. In the 1960s scientists found that the ANS had an afferent as well as a motor system, and control of its functions was possible with instrumentation and conditioning. Katkin and Goldband (1980) selected a skills acquisition model as the basis for teaching biofeedback. Following this model, persons determine the relationship between their voluntary muscle or cognitive/affective activities and ANS functioning. They learn skills to control muscular and cognitive activities, which can then be reinforced to control ANS responses. The biofeedback instrument has a visual and/or auditory display that informs the person whether control has been achieved; thus, learning is reinforced.

Providing behavioral strategies to modify physiological activity is an integral part of using biofeedback (Nakagawa-Kogan, 1994). Biofeedback can be used with relaxation strategies to control ANS responses that affect brain waves, peripheral vascular activity, heart rate, blood glucose, and skin conductance. Biofeedback combined with exercise can strengthen muscles weakened by conditions such as chronic pulmonary disease, knee surgery, or age and can recruit auxiliary motor nerves in hemiplegia. In combination with positioning and biomechanics, biofeedback can reduce injury from repetitive activities such as typing.

INTERVENTION

Nurses are ideal professionals to provide biofeedback because of their knowledge of physiology, psychology, and health and illness states. However, nurses need to acquire special information and skills to use biofeedback. It is recommended that information be gained from classes and workshops available in many locations and that nurses using biofeedback become certified. The Association for Applied Psychophysiology and Biofeedback (AAPB) is an excellent resource for information and certification and can be contacted at 10200 W. 44th Avenue, Wheat Ridge, CO 80033 (303-422-8436). Although state practice acts differ, the nurses network of AAPB is working toward nationwide acceptance of autonomous nursing biofeedback practice and inclusion of biofeedback principles in basic nursing education programs (Smart, 1990). This chapter provides an overview of biofeedback, the health conditions in which it is useful, and a protocol that can be used by nurses trained in biofeedback techniques.

TECHNIQUES

A biofeedback unit consists of a sensor that monitors the patient's physiological activity and a transducer that converts what is measured into an electronic visual or auditory display to the patient. Frequently measured physiological parameters include muscle depolarization that is monitored by electromyogram (EMG) and peripheral temperature.

Biofeedback provides information about changes in a physiological parameter when behavioral treatments such as relaxation or strengthening exercises are used for a health problem. For example, a relaxation tape helps persons relax muscles to reduce blood pressure, while the EMG biofeedback instrument informs the learner of progress. Peripheral temperature feedback is also used with relaxation; as muscles relax, circulation improves and the fingers and toes get warmer. When exercises are used to strengthen perineal muscles in preventing urinary incontinence, success in contracting the correct muscles may be monitored by a pressure sensor inserted into the vagina. In health conditions exacerbated by stress, biofeedback is often combined with stress-management counseling.

Biofeedback is most frequently used in an office or clinic setting. Brown (1977) advocated using seven to twelve 30-minute training sessions. The number of sessions should be decided upon by the therapist and patient during the initial session prior to beginning training. If the patient has not achieved mastery or control of a function at the end of the agreed-upon number of sessions, the reasons and the need for further sessions should be discussed.

The first session is devoted to assessing the patient, choosing the appropriate mode of feedback, discussing the roles of the nurse and patient, and obtaining baseline measurements. Measuring several parameters helps in getting valid baseline data. Because success will be determined by changes from baseline, it is essential that these be accurate and reflect the true status of the parameter being used. The first session will be longer than subsequent ones, perhaps lasting 1 to 2 hours. Behavioral exercises are provided. It is important that patients understand the content of this session because it is necessary for using the equipment.

The therapist plays a key role in the success of biofeedback. It is helpful for the nurse to have advanced training in relaxation, imagery, and stress-management counseling. Because practice of the behavioral techniques is vital, the nurse who succeeds in motivating patients to practice at home will have patients who achieve their goals.

The final sessions focus on integration of the learning into the person's life. The patient is connected to the machine but does not receive feedback while practicing the technique; the nurse monitors the degree of control achieved. Descriptions of stressful situations are provided, and the person is asked to practice the procedure as if in that situation. Final measurements are taken. Follow-up sessions at 1 month and 6 months are advocated.

Biofeedback-Assisted Relaxation

Table 9.1 outlines a protocol for using biofeedback with cognitive-behavioral interventions for relaxation and stress management. This technique could be used for hypertension, anxiety, asthma, irritable bowel syndrome, headache, or chronic pain because muscle relaxation improves them. The protocol should be tailored to the patient, condition, and type of feedback.

Various types of relaxation exercises such as autogenic phrases or systematic relaxation may be used. To increase patient awareness of the relaxed state, progressive muscle relaxation may be helpful. Imagery may relax patients by distracting and reducing negative or stressful thoughts. Hypnosis and self-hypnosis produce an alternative state of mind. Music relaxes and distracts and may be used with relaxation or imagery.

It is important to keep the requirements for home practice simple, interesting, and meaningful. Boredom with the same relaxation tape, failure to find a convenient time to practice, and lack of noticeable improvements may decrease adherence to home practice. Providing a new relaxation technique can revive interest. To integrate new skills into daily life, patients can progress to mini-relaxation and use of cues (thoughts, positions, or activities) to signal relaxation. Other intervention protocols are found in the literature (Coxe, 1994; King, 1992; Schwartz & Associates, 1995).

Although some patients have multiple symptoms requiring treatment, training should only address one symptom at a time. Other symptoms can be treated sequentially after mastery of the first one is attained. The patient decides which symptom will be treated first.

MEASUREMENT OF OUTCOME

Table 9.2 lists feedback parameters that reflect mastery of the behavioral intervention or control of the health problem. Frequently used parameters include heart rate, muscle tension, peripheral temperature, and blood pressure. EMG monitoring demonstrates changes more quickly than temperature or galvanic skin response, but the choice may depend on the appropriateness to the health condition. Temperature feedback is used in peripheral vascular problems, but health care outcomes may be fewer episodes of painful vasoconstriction. EMG feedback and temperature feedback are used in persons with diabetes mellitus, tension headache, and chronic pain. Outcomes may include decreased glycoslated hemoglobin, headaches, or pain.

TABLE 9.1 Biofeedback Protocol

1. Before first session
   - Determine health problem for which biofeedback treatment is sought.
   - Ask for physician's name so care can be coordinated.
   - Give information on location, time commitment, and cost.
   - Request a 2-week patient log of medications and the frequency and severity of the health problem, such as the number, intensity, and time of headaches.
   - Answer questions.

2. First session
   - Interview patient for a health history; include the specific health condition.
   - Assess abilities for carrying out current medical regimen and behavioral intervention.
   - Discuss rationale for using biofeedback, type of feedback, and behavioral intervention.
   - Explain that the role of the nurse is to provide ten 50-minute sessions once a week, using the biofeedback instrument to supply physiological information.
   - Explain that the patient is the major factor in the successful use of biofeedback; that it is important to continue to keep a log of the health problem and also to include home practice sessions. The patient should consult the physician if health problems occur.
   - Explain the procedure. If using frontal muscle tension feedback, apply 3 sensors to the forehead after cleaning the skin with soap and water and applying gel. Set the biofeedback machine and operate according to instructions.
   - Obtain baseline EMG readings of frontal muscle tension for 5 minutes while the patient sits quietly with closed eyes.
   - Instruct the patient to practice taped relaxation instructions for 20 minutes while the EMG sensors are on the forehead. Ask the patient to watch the biofeedback display for information on the decreasing level of muscle tension.
   - Review 2-week record of the health problem and set mutually determined goals.
   - Give a tape and instructions for practicing relaxation at home. Provide a log to record practice and responses. Discuss timing, frequency, length, and setting for practice.
   - Discuss self-care for any possible side effects to the behavioral intervention.

3. Subsequent sessions
   - Open session with a 20-minute review of the health-problem log, stressors, and ways used for coping in past week; provide counseling for adaptive coping.
   - Apply sensors and earphones and let the patient practice relaxation for 20 minutes while watching the display. Quietly leave room after patient masters the technique.
   - Vary relaxation techniques to maintain interest and increase skill.
   - Give instructions for incremental integration of relaxation into daily life. For example, add 30-second mini-relaxation exercises for busy times of the day.

4. Final session
   - Conduct session as above; obtain final EMG readings.
   - Discuss plan for ongoing practice and management of stress after end of treatment.

TABLE 9.2   Parameters Used for Feedback to Patient

Airway resistance	EMG muscle depolarization	Peripheral skin temperature
Blood pressure	Forced expiratory volume	Tidal volume
Blood volume	Galvanic skin response	Tracheal noise
Bowel sounds	Gastric pH	Vaginal pressure
Brain waves	Heart rate	

USES

CONDITIONS/POPULATIONS

Biofeedback has been used in the treatment of many medical and psychological problems. For example, a review of research on the use of biofeedback in Raynaud's disease indicated evidence that biofeedback is often efficacious in treating this condition (Surwit & Jordan, 1987). Biofeedback-assisted relaxation has been more successful in the treatment of tension headache than in migraine (Andrasik & Blanchard, 1987; Blanchard & Andrasik, 1987). Patients with advanced heart failure who use biofeedback can voluntarily decrease vascular resistance, increasing cardiac output (Dracup, Woo, & Stevenson, 1993; Moser, Stevenson, Woo, & Dracup, 1992). Persons with cystic fibrosis used biofeedback with pursed-lip breathing to improve forced expiratory volume (Delk, Gevertz, Hicks, Carden, & Rucker, 1994). Other conditions and populations treated with biofeedback are described in Table 9.3.

Hypertension

When Westerners noted that yogis and shamans were able to lower their blood pressure by meditating and relaxing, they began to study the use of biofeedback to lower blood pressure. A review of studies of biofeedback for hypertension, noted that systolic reductions of 4 to 22 mm Hg and diastolic decreases of 1 to 15 mm Hg were achieved and maintained for periods of 6 to 48 months (Glasgow & Engel, 1987). Such reductions might allow reduction in dosages of antihypertensive medications. Recently, research has focused on the effects of biofeedback assisted relaxation on blood pressure and immune factors, and has examined the physical and psychological predictors of those who reduced their blood pressure (Blanchard et al.,1989; McGrady, 1994; Nakagawa-Kogan, Garber, Jarrett, Egan, & Hendershot, 1988).

TABLE 9.3   Conditions and Populations in Which Biofeedback Has Been Used

Anxiety (Scandrett, Bean, Breedan, & Powell, 1986)

Children (Olness & Kohen, 1996)

Chronic pain (Spence, Sharpe, Newton-John, & Campion, 1995; Strong et al., 1989)

Chronic pulmonary disease (Delk, Gevertz, Hicks, Carden, & Rucker, 1994)

Diabetes mellitus (McGrady, Bailey, & Good, 1992)

Headaches (Engel & Rapoff, 1990; King, 1992)

Heart disease (Dracup et al., 1993; Nakagawa-Kogan, Garber, Jarrett, Egan, & Hendershot, 1988)

Hypertension (Blanchard et al., 1989; McGrady, 1994; Nakagawa-Kogan et al., 1988)

Irritable bowel (Radnitz & Blanchard, 1988)

Older adults (Arena, Hannah, Bruno, & Meador, 1991; Burns et al., 1993)

Raynaud's disease (Surwit & Jordan, 1987; Schwartz & Kelly, 1995)

Urinary incontinence (Beckman, 1995; Coxc, 1994)

Chronic Pain

Biofeedback along with relaxation, imagery, music, or hypnosis can be used for cancer or back pain, as a complementary therapy to medication. Such use can teach patients control over their pain and may reduce the side effects of analgesic medication. Jacox and colleagues (1994) reported that well-designed quasi-experimental studies show the efficacy of biofeedback in reducing chronic pain.

Urinary Incontinence

Urinary incontinence is a major problem in an aging population. It is embarrassing and restrictive and is a major reason for institutionalization. Interventions to manage incontinence would significantly reduce health care costs. The Urinary Incontinence Guideline Panel (1992) reports 54% to 95% improvement in incontinence when the combination of biofeedback and behavioral treatments is used. The panel suggests that therapists become familiar with the anatomic and physiological basis for different forms of bladder dysfunction and learn strengthening exercises and special measurement methods. The goal is to optimize use of striated pelvic floor muscles to control bladder function (Tries & Eisman, 1995).

Diabetes Mellitus

Research has shown that biofeedback-assisted relaxation has been useful in reducing blood glucose in both insulin-dependent and non-insulin-dependent diabetes mellitus (McGrady, Bailey, & Good, 1992; Surwit & Feinglos, 1983). It is suggested that this intervention be used with persons who are adherent to their diabetic regimen, yet present stress-related symptoms that seem to affect their glycemic control. It has reduced average blood glucose, glycoslated hemoglobin, and fasting values (McGrady, Graham, & Bailey, 1996).

Children and Older Adults

Olness and Kohen (1996) describe many conditions in children, such as migraine, hypertension, and fecal incontinence, in which biofeedback combined with hypnotherapy teaches them to change their thoughts in order to bring about changes in their bodies. The authors describe special biofeedback equipment and techniques that appeal to children. Biofeedback has also been successfully used with older adults (Middaugh, Woods, Kee, Hardin, & Peters, 1991). Modifications in biofeedback sessions may be needed for older adults to increase comprehension and retention (Arena, Hannah, Bruno, & Meador, 1991). Because of sensory changes in elders, visual feedback should be large enough for them to see and auditory feedback loud enough to hear.

PRECAUTIONS

Biofeedback should be used cautiously, if at all, in persons with depression psychosis, seizures, and hyperactive conditions. Those with rigid personalities may be unwilling to change their mode of functioning (Williams et al., 1981). However, negative reactions may be related to relaxation rather than to biofeedback, and may be avoided by means of patient education and the type of relaxation used (Schwartz & Schwartz, 1995).

Biofeedback-assisted relaxation is expected to lower blood pressure, heart, and respiratory rates. Excessive decreases should be avoided in patients with cardiac conditions, hemodynamic instability, or multiple illnesses.

Use of relaxation therapies might also result in a need for reduced medication in diabetes mellitus, hypertension, and asthma. This should be discussed with patients and physicians; responses should be carefully monitored. For example, relaxation exercises in persons with diabetes can beneficially reduce blood glucose, but hypoglycemic reactions may occur if adjustments in insulin or diet are not made. McGrady and Bailey (1995) suggest a team approach that includes the physician, a certified diabetic educator, a certified biofeedback practitioner, and the patient. Patients should be taught to manage hypoglycemia because reactions can occur at a single relaxation session or over time as the program lowers blood glucose. The nurse should also keep simple carbohydrates, glucagon, and a blood glucose monitor in the office and maintain expertise to administer them. Home practice can be scheduled to avoid times of low blood glucose (McGrady & Bailey, 1995).

Electric shock is a hazard when any electrical equipment is used. Dangerous levels of current flow may arise from equipment malfunction or operator error (Katkin & Goldband, 1980). The AAPB publishes a list of companies whose products have passed their safety code.

Although biofeedback is noninvasive, cost-effective, and very promising in the treatment of many conditions, it is not a miracle intervention. It requires that the therapist be knowledgeable about the health problem, intervention, and medication effects and that they have a sincere interest in the patient outcome. Considerable patient time, attention, and motivation are needed for success. To control the condition, ongoing use of the behavioral technique may be needed after biofeedback sessions end. This should be made very clear before training is initiated.

FUTURE RESEARCH

There is great need for controlled clinical trials to determine the effectiveness of biofeedback in treating physiological and psychological conditions (Hatch, Fisher, & Rugh 1987). Nurses employing biofeedback can address the following questions:

1. What are the self-care characteristics of persons who benefit most from biofeedback?

2. Does autogenic training with peripheral temperature feedback improve diabetic foot ulcers?

3. What is the effect of biofeedback-assisted relaxation on chronic back pain?

4. Do persons who lower their blood pressure with biofeedback-relaxation continue home practice and maintain the lower level when the sessions are completed?

5. Does biofeedback plus medication result in better health outcomes than medication alone?

6. Does a biofeedback-assisted intervention reduce the amount of medication and side effects?

REFERENCES

Andrasik, F., & Blanchard, E. B. (1987). The biofeedback treatment of tension headache. In J. Hatch, J. Fisher, & J. Rugh (Eds.), *Biofeedback—Studies in clinical efficacy* (pp. 281–321). New York: Plenum.

Arena, J. G., Hannah, S. L., Bruno, G. M., & Meador, K. J. (1991). Electromyographic biofeedback training for tension headache in the elderly: A prospective study. *Biofeedback and Self Regulation 16*, 379–390.

Beckman, N. J. (1995). An overview of urinary incontinence in adults: Assessments and behavioral interventions. *Clinical Nurse Specialist 9*, 241–247.

Blanchard, E. B., & Andrasik, F. (1987). Biofeedback for vascular headache. In J. Hatch, J. Fisher, & J. Rugh (Eds.), *Biofeedback—Studies in clinical efficacy* (pp. 1–48). New York: Plenum.

Blanchard, E. B., McCoy, G. C., Berger, M., Musso, A., Pallmeyer, T. P., Gerardi, R., Gerardi, M. A., & Pangburn, L. (1989). A controlled comparison of thermal biofeedback and relaxation training in the treatment of essential hypertension, IV: Prediction of short-term clinical outcome. *Behavior Therapy, 20*, 405–415.

Brown, B. (1977). *Stress and the art of biofeedback.* New York: Bantam Books.

Burns, P., Pranikoff, K., Nochajski, T., Hadley, E., Levy, K., & Ory, M. (1993). A comparison of effectiveness of biofeedback and pelvic muscle exercise treatment of stress incontinence in older community-dwelling women. *Journal of Gerontology: Medical Sciences, 48*, M167–M174.

Coxe, J. (1994). Assessment for biofeedback and behavioral therapy for urinary incontinence. *Urologic Nursing, 14*, 82–84.

Delk, K. K., Gevertz, R., Hicks, D. A., Carden, F., & Rucker, R. (1994). The effects of biofeedback-assisted breathing retraining on lung function in patients with cystic fibrosis. *Chest, 105*, 23–28.

Dracup, K., Woo, M., & Stevenson, L. (1993). Use of BF in patients with advanced heart failure to reduce systemic vascular resistance. *AACN Clinical Issues in Critical Care, 3*, 30.

Engle, J. M., & Rapoff, M. A. (1990). Biofeedback-assisted relaxation training for adult and pediatric headache disorders. *Occupational Therapy Journal of Research, 10*, 283–299.

Glasgow, M. S., & Engel, B. T. (1987). Clinical issues in biofeedback and relaxation therapy for hypertension: Review and recommendations. In J. P. Hatch, J. G. Fisher, & J. D. Rugh (Eds.), *Biofeedback—Studies in clinical efficacy* (pp. 81–121). New York: Plenum.

Jacox, A., Carr, D. B., Payne, R., et al. (1994, March). *Management of cancer pain clinical practice guideline No. 9.* AHCPR Publication No. 94-0592. Rockville, MD: U.S. Department of Health and Human Services, Agency for Health Care Policy and Research, Public Health Service.

Katkin, E., & Goldband, S. (1980). Biofeedback. In F. Kanfer & A. Goldstein (Eds.), *Helping people change* (pp. 537–558). New York: Pergamon Press.

King, T. I. (1992). The use of electromyographic biofeedback in treating a client with tension headaches. *The American Journal of Occupational Therapy, 46,* 839–842.

McGrady, A. (1994). Effects of group relaxation training and thermal biofeedback on blood pressure and related physiological and psychological variables in essential hypertension. *Biofeedback and Self-Regulation, 19,* 51–66.

McGrady, A., & Bailey, B. K. (1995). Biofeedback-assisted relaxation and diabetes mellitus. In M. S. Schwartz & Associates (Eds.), *Biofeedback: A practitioner's guide* (2nd ed., pp. 471–489). New York: Guilford Press.

McGrady, A., Bailey, B. K., & Good, M. (1992). Biofeedback-assisted relaxation in insulin dependent diabetes mellitus: A controlled study. *Diabetes Care, 14,* 160–165.

McGrady, A., Graham, G., & Bailey, B. (1996). Biofeedback-assisted relaxation in insulin-dependent diabetes: A replication and extension study. *Annals of Behavioral Medicine, 18(3),* 185–189.

Middaugh, S. J., Woods, S. E., Kee, W. G., Harden, R. N., & Peters, J. R. (1991). Biofeedback-assisted relaxation training for the aging chronic pain patient. *Biofeedback and Self Regulation, 16,* 361–377.

Moser, D., Stevenson, L., Woo, M., & Dracup, K. (1992). Voluntary control of regional blood flow with biofeedback in advanced heart failure patients. *Heart & Lung, 21,* 292.

Nakagawa-Kogan, H. (1994). Self-management training: Potential for primary care. *Nurse Practitioner Forum, 5,* 77–84.

Nakagawa-Kogan, H., Garber, A., Jarrett, M., Egan, K. J., & Hendershot, S. (1988). Self-management of hypertension: Predictors of success in diastolic blood pressure reduction. *Research in Nursing and Health, 11,* 105–115.

Olness, K., & Kohen, D. P. (1996). *Hypnosis and hypnotherapy with children* (3rd ed.). New York: Guilford Press.

Radnitz, C. L., & Blanchard, E. B. (1988). Bowel sound biofeedback as a treatment for irritable bowel syndrome. *Biofeedback and Self-Regulation, 13,* 169–179.

Scandrett, S. L., Bean, J. L., Breedan, S., & Powell, S. (1986). A comparative study of biofeedback and progressive relaxation in anxious patients. *Issues in Mental Health Nursing, 8,* 255–271.

Schwartz, M. S., & Associates. (1995). *Biofeedback: A practitioner's guide* (2nd ed.). New York: Guilford Press.

Schwartz, M. S., & Kelly, M. F. (1995). Raynaud's disease: Selected issues and considerations in using biofeedback therapies. In M. S. Schwartz & Associates (1995). *Biofeedback: A practitioner's guide* (2nd ed., pp. 429–444). New York: Guilford Press.

Schwartz, M. S., & Schwartz, N. M.(1995). Problems with relaxation and biofeedback: Assisted relaxation and guidelines for management. In M. S. Schwartz & Associates (Eds.), *Biofeedback: A practitioner's guide* (2nd ed., pp. 288–300). New York: Guilford Press.

Smart, S. (1990). Empowering patients through biofeedback. *California Nurse, 86(7),* 13.

Spence, S. H., Sharpe, L., Newton-John, T., & Champion, D. (1995). Effect of EMG biofeedback compared to applied relaxation training with chronic upper extremity cumulative trauma disorders. *Pain, 63,* 199–206.

Strong J., Cramond, T., & Maas, F. (1989). Effectiveness of relaxation techniques with patients who have chronic low back pain. *Occupational Therapy Journal of Research, 1,* 184–192.

Surwit, R. S., & Feinglos, M. N. (1983). The effects of relaxation on glucose tolerance in non-insulin-dependent diabetes mellitus. *Diabetes Care, 6,* 176–179.

Surwit, R. S., & Jordan, J. S. (1987). Behavioral treatments for Raynaud's syndrome. In J. Hatch, J. Fisher, & J. Rugh (Eds.), *Biofeedback—Studies in clinical efficacy* (pp. 255–279). New York: Plenum.

Tries, J., & Eisman, E. (1995). Urinary incontinence: Evaluation and biofeedback treatment. In M. S. Schwartz & Associates (Eds.), *Biofeedback: A practitioner's guide* (2nd ed., pp. 597–632). New York: Guilford Press.

Urinary Incontinence Guideline Panel (1992). *Urinary incontinence in adults: Clinical practice guideline.* (AHCPR Pub. No. 92-0038). Rockville, MD: U.S. Department of Health and Human Services, Agency for Health Care Policy and Research, Public Health Service.

Williams, M., Nigl, A., & Savine, D. (1981). *A textbook of biological feedback.* New York: Human Science Press.

10

Meditation

Mary Jo Kreitzer

Meditation is a self-directed practice for relaxing the body and calming the mind that has been used by people in many cultures since ancient times. The practice of meditation is frequently viewed as a religious practice, although its health benefits have been long recognized. It is a recommended intervention for stress reduction, anxiety and anxiety-related disorders, for expanding awareness, and for improvement in well-being.

The resurgence in interest in meditation has drawn largely from Eastern religious practices, particularly those of India, China, and Japan. Records substantiate the use of meditation by Hindus in India as early as 1500 B.C. Taoists in China and Buddhists in India included meditation as an integral part of their religious life. Zen Buddhists in Japan developed a special form of meditation called *zazen,* a sitting meditation in which a quiet awareness is maintained of whatever is happening at the time.

Meditation has also been an important aspect of the Western world and Judeo-Christian tradition. Christian monks and hermits went to the desert to meditate and meditation remains a key element of monastic life. Christian contemplation, centering prayer, and praying the rosary or repeating the Hail Mary are forms of meditation. West (1979) noted the use of meditation in the American Indian culture, the Kung Zhu/twasi of Africa, and the Native Americans of Alaska of North America. In the United States, the most common forms of meditation are sedentary, though there is an increasing interest in many moving meditations such as the Chinese martial art tai chi, the Japanese martial art of aikido, and walking meditation in Zen Buddhism. Although specific meditative practices vary considerably, the outcomes are similar for all techniques.

This chapter provides an overview of mediation in general and will highlight the meditative approaches of *transcendental mediation* (TM), *centering prayer*, the relaxation response, and mindfulness meditation in more detail.

DEFINITION

Many definitions of meditation can be identified in the literature. West (1979) defined meditation as an exercise in which the individual focuses attention or awareness in order to dwell upon a single object. The definition proposed by Goleman and Schwartz (1976) is similar, in that attention is focused on a single percept. They defined meditation as follows:

> The systematic and continued focusing of the attention on a single target percept—for example, a mantra or sound—or persistently holding a specific attentional set toward all percepts or mental contents as they spontaneously arise in the field of awareness. (p. 457)

Welwood's definition (1979) is broader than the previous two; he viewed meditation as a technique that allows a person to investigate the process of his or her consciousness and experiences and to discover the more basic underlying qualities of one's existence as an animate reality. Intense concentration blocks other stimuli, allowing the person to become more aware of self.

Everly and Rosenfeld (1981) divided meditation techniques into four forms: mental repetition, physical repetition, problem concentration, and visual concentration. In mental repetition the person concentrates on a word or phrase, commonly called a mantra. Concentration on breathing is frequently the focus in physical repetition techniques; however, dance or other body movements can be the object of concentration. Jogging, for example, allows for concentrating on a physical activity, repetitive breathing, and the sound of one's feet hitting the ground. In *samatha* Buddhist meditation, the person watches or concentrates on the breath entering and flowing from the tip of the nostrils. In problem-contemplation techniques, an attempt is made to solve a problem that contains paradoxical components, which Zen terms the *koan*. Visual concentration techniques are akin to imagery.

Borysenko (1988) defines meditation simply as any activity that keeps the attention pleasantly anchored in the present moment. It is the way we learn to access the relaxation response. Kabat-Zinn et al. (1998) note that meditation is fundamentally different from relaxation techniques in both methods and objectives. A common but erroneous assumption is that the goal of meditation is to achieve a specific, highly pleasant meditative state akin to deep relaxation. According to Kabat-Zinn et al., there is no single meditative state and the overall orientation is one of non-striving and non-doing.

SCIENTIFIC BASIS

An understanding of the scientific basis for meditation is emerging. In 1979, West noted that there were few theoretical explanations for meditation's effectiveness, though various explanations had been proposed, including adaptive regression (Shafii, 1973) and desensitization, as meditating allows the person to deal with unfinished psychic material (Tart, 1971). Another hypothesis for the effectiveness of meditation was that it was a way of learning to experience without categorizing or predetermining (Goleman, 1977). Everly and Rosenfeld (1981) suggested that the role of the focal device used in meditation is to allow the intuitive, non-ego-centered mode of thought processing to dominate consciousness in place of the normally dominant analytic, ego-centered style. When the left (rational, analytic) hemisphere of the brain is silenced, the intuitive mode produces extraordinary awareness, a state frequently called *nirvana*. A positive mood, an experience of unity, an alteration in time-space relationships, an enhanced sense of reality and meaning, and an acceptance of things that seem paradoxical are experienced in this superconscious state. A serious meditator may progress through a continuum from the beginning meditation to this superconscious state.

In a report to the National Institutes of Health (1992) on alternative medical systems and practices in the United States, research on meditation was summarized as one of several mind-body interventions. In describing how and why meditation may work, Kenneth Walton, director of the neurochemistry laboratory at Maharishi International University, was quoted as follows:

> The frequently striking results of [studies of transcendental meditation] have not been widely discussed in the medical literature, purportedly because there is no reasonable mechanism which could explain such a spectrum of health effects from a simple mental technology. . . . Only in the last year has the stress connection emerged with the degree of clarity it now has. The . . . bottom line is the proposed vicious circle linking chronic stress, serotonin metabolism, and hippocampal regulation of the hypothalamic-pituitary-adrenocortical (HPA) axis. (p. 16)

A similar theory has been advanced by Everly and Benson (1989), who suggest that meditation is effective with a wide variety of conditions that may be called "disorders of arousal" in which the limbic system of the brain has become overstimulated. It is possible that relaxation and meditation work by "retuning" the nervous system by damping the production of adrenergic catecholamines, which stimulate limbic activity. They further suggest that excessive limbic activity may also account for the association of chronic stress and increased susceptibility to infection.

INTERVENTION

While there are a wide variety of meditation techniques described in the literature (Carrington, 1984; Goleman, 1977; LeShan, 1974; Lichstein, 1988), the following four techniques will be described: transcendental meditation, centering prayer, relaxation response, and mindfulness meditation.

TECHNIQUES

Transcendental Meditation

A much-publicized technique, transcendental meditation (TM), was developed and introduced into the United States in the early 1960s by the Indian leader Maharishi Mahesh Yogi. It is estimated that there are now well over 2 million practitioners. The concept of TM is relatively simple. Students are given a mantra (a word or sound) to repeat silently over and over again while sitting in a comfortable position. The mantra is selected not for its meaning but strictly for its sound. It is the understanding that this sound alone attracts the mind and leads it effortlessly and naturally to a slightly subtler level of the thinking process. If thoughts other than the mantra come to mind, the student is asked to notice them and return to the mantra. It is suggested that practitioners mediate for 20 minutes in the morning and again in the evening. TM is easily learned and is practiced by people of every age, education, culture, and religion. It is not a philosophy and does not require specific beliefs or changes in behavior or lifestyle (Russel, 1976).

Centering Prayer

Though similar to TM in several respects, centering prayer is based in Christianity and is designed to reduce the obstacles to contemplative prayer and union with God. Thomas Keating (1995), the founder of the centering prayer movement, describes centering prayer as a discipline designed to withdraw our attention from the ordinary flow of thoughts. The understanding is that people tend to identify with their thoughts—the debris that floats along the surface of the river—rather than being in touch with the river itself—the source from which these mental objects are emerging. Keating suggests that like boats or floating debris, our thoughts and feelings must be resting on something. They are resting, he asserts, on the inner stream of consciousness, which is our participation in God's being. In centering prayer, as with TM, people are encouraged to find a comfortable position, to close their eyes, and, to focus on a sacred word. Keating notes that 20 to 30 minutes is the minimum amount of time necessary for most people to establish interior silence and to get beyond their superficial thoughts.

Relaxation Response

This response incorporates four elements that are common in many of the other relaxation techniques: a quiet environment, a mental device, a passive attitude, and a comfortable position.

A quiet environment, which is an element of Benson's technique (1975), eliminates outside stimuli and allows the person to concentrate on the mental device. Some people prefer a church or chapel for meditating, but such a place may not be readily accessible. Playing music while meditating is not advocated because it may draw the person's attention away from the internal processes. People should select the place they wish to use for meditation and continue to use that place. This eliminates adjusting to new surroundings and stimuli each time a person meditates.

Use of a mental device helps shift the mind from logical, externally oriented thought to inner rumination. The purpose of the mental device is to preoccupy oneself with an emotionally neutral, repetitive, and monotonous stimulus (Lichstein, 1988). Unlike TM, in which the teacher gives the student a mantra, Benson's technique requires the person to select the mental device that will be used whenever the person meditates. It may be a sound, word, or phrase that is repeated silently or aloud, a phrase or portion of a religious prayer or psalm. Fixation on an object is also sometimes used as the mental device.

Mindfulness Meditation

Mindfulness, awareness, or insight meditation are Western terms used interchangeably to describe the Buddhist practice of *vipassana* meditation. The goal of this meditative practice is to increase insight by becoming a detached observer of the stream of changing thoughts, feelings, drives, and visions until their nature and origin is recognized. The process includes eliciting the relaxation response, centering on breath, and then focusing attention freely from one perception to the next. In this form of meditation, no thought or sensation is considered an intrusion. When they drift into consciousness, they become the focus of attention (Kutz et al., 1985).

An extension of the practice of mindfulness meditation is what Borysenko (1988) calls "meditation in action" (p. 91). It involves a "be here now" approach that allows life to unfold without the limitation of prejudgement. Using this approach, mindfulness exercises are carried out during normal, daily activities. It requires being open to an awareness of the moment as it is and to what the moment could hold. It produces a relaxed state of attentiveness to both the inner world of thoughts and feelings and the outer world of actions and perceptions. Borysenko notes that mindfulness requires a change in attitude: joy is not sought in finishing an activity, but rather in doing it.

Mindfulness-based stress reduction programs (MBSR) originated with the Stress Reduction Clinic at the University of Massachusetts Medical Center and are currently used in more than 80 clinics, hospitals, and HMOs in the U.S. and abroad (Kabat-Zinn et al., 1998). It is generally understood that in MBSR training, participants receive training in three formal meditation techniques: a body scan meditation, a sitting meditation, and mindful hatha yoga, which involves simple stretches and postures.

GUIDELINES

Borysenko (1988) describes a simple step-by-step process of meditation incorporating many of the concepts previously described that can be used to teach meditation to patients:

1. Choose a quiet place where you will not be disturbed by other people or by the telephone.
2. Sit in a comfortable position with back straight and arms and legs uncrossed, unless you choose to sit cross-legged on the floor.
3. Close your eyes.
4. Relax your muscles sequentially from head to feet.
5. Focus on your breathing, noticing how the breath goes in and out, without trying to control it in any way.
6. Repeat your focus word silently in time with your breathing.

Borysenko advises meditators to not worry about how they are doing. It is helpful to maintain a passive attitude and allows relaxation to occur at its own pace. When distracting thoughts intrude, meditators are encouraged to ignore them by not dwelling on them and return to repeating the chosen word. Successful meditation usually takes practice—at least once a day for 10 to 20 minutes.

Benson (1975) suggests that people wait for 2 hours after any meal before meditating, as the digestive processes seem to interfere with the elicitation of the relaxation response. He also emphasizes the importance of fitting the technique to the individual and making modifications as necessary. Therefore, before any teaching is initiated, an assessment of the individual is needed to determine what might be the most appropriate technique for a particular person or a specific condition. This requires that nurses have knowledge about specific meditation techniques.

USES

There is a substantial body of research supporting the use of meditation for a wide variety of conditions. Table 10.1 lists conditions for which meditation

TABLE 10.1   Conditions In Which Meditation Has Been Used

Anxiety (Kabat-Zinn & Massion, 1992; Miller et al., 1995)

Asthma (Wilson, Hansberger, Chin, & Novey, 1975)

Carotid atherosclerosis (Castillo-Richmond et al., 2000)

Chronic pain (Kabat-Zinn & Massion, 1982; Kabat-Zinn, Lipworth & Burney, 1985)

Coronary artery disease (Zamarra, Schneider, Bessaghini, Robinson, & Salerno, 1996)

Coronary care units (Guzzetta, 1989)

Diagnostic procedures (Frenn, Fehring, & Kartes, 1986)

Drug abuse (Shafii, 1973)

Headache (Benson, Klemchuk, & Graham, 1974)

Hypertension (Schneider et al., 1996)

Psoriasis (Kabat-Zinn et al., 1998)

Psychotherapy (Bogart, 1991)

has been used. Use of meditation for patients with chronic pain, hypertension, and anxiety and generalized stress will be discussed.

In addition to being a low-cost intervention with demonstrated efficacy, there are some data that suggest meditative practices may also impact overall use of health care services. In a study comparing 2,000 people who meditated with a group of non-meditators of comparable age, gender, and profession, it was found that over a 5-year period, use of medical services (visits to the doctor and hospitalizations) by the group who meditated was 30% to 87% less than the group of non-meditators (Orme-Johnson, 1987). The difference was greatest for individuals over 40 years of age.

CONDITIONS/POPULATIONS

Chronic Pain

Use of meditation for patients experiencing chronic pain has been well documented experientially and empirically. Early studies of mindfulness-based stress reduction examined the impact of MBSR on patients with chronic pain. In a study of 51 patients with chronic pain who had been unsuccessfully treated by conventional methods, Kabat-Zinn (1982) reported significant decreases in pain and in the number of medical symptoms reported by patients enrolled in a 10-week training program. Significant reductions in mood disturbances and psychiatric symptomatology were also noted. One methodological limitation of this study was the lack of a comparison or control group.

A larger clinical trial by Kabat-Zinn, Lipworth, and Burney (1985) examined the impact of mindfulness meditation on 90 chronic-pain patients. Statistically significant reductions were reported in present-moment pain, negative body image, inhibition of activity by pain, symptoms, mood disturbance, and psychological symptomatology including anxiety and depression. A comparison group of chronic-pain patients did not show significant improvement on these measures. Improvements reported by the patients who received the 10-week mindfulness meditation training were maintained up to 15 months postmeditation training for all measures except present-moment pain.

A 4-year follow-up of 225 chronic-pain patients (Kabat-Zinn et al., 1987) enrolled in an 8-week mindfulness meditation training program documented that improvements in physical and psychological status were maintained: 93% of patients reported the present use of at least one of the three meditation practices taught in the initial training.

Hypertension

Because of the decreases in blood pressure experienced by persons who had practiced TM, Benson (1975) explored the effectiveness of the relaxation response in persons with hypertension. Statistically significant changes between the experimental and control groups were found in his initial study. Mean systolic pressures decreased from 146 to 137 mm Hg, and mean diastolic pressures from 93.5 to 88.9 mm Hg in subjects who were taught and who practiced Benson's technique. Blood pressure was not measured immediately after the person had meditated, but rather readings were taken at random times throughout the day. It is hypothesized that meditation counteracts the sympathetic responses of the flight-or-fight reaction to stressors. Other studies (Benson, Rosner, Marzetta, & Klemchuk, 1974; Blackwell et al., 1976; Pollock, Weber, Case, & Laragh, 1977) likewise found decreases in blood pressure in people who regularly meditated. However, only short-term (3-month) effects occurred in the Blackwell and Pollock studies. West (1980) attributes this to the placebo effects showing diminishing returns with the passage of time. Conversely, the influence of the instructor may have prompted some persons to practice initially, but the motivation to practice decreased with passing time. Benson (1975) stated that the relaxation response in and of itself probably will not be sufficient to lower severe or moderately high blood pressure, but its continued use will result in fewer or reduced doses of antihypertensive medications. The practice of meditation could potentially help to prevent the occurrence of hypertension.

A recent study of hypertensive African Americans (Castillo-Richmond et al., 2000) was designed to measure the impact of a TM program on carotid atherosclerosis. In a randomized controlled trial comparing a TM program with a health education program, groups were matched for teaching format, instructional time, home practice, and expectations of health outcomes. Preliminary findings revealed that the TM program was associated with reduced carotid atherosclerosis. This study is encouraging given the high incidence of hypertension and cardiovascular disease in the African American population.

Anxiety and Generalized Stress

Two studies have examined the effect of a group mindfulness-based meditation program on patients with anxiety disorders. In a study of 22 patients diagnosed with generalized anxiety disorder or panic disorder with or without agoraphobia, Kabat-Zinn (1992) reported significant reductions in anxiety and depression. These improvements were maintained at a 3-month follow-up. A follow-up study of this same patient population at 3 years (Miller, Fletcher, & Kabat-Zinn, 1995) revealed maintenance of the gains reported in the original study on the following measures: anxiety, depression, number and severity of panic attacks, mobility, and fear.

Astin (1997) conducted a study of the effect of an 8-week mindfulness-based stress reduction program on 28 medical students who were randomized to an experimental group or a nonintervention control group. Participants in the mindfulness meditation training evidenced significant reductions in overall psychological symptomatology (depression and anxiety), increases in a perceived sense of control, and higher scores on a measure of spiritual experiences. Astin concluded that mindfulness meditation might serve as a powerful cognitive behavioral coping strategy for transforming the ways in which people respond to life events.

The impact of a mindfulness-based stress reduction program on English- and Spanish-speaking patients cared for in a bilingual inner-city primary care clinic was conducted by Roth and Creaser (1997). Data revealed that patients who completed the 8-week training program reported statistically significant decreases in medical and psychological symptoms and improvement in self-esteem. Anecdotal reports of the 79 patients who completed the training program indicated that many experienced changes far more profound than the documented reduction in physical and psychological symptoms.

Changes reported included greater peace of mind, more patience, less anger and temper outbursts, better interpersonal communication, more harmonious relationships with family members, improved parenting skills, more restful sleep, decreased use of medications for pain, sleep, and anxiety; decrease or cessation of smoking, weight loss, greater acceptance of aspects of life over which they have no control, greater self-knowledge, and a marked improvement in the overall sense of well-being.

MEASUREMENT OF OUTCOMES

The purpose for which meditation is used will dictate the parameters for evaluating its effectiveness. Commonly used measures include heart rate, blood pressure, respiratory rate, oxygen consumption, skin conductance, EEG and EMG recordings, scores on anxiety scales, and subjective reports. Benson (1975) reported that subjects practicing the relaxation response were calmer, more receptive to ideas, more patient, committed to daily exercise, less likely to use alcohol, and were happier overall. Although Credidio (1982) found no changes on the scores of the Eysenck Personality Inventory between persons who were taught meditation and those in the control group, subjective reports indicated a positive reaction to the use of meditation. Because subjective reporting is a predictor of whether or not a person will continue to practice an intervention, how the person feels about the effects of meditation is important.

To document the efficacy of meditation, nurses in clinical areas can use blood pressure readings, heart rate, and respiratory rate as indicators of the effectiveness of meditation. Measures should not only be taken before and immediately after practicing meditation, but also at other times during the day, and records should be kept to determine if changes occur over time. Because the person is resting while meditating, it would be expected that the readings would be lower after practice. It is also important that continued follow-up be done to determine if the effect persists over time.

PRECAUTIONS

Meditation is not a benign intervention. The nurse must be aware of side effects of the intervention, persons for whom it should not be used, and assessments to be made as the person practices meditation. Careful monitoring of reactions to medications is necessary, as doses may need to be altered. Everly and Rosenfeld (1981) noted problems of overdosage with insulin, sedatives, and cardiovascular medications in people who meditated. Because of the effect meditation can have on the cardiovascular system, the blood pressure should be checked before meditation begins. It if is below 90 mm Hg, meditation should not be practiced. Patients should be instructed not to meditate if there is light-headedness or dizziness. Also, the person should not stand immediately after meditating because a hypotensive state is frequently present.

Benson (1975) notes that hallucinations can occur if the person meditates for several hours at a time. Loss of contact with reality is a possibility, and continued assessment is needed to determine if this is occurring. Lazarus (1976) reported cases of attempted suicide, schizophrenia, and severe depression after the continued practice of meditation. While meditation perhaps should not be prescribed for some people, the characteristics of people who would be harmed by meditation are unclear.

FUTURE RESEARCH

Although nurses are increasingly using meditation in their practice, the research base for the use of meditation in nursing is sparse. Much of the current research is being conducted by interdisciplinary teams. Because meditation holds great promise as a therapeutic nursing intervention, nurses should be encouraged to contribute to whatever research is being done. Questions and areas that merit further investigation include:

1. What are the characteristics of people who benefit from meditation? Do people who continue to practice meditation differ significantly from those who abandon it?

2. How easily generalized are the effects of meditation? Does its use affect other areas of the person's life than those for which it was taught? If the person is taught meditation as a means of decreasing hypertension, is there also an improvement in sleep or other areas?

3. How does meditation differ from other forms of self-regulation such as hypnosis, relaxation, and guided imagery in process and outcome?

REFERENCES

Astin, J. (1997). Stress reduction through mindfulness meditation: Effects of psychological symptomatology, sense of control, and spiritual experiences. *Psychotherapy and Psychosomatics, 66*, 97–106.

Benson, H. (1975). *The relaxation response.* New York: Avon.

Blackwell, B., Bloomfield, S., Gartide, P., Robinson, A., Hanenson, I., Magenheim,

H., Nidich, S., & Zigler, R. (1976). Transcendental meditation in hypertension. Individual response patterns. *Lancet, 1*(7953), 223–226.

Borysenko, J. (1988). *Minding the body, mending the mind.* New York: Bantam Books.

Carrington, P. (1984). Modern forms of meditation. In R. Woolfolk & P. Lehrer (Eds.), *Principles and practice of stress management* (pp. 108–141). New York: Guilford Press.

Castillo-Richmond, A., Schneider, R., Alexander, C., Cook, R., Myers, H., Nidich, S., Haney, C., Rainforth, M., & Salerno, J. (2000). Effects of stress reduction on carotid atherosclerosis in hypertensive African Americans. *Stroke, 31*(3), 568–573.

Credidio, S. (1982). Comparative effectiveness of patterned biofeedback vs. meditation training on EMG and skin temperature changes. *Behavior Research and Therapy, 20,* 233–241.

Everly, G. S., & Benson, H. (1989). Disorders of arousal and the relaxation response: Speculations on the nature and treatment of stress-related diseases. *International Journal of Psychosomatics, 36,* 15–21.

Everly, G., & Rosenfeld, R. (1981). *The nature and treatment of the stress responses.* New York: Plenum Press.

Frenn, M., Fehring, R., & Kartes, S. (1986). Reducing stress of cardiac catheterization by teaching relaxation. *Dimensions of Critical Care Nursing, 5,* 108–116.

Goleman, D. (1977). *The varieties of the meditative experience.* New York: E.P. Dutton.

Goleman, D., & Schwartz, G. (1976). Meditation as an intervention in stress reactivity. *Journal of Consulting and Clinical Psychology, 44,* 456–466.

Guzzetta, C. E. (1989). Effects of relaxation and music therapy on patients in a coronary care unit with presumptive acute myocardial infarction. *Heart & Lung, 18,* 609–618.

Kabat-Zinn, J. (1982). An outpatient program in behavioral medicine for chronic pain based on the practice of mindfulness meditation. *General Hospital Psychiatry, 4,* 33–47.

Kabat-Zinn, J., Lipworth, L., & Burney, R. (1985). The clinical use of mindfulness meditation for the self-regulation of chronic pain. *Journal of Behavioral Medicine, 8*(2), 163–190.

Kabat-Zinn, J., Lipworth, L., Burney, R., & Sellers, W. (1987). Four-year follow-up of a meditation program for the self-regulation of chronic pain: treatment outcomes and compliance. *Clinical Journal of Pain, 2,* 159–173.

Kabat-Zinn, J., Massion, A. O., Kristeller, J., Peterson, L. G., Fletcher, K. E., Pbert, L., Lenderking, W. R., & Santorelli, S. F. (1992). The effectiveness of a meditation-based stress reduction program in the treatment of anxiety disorders. *American Journal of Psychiatry, 149,* 936–943.

Kabat-Zinn, J., Wheeler, E., Light, T., Skillings, A., Scharf, M. J., Cropley, T. G., Hosmer, D., & Berhard, J. D. (1998). Influence of a mindfulness meditation-based stress reduction intervention on rates of skin clearing in patients with moderate to severe psoriasis undergoing phototherapy (UVB) and photochemotherapy (PUVA). *Psychosomatic Medicine, 60,* 625–632.

Keating, T. (1995). *Open mind, open heart.* New York: Continuum.

Kutz, I., Leserman, J., Dorrington, C., Morrison, C., Borysenko, J., & Benson, H. (1985). Meditation as an adjunct to psychotherapy. *Psychotherapy and Psychosomatics, 43*(4), 209–218.

Lazarus, A. A. (1976). Psychiatric problems precipitated by transcendental meditation. *Psychological Reports, 39,* 601–602.

LeShan, L. (1974). *How to meditate.* Boston: Little, Brown.

Lichstein, K.L. (1988). *Clinical relaxation strategies.* New York: John Wiley & Sons.

Miller, J. J., Fletcher, K., & Kabat-Zinn, J. (1995). Three-year follow-up and clinical implications of a mindfulness meditation-based stress reduction intervention in the treatment of anxiety disorders. *General Hospital Psychiatry, 17,* 192–200.

National Institutes of Health. (1992). *Alternative medicine: Expanding medical horizons.* Washington, DC: U.S. Government Printing Office.

Orme-Johnson, D.W. (1987). Medical care litigation and the transcendental meditation program. *Psychosomatic Medicine, 49,* 493–507.

Pollack, A. A., Case, D. B., Weber, M. A., & Laragh, J. H. (1977). Limitations of transcendental meditation in the treatment of essential hypertension. *Lancet,* 1(8002), 71–73.

Roth, B., & T. Creaser (1997). MBSR: Experience with a bilingual inner-city program. *The Nurse Practitioner, 20,* 150–176.

Russel, P. (1976). *The TM technique.* Boston: Routledge and Kegan PAUI.

Shafii, M. (1973). Adaptive and therapeutic aspects of meditation. *International Journal of Psychoanalysis and Psychotherapy, 2,* 431–443.

Tart, C. (1971). A psychologist's experiences with transcendental meditation. *Journal of Transpersonal Psychology, 3,* 135–143.

Welwood, J. (1979). *The meeting of the ways: Explorations in east/west psychology.* New York: Schocken Books.

West, M. (1979). The psychosomatics of meditation. *Journal of Psychosomatic Medicine, 24,* 265–273.

West, M. (1980). Meditation. *British Journal of Psychiatry, 135,* 457–467.

11

Prayer

Mariah Snyder

Prayer has been identified as a complementary therapy by the National Center for Complementary and Alternative Medicine (2000). According to a survey published in *Time* magazine, 82% of Americans believe in the healing power of personal prayer, and 73% of the respondents stated that prayers for others could help in curing illnesses (Kaplan, 1996). Prayer is ubiquitous, having been used by persons of all cultures throughout time. However, it is only within recent years that official studies have begun to document the effect prayer has on health outcomes. Physicians like Larry Dossey (1993, 1999) and Rachel Remen (1996, 2000) have done much to publicize the positive results of prayer in the popular press. Despite the wide acceptance of the impact prayer can have on promoting health and healing, skeptics continue to question the value of prayer in bringing about positive health outcomes.

Prayer has been an integral part of nursing for centuries. The holistic perspective of nursing mandates that nurses assess the spiritual needs of a patient along with the physical, psychological, and social elements. Many early schools of nursing in the United States were affiliated with specific Christian religious organizations. Within this context, student nurses were taught to include prayer as part of their care. With the increasing cultural diversity and the emergence of public and nonsectarian hospitals and care facilities, "official" prayer essentially vanished from most nursing curricula. In recent years courses on spirituality in nursing have begun to reemerge.

A growing body of knowledge is providing evidence that prayer is used extensively by persons in all cultures in times of need such as during an illness (Fontaine, 2000). People often equate prayer with religion, yet prayer, like spirituality, transcends religion. Prayer and spirituality acknowledge the

---

Content includes material found in the prayer chapter in earlier editions contributed by Dr. Marilyne Gustafson.

existence of a Greater Being and that we as humans have an connectedness with this Being. Cultural and religious groups have different names for this Higher Being: God, Supreme Being, Mother Earth, Master of the Universe, Creator, Absolute, El, or Great Spirit.

DEFINITION

"Prayer" is from the Latin *precarius*, which means to obtain by begging, and from *precari*, which means to entreat. Gustafson (1998) defined prayer as "a solemn and humble approach to a divinity in work or thought" (p. 259). Prayer has also been defined as communication with the Absolute (Dossey, 1993). Brown (1996) defined prayer as "what happens when the soul cries out to its Maker and no matter what the words, no matter what the feelings, no matter what the method, when it happens, this is prayer" (p. 6) According to Dossey (1993), since prayer has its roots in the unconscious it is impossible for us to grasp the entire meaning of prayer.

Prayer and meditation (chapter 10) share many commonalities. Prayer is distinguished from meditation in that it is a communication with a Higher Being. While the object of meditation is to focus attention on a word or object so as to become more attentive and aware, the focus of prayer is on communication with a Higher Being. There are many forms of meditation and some of these, such as centering, incorporate prayer.

Many different types of prayer have been described in the literature. Table 11.1 lists the types of prayer that are commonly used. Prayer may be done on an individual basis, within a group, or as part of a faith or religious community. In the latter context, prayer often has prescribed words and rituals. One exception to this is the Quaker prayer meeting that does not use prescribed words. Prayer, however, is unique to an individual in that each person has established his or her relationship with the Absolute or Higher Being. Dossey (1993) makes a distinction between prayer and prayerfulness. The former, Dossey states, is associated with the traditions of specific religious groups while prayerfulness is "a feeling of unity with the All" (p. 24). Others contend, however, that prayer is not denomination-specific but rather a communication that persons have with a Higher Being.

SCIENTIFIC BASIS

Some may suggest that it is oxymoronic to explore the scientific basis of prayer because religion and science are based on different principles. Dossey

TABLE 11.1   Types of Prayer

Adoration or praise: acknowledging the greatness of a Higher Being
Colloquial: informal communication with Higher Being
Directed: requesting a specific outcome
Intercessory: communicating with a Higher Being for another who has a need
Lamentation: communicating to a Higher Being for bereavement
Nondirected: requests for the best thing to occur in a given situation
Petition: asking a Higher Being for a personal request
Ritual: Using set words or rituals
Thanksgiving: offering gratitude to a Higher Being for a request or gift received

(1993) has proposed a number of strategies that may underlie the positive impact prayer has had on illness. Prayer in groups provides social support. Likewise, knowing that others care for you and are praying for you may promote a sense of belonging. Research has documented the positive effects that social support and a sense of belonging have on health outcomes (Dossey, 1999). Another possible cause for the positive effects of prayer is that it often produces positive emotions, which in turn may have a positive impact on the immune system. At this point in time, these are all hypotheses.

Since the seminal research by Joyce and Welldon (1965), numerous research studies have been conducted, and the findings from many of these studies support the benefits of prayer on health. Byrd (1997) randomized patients who were admitted to a critical care unit into a group who received intercessory prayer by Christians and a control group. Findings showed that patients in the intercessory prayer group required less ventilatory assistance and fewer antibiotics and diuretics than did patients in the control group. Harris and colleagues (1999) reported that patients in a coronary care unit who received intercessory prayer had an 11% reduction in critical care outcome scores, contrasted with a 4% reduction in the control group. In both of these studies, the length of hospital stay was not affected by prayer. In the mantra project conducted at Duke University (Mitchell & Krucoff, 1999), findings showed a 50% to 100% reduction in adverse outcomes in subjects undergoing cardiac catheterization who were prayed for compared with patients who had received the standard treatment.

Studies have also been conducted on the use of prayer with persons having chronic conditions. Sicher, Targ, Moore, and Smith (1998) found that the use of distant healing prayer with persons with AIDS resulted in the experimental group having a lower severity index after 6 months than subjects in the control group. Subjects in the prayer group showed improved mood; however, no differences in CD4$^+$ counts was found between the two groups. O'Laire (1997) found differences between the control and experimental groups on depression, self-esteem, or mood. Positive results from prayer have not been found in all of the reported studies. Walker, Tonigan, Miller, Comer, and Kahlich (1997) did not find any differences in alcohol consumption in chronic alcoholics between the group receiving intercessory prayer and the control group. In a review of studies on intercessory prayer, Roberts, Ahmed, and Hall, (2000) concluded that the findings from their review provided no guidance to either uphold or refute the effects of intercessory prayer on health outcomes.

In the aforementioned studies, praying was done by persons other than the patients. A number of studies have documented the effectiveness of prayer as a coping strategy. Ai, Dunkle, Peterson, and Bolling (1998) found that patients who prayed following cardiac surgery had a significant decline in depression at 1 year compared to immediately after surgery and that they had less overall distress. The relationship between church attendance and health was examined by Strawbridge, Cohen, Shema, and Kaplan (1997). They found that people who frequently attended church had lower mortality rates than those who attended on an infrequent basis. Persons who went to church regularly also were more likely to engage in health-promoting behaviors such as exercising and not smoking.

The mechanism of how prayer works, whether intercessory on behalf of others or for oneself, is not known. Dossey has proposed that prayer is one of a number of nonlocal phenomena, that is, prayer is not constrained by space or time. The person praying does not have to be in proximity to the person being prayed for in order to be effective. A question also exists about whether the person being prayed for must believe in it or be receptive to it. In research studies, patients have given consent to be the recipient of prayers. However, in daily life, prayers are said for others without their knowledge. Meditation by mediators for the purpose of lowering crime in communities has produced positive results even though the many citizens were unaware of the project (Mason, personal communication, May 2000). Roberts et al. (2000) noted that the understanding of prayer may be beyond our present scientific methods, and if the effects occur because of a Higher Being, determining the mechanism may be beyond our ability to prove or disprove the effects.

INTERVENTION

When prayer is discussed in terms of health, intercessory prayer (that is, prayer for others or for self related to a particular problem) is often the type of prayer being used. Less attention has been given to exploring the impact of overall prayerfulness on the lives of individuals. As noted in the previous section, studies have documented positive effects resulting from the use of prayer as a coping strategy.

ASSESSMENT

Spiritual assessment should be part of a patient's health history obtained by nurses or other health professionals. Many spiritual assessments include information about the beliefs people hold, how they address the Higher Being, and things that are important to them in order to pray. The latter might include books or objects. A number of assessment guides have been developed (Kerrigan & Harkulich, 1993; O'Brien, 1999; Reed, 1991; Stoll, 1979). The spiritual assessment guide developed by O'Brien gathers information about beliefs in a Higher Being, religious practices, and spiritual contentment by using questions like the following:

- I receive strength and comfort from my spiritual beliefs.
- My relationship with God is strengthened by personal prayer.
- I feel far away from God (pp. 66–67).

Information from the spiritual assessment will guide nurses in developing a plan of care. Possible actions include providing an environment that will assist them in praying; obtaining resources for the person; contacting a minister, rabbi, priest, or spiritual guide; or praying with the person if appropriate.

Findings from the spiritual assessment will guide the nurse in the use of prayer. The times for discussing the use of prayer include when a diagnosis is given, when the person is fearful or anxious, before and after surgery, when giving birth, and at the end of life. Prayers of thanksgiving should not be forgotten in times of recovery or when the findings from a diagnostic test show no serious condition.

Increased attention is being paid to health professionals praying for their patients (Post, Puchalski, & Larson, 2000). Praying is closely linked to caring for a person. Praying for patients can be as simple as asking God (or the name you give to your Higher Being) to bless the patients and families you meet during the day, or it may be a short prayer as one enters a room. (We have little information about prayer dosage! Are long prayers better than short ones?) Remen (2000) commented that caring for the souls of our patients is as important as caring for their bodies.

While prayer can be used separately from a religious context, knowledge about the beliefs and practices of the major religions is helpful.

Knowledge about prayer and religious rituals will help the nurse make the patient feel comfortable in using practices that are part of their tradition. (It is beyond the scope of this chapter to provide this information.) Many excellent resources are available, such as *Religions of the World* (Smith, 1995), that will provide nurses with information about religious traditions that will be helpful in caring for the spiritual needs of persons from diverse cultures.

TECHNIQUE

The prayer form should take the form that the patient desires. If nurses feel comfortable doing so, they can ask if patients would like the nurse to join them in praying. Reading scripture or from a holy book is one way to pray with a person; otherwise, provide an environment in which the person can pray. Many hospitals, nursing homes, and clinics have a chapel or room for prayer and meditation. Accompanying a patient to the chapel or prayer room acknowledges one's intent to help the patient. The health status of many patients in acute care settings does not allow them to go to a chapel; however, family members may find it helpful. Those with a religious affiliation may wish to use the formal prayers of their faith tradition. For example, Christians may find the Lord's Prayer comforting. Patients of the Jewish faith may want to read the psalms or have them read to them, and Muslims may choose to read from the Qur'an (Koran). Giving praise to the four directions may be a prayer form used by people of Native American ancestry. Nurses need to respect whatever form or ritual the prayer takes.

Prayer circles or chains are becoming more common. These provide a vehicle for intercessory prayer to be offered for a particular person or family. If a nurse knows about the existence of a prayer circle, he or she could ask a patient or family member if they would like to have the group pray for them. The following is a message of thanks from a family member to prayer circles who had prayed for his father when he was hospitalized:

> I wish to extend my thanks and that of my family to all of you who prayed for my father, Andy, during these past weeks. It has been a time filled with many ups and downs, highs and lows, and many emotions. Many of you received an e-mail message requesting prayers for my father after he had suffered a heart attack and subsequently had heart bypass surgery. Some of you contacted prayer circles who then prayed for my father, many of whom have never met my father. This is an occurrence that humbles a person. My father suffered many complications following surgery. The doctors and critical care staff recognized that something more was occurring than their interventions and treatment. That something was prayer. The doctors and staff returned to the family room to tell us that miracles were occurring in the ICU where my father was a patient. I am confident that these were due to your prayers.

MEASUREMENT OF OUTCOMES

The purpose for which prayer has been used will dictate what outcomes to measure. Because of the mind-body-spirit interactions, nurses may want to include more holistic measures than simply measurement of physiological or psychological statuses. For example, other indicators of effectiveness that could be pursued are the contentment of a person, overall well-being, and the person's relating that they are more at peace. The effect of prayer may be healing rather than curing an illness which presents a challenge to Western measurement indices.

PRECAUTIONS

Because of the highly personal nature of faith, spirituality, religious beliefs and practices, it is important for the nurses to assess both the prayer preferences of patients and their own personal beliefs and comfort with using prayer. Knowledge about the beliefs and practices of other faith traditions is imperative in our pluralistic society. Used improperly prayer may offend others, awaken old antipathies, and make patients uncomfortable. Assessment and then offering possibilities is paramount.

The nurse should not be surprised when patients request prayers that the nurse may view as manipulative or magical. Prayers for cures in what might be considered impossible situations would be requests that the nurse needs to consider thoughtfully. One of the rules used by hospital chaplains is to pray as directed by patients and support the patient's prayer even when the desired outcome is seemingly impossible (Leonard, 2000). Post and colleagues (2000) noted that prayer should be viewed as a complementary therapy and not used to the exclusion of biomedical therapies.

USES

Prayer has been used with persons having every type of illness, of any age group, and from all cultures. Table 11.2 lists selected conditions for which studies on the use of prayer have been conducted. The literature also contains many anecdotal accounts about the efficacy of prayer. For instance, in a survey of women with breast cancer, VanderCreek, Rogers, and Lester (1999) found that 76% of the women prayed, which was the most frequently used complementary therapy.

TABLE 11.2   Selected Studies Documenting the Effectiveness of Prayer

Addictive behaviors (Walker, Tonigan, Miller, Comer, & Kahlich, 1997)

Cancer (VanderCreek, Rogers, & Lester, 1999)

Cardiac conditions (Ai, Dunkle, Peterson, & Bolling, 1998; Byrd, 1988; Harris, et al., 1999)

Caregivers (Stolley, Buckwalter, & Koenig, 1999)

Depressive symptoms (Ellison, 1995)

Immunosufficiency syndrome (Sicher, Targ, Moore, & Smith, 1998)

FUTURE RESEARCH

The growing public interest in prayer and the increasing inclusion of content about spirituality and prayer in the curricula of health professional schools should result in increased research on prayer. Conducting research on prayer is fraught with challenges and the following are several areas in which research is needed:

1. Most of the reported studies have been from a Judeo-Christian perspective. Explorations of the impact prayer has on health outcomes need to reflect the many cultures and religions of the world.

2. Studies are needed on the efficacy of prayer in health promotion. Most studies to date have examined prayer in acute and chronic illness situations.

3. What are the methods that are best suited for studying the outcomes of prayer? Can it be studied within the context of Western scientific methods? If these methods are used, how can the essential elements of prayer be preserved? How can researchers know that the intercessory prayer being tested is the only prayer that is being said for the patient?

REFERENCES

Ai, A. L., Dunkle, R. E., Peterson, C., & Bolling, S. F. (1998). The role of private prayer in psychological recovery among midlife and aged patients following heart surgery. *The Gerontologist, 38,* 591–601.

Brown, S. (1996). *Approaching God.* Nashville, TN: Moorings.

Byrd, R. C. (1988). Positive therapeutic effects of intercessory prayer in a coronary care unit population. *Southern Medical Journal, 81,* 826–829.

Dossey, L. (1993). *Healing words.* New York: HarperSanFrancisco.

Dossey, L. (1999). *Reinventing medicine*. New York: HarperSanFrancisco.

Ellison, C. (1995). Race, religious involvement, and depressive symptomatology in a southeastern U.S. community. *Social Science and Medicine, 40*, 1561–1572.

Fontaine, K. L. (2000). *Healing practices: Alternative therapies for nursing*. Upper Saddle River, NJ: Prentice Hall.

Gustafson, M. B. (1998). Prayer. In M. Snyder and R. Lindquist (Eds.), *Complementary/Alternative Therapies in Nursing* (pp. 259–268). New York: Springer Publishing Co.

Harris, W. S., Gowda, M., Kolb, J. W., Strychacz, C. P., Vacek, J. L., Jones, P. G., Forker, A., O'Keefe, J. H., & McCallister, B. D. (1999). A randomized, controlled trial of the effects of remote, intercessory prayer on outcomes in patients admitted to the coronary care unit. *Archives of Internal Medicine, 159*, 2273–2278. [On-line], http://www.jesuit.ie/prayer.

Joyce, C. R., & Welldon, R. M. (1965). The objective efficacy of prayer. *Journal of Chronic Disease, 18*, 367–376.

Kaplan, M. (1996). Ambushed by spirituality. *Time, 147*(26), 62.

Kerrigan, R., & Harkulich, J. T. (1993). A spiritual tool. *Health Progress, 74*(5), 46–49.

Leonard, B. J. (2000). Personal communication. August, 2000.

Mitchell, W., & Krucoff, M. D. (1999). The MANTRA study project. *Alternative Therapies in Health & Medicine, 5*(3), 74–82.

O'Brien, M. E. (1999). *Spirituality in nursing: Standing on holy ground*. Sudbury, MA: Jones and Barlett.

O'Laire, S. (1997). An experimental study of the effects of distant, intercessory prayer on self-esteem, anxiety, and depression. *Journal of Alternative Therapies, 38*–53.

[On-line] National Center for Complementary/Alternative Medicine. http://www.nih.gov.

Post, S. G., Puchalski, C. M., & Larson, D. B. (2000). Physicians and patient spirituality: Professional boundaries, competency, and ethics. *Annals of Internal Medicine, 132*, 578–583.

Reed, P. G. (1991). Preferences for spirituality-related nursing interventions among terminally ill and non-terminally ill hospitalized adults and well adults. *Applied Nursing Research, 4*, 122–128.

Remen, R. N. (1996). *Kitchen table wisdom*. New York: Riverhead Books.

Remen, R. N. (2000). *My grandfather's blessings*. New York: Riverhead Books.

Roberts, L., Ahmed, I., & Hall, S. (2000). Intercessory prayer for the alleviation of ill health. *The Cochrane Library, (3)* (Update 2/23/00).

Sicher, F., Targ, E., Moore, D., & Smith, H. S. (1998). A randomized double-blind study of the effect of distant healing in a population with advanced AIDS: Report of a small scale study. *Western Journal of Medicine, 169*, 356–363.

Smith, H. (1995). *Religions of the World*. Boulder, CO: Sounds True.

Stoll, R. (1979). Guidelines for spiritual assessment. *American Journal of Nursing, 79*, 1574–1577.

Stolley, J. M., Buckwalter, K. C., & Koenig, H. G. (1999). Prayer and religious coping for caregivers of persons with Alzheimer's disease and related disorders. *American Journal of Alzheimer's Disease, 14*, 181–191.

Strawbridge, W. J., Cohen, R. D., Shema, S. J., & Kaplan, G. A. (1997). Frequent attendance at religious services and mortality over 28 years. *American Journal of Public Health, 87,* 957–961.

VanderCreek, L., Rogers, E., & Lester, J. (1999). Use of alternative therapies among breast cancer patients outpatients compared with the general population. *Alternative Therapies, 5,* 71–76.

Walker, S. R., Tonigan, J. S., Miller, W. R., Comer, S., & Kahlich, L (1997). Intercessory prayer in the treatment of alcohol abuse and dependence: A pilot investigation. *Journal of Alternative Therapies, 3,* 79–85.

12

Storytelling As a Healing Tool

Roxanne Struthers

Storytelling, a natural and common component of everyday conversation, is utilized by all age groups as an ordinary, powerful tool to communicate with others (Witherell & Noddings, 1991). Stories are constructed to teach religion and values (Lawlis, 1995), tell a tale, impart information to others, and explain views and share experiences. The ancient art of storytelling predated writing and was used by preliterate societies (Bowles, 1995; Wenckus, 1994). In fact, storytelling is described as one of the oldest arts, having its roots in the beginning of articulate expression.

Storytelling is an intrinsic part of many cultures (Lindesmith & McWeeny, 1994). To date, indigenous peoples tell stories as oral tradition (Diekelmann, 1994/1995), and storytelling takes precedence over written tradition within these cultures. Something does not have to be written down to be true (Jones, 1995). Representatives of many indigenous cultures argue that writing absolves individuals from remembering and therefore dilutes the complexity of knowledge that can be kept alive in any society (Thorne, 1993). Furthermore, the act of imparting oral knowledge and telling the story brings about a metaphysical presence, and a natural, holistic, intuitive, and spiritual order to communication (Crazy Bull, 1997).

Nurses have been telling stories forever (Bowles, 1995) and listening to stories even longer. Whether we are the nursed or the nurse, we are the stories we tell (Sandelowski, 1994). It is in the unfolding and intertwining of the story that it becomes my story, your story, our story. We are all connected on a deeper, higher level and storytelling can take us to these levels.

DEFINITION

Storytelling, an art and a science (Lawlis, 1995), is an individual account of an event that creates a memorable picture in the mind of the listener

(Kirkpatrick, Ford, & Castelloe, 1997). There are many forms of story, including the fairy tale, the legend, the personal incident, and the personal myth (Lawlis, 1995). Nevertheless, a factual or fictional story always has certain characteristics. Labov, a sociolinguist, states that a complete story typically comprises

- an abstract—what the story is about
- an orientation—the "who, when, where, what" of the story
- complicating action—the "then-what-happened" part of the story
- evaluation—the "so-what"of the story
- resolution—the "what-finally-happened" portion of the story
- the coda—the signal a story is over
- return to the present (Sandelowski, 1994, p. 25).

M. A. Newman, a nursing theorist, defines stories or narratives as expressions of human consciousness and a means to expand this consciousness (1994); thus, they help a person move towards wholeness that defines health. Storytelling has been defined by Bowles (1995) as descriptive and a medium by which personal experience may be communicated to others with immediacy and relevancy that is capable of affecting changes in the narrator as well as the audience. In other words, storytelling is an age-old healer.

According to a indigenous Canadian teacher, natural forms of indigenous healing include song, dance, ritual, and storytelling (C. Bird, personal communication, August 3, 2000). In indigenous healing workshops and retreats, storytelling is a major framework utilized to assist with the healing process. Usually these storytelling sessions occur with the participants sitting in a talking circle, also known as a healing circle or sharing circle. According to Lee (1995) the circle is the most universally occurring shape, therefore all healing ceremonies take place in a circle. The circle is significant in how things are perceived by a person and how the mind is guided by intuition. From this vantage point, process is crucial, the mind can exclaim with wonder and delight at what is revealed through the eyes of the heart, and intuitive knowledge discerns that things will occur when and how they are intended to happen.

SCIENTIFIC BASIS

Storytelling is routinely thought of as an act or tool for prompting and influencing the health status of individuals and groups. Some of the attributes of health that storytelling affects include (a) providing a connection to other people; (b) rendering a sense of connection between life events; (c) unlocking an opportunity for healing to occur; (d) aiding one to achieve the fullness of human potential; and (e) an integrated sense of self (Sandelowski, 1994). Storytelling also changes people's sense of time and place, stimulates strong emotions, encourages communication, and helps them resolve problems (Snyder, 1992). According to Lawlis (1995), anxiety is lowered in the listener, imagery is created and accommodated, relaxation ensues, pain may be relieved, and patients can become empowered. Nagai-Jacobson and Burkhardt (1996) state that storytelling can awaken spiritual forces and facilitate the release of energy, resulting in the healing of ourselves and others. Teachers know that students come alive when the teacher digresses and tells a story (Noddings, 1994). It is also known that whenever an individual wants to report "what really happened," the natural impulse is to tell a story (Bowman, 1995, p. 35).

A nurse-orator made a tape addressing how she personally demonstrated caring as a school nurse on an American Indian Reservation in North Dakota. Someone who listened to the tape wondered if this nurse ever wrote and published. Responding to this comment, the school nurse replied, "When you write it down, it loses something" (V. Allen, personal communication, June 17, 1996).

RESEARCH

Although storytelling is utilized as a therapeutic and every-day tool, research on its effectiveness as a nursing intervention is scant. In current intervention research studies of utilizing storytelling, various methods of storytelling have been used alone or in conjunction with other interventions, and there are multiple instruments to measure the effectiveness of storytelling.

In a study by Walker (1988), cartoon storytelling was one assessment strategy employed with the 7- to 11-year-old siblings of pediatric cancer patients. Other intervention tactics included puppet play, drawing, sentence completion, and open-ended interviews. The research goal was to identify and describe cognitive and behavioral coping strategies used by siblings of pediatric cancer patients. A selected non-random Caucasian sample of 26 siblings (16 male and 10 female) from 15 families at a regional children's hospital participated in the research study. Content analysis of the data revealed major stressor themes of loss, fear of death, and change among the siblings.

In a descriptive correlation study, Collins (1991) described stress levels in fourth-grade children from three diverse living environments. Spontaneous storytelling was used and measured according to a newly developed Spontaneous Storytelling Tool and an adapted Life Events Questionnaire (LEQ). Sixty five non-random subjects, 27 boys and 38 girls, participated in the research study. Of these research subjects, 48 were White and 19 non-White. Results showed that the LEQ stress scores were the same for children from all the environments. There were differences in story themes demonstrated by low, moderate, or high stress levels in accounts told by the fourth-graders.

In a quasi-experimental pre-post test study, reminiscent storytelling was used with older adults to investigate storytelling as a therapeutic modality to enhance a sense of power. The group consisted of 81 voluntary non random-selected independent-living adults over the age of 60 (81% were female). The experimental group participated in three sessions of reminiscent storytelling in a week's time. The control group did not participate in reminiscent storytelling. Research results showed that reminiscent storytelling did not increase power in the experimental group. In fact, both groups exhibited a small decrease in power between the pretest and first posttest. However, both groups showed a significant increase in power between the two posttests. It is hypothesized that the act of administering the three tests simulated an act of social exchange strong enough to increased the power in this isolated older population (Bramlett & Gueldner, 1993).

Banks-Wallace (1998) found storytelling useful for learning more about the historical and contextual factors affecting the well-being of women of African descent and improving their lives. A secondary narrative analysis of 115 stories from a convenience sample of 28 women of African descent revealed six major functions of storytelling: (a) contextual grounding, (b) bonding with others, (c) validating and affirming experiences, (d) venting and catharsis, (e) resisting oppression, and (f) educating others.

Howard (1991) states that culture shapes our stories. A contemporary example of culture-specific storytelling and conveyance of oral knowledge is the talking circle exercised by indigenous American Indians. In an intervention study, 88 sites in California were randomly assigned to either the intervention or the control intervention ($n = 414$). Hodge, Fredericks, and Rodriguez (1996) discovered that American Indian women responded favorably to the use of the talking circle, coupled with traditional stories, as a vehicle to disseminate cancer education and improve adherence to cancer screening. Hodge, Stubbs, Gurgin, and Fredericks (1998), showed that the talking circle was effective for teaching about cancer prevention. In a participatory action research study in Washington, Yakima Indian women ($n = 10$) also preferred storytelling as a natural pattern of communication when learning about health promotion relating to cervical cancer prevention (Strickland, Squeoch, & Chrisman, 1999). Research shows conclusively that culturally appropriate communication methods, such as storytelling, are effective in health promotion activities.

Thus, findings exist demonstrating that storytelling is an efficacious intervention.

INTERVENTION

Inherent in each person's story is a key to healing (Roche, 1994) and an opportunity for personal growth (Heiney, 1995). However, it is only recently in America and the Western world that telling one's personal story is recognized as a therapeutic healing modality (Larkin & Zabourek, 1988; Sandelowski, 1994). There is power in articulating a personal story and certain outcomes happen when this occurs.

Storytelling within the talking circle is one format in which the art of storytelling occurs. Indigenous Ojibwa and Cree women healers used talking circles (also called healing circles or sharing circles) and storytelling in their everyday traditional healing practice (Struthers, 1999) as an instrument of healing. This format was also used to teach culture, traditions, and health education and promotion.

TECHNIQUES

To conduct a talking circle, usually 5 to 10 participants sit in chairs placed in a circle in an environment that is conducive to healing. A facilitator opens the session by welcoming everyone and sharing a story. The information disclosed usually centers around a selected topic or reason for the talking circle. Then the circle is opened to all and each person is accorded the opportunity to talk. Typically, a feather, rock, or other item is passed from one talking circle participant to the next speaker-talker, who holds the item while speaking. During this time, that particular person takes the lead and shares their story with the group. While the person is speaking, the facilitator and the other talking circle participants respect and support the person who is sharing their story by honoring them, being present, and listening to the essence of their story. After each person has had a chance to contribute, the facilitator summarizes the events and the circle closes. The group can be small, with only two people present, or larger than 10 if the facilitator is experienced.

When one tells their story within a talking circle, several things happen simultaneously. A "place" is created where the following elements come together:

1. A *healing environment*: The first step necessary for healing to take place from storytelling is to create an environment conducive to storytelling

(Lindesmith & McWeeny, 1994). It is not possible to expect healing without a conducive healing atmosphere. Therefore, it is imperative that a comfortable physical environment be sought out, away from other distractions. With chairs placed in a circle, everyone can view everyone else and experience their presence. The environment can be cleansed and kept clear with the assistance of purification rituals. Some persons may use candles, crystals, or feathers, for instance. In the Native American tradition sage, cedar, or sweet grass are commonly utilized for this purpose.

2. *Nonjudgment:* Individuals and groups must feel safe and supported in their surroundings in order to facilitate the healing process (Bowman, 1995). When speaking we are often reluctant to reveal too much about ourselves because it makes us vulnerable. However, we cannot tell a story without self-disclosure (Kelly, 1995). Therefore, an atmosphere free from criticism, exploration, interpretation, or judgement must prevail (Heinrich, 1992; Kuhrik, 1995; Lindesmith & McWeeny, 1994) and confidentiality must be emphasized.

3. *Listening:* It is of utmost importance that others listen to the story. More than anything, we need to cultivate the quality of listening carefully, patiently, attentively, and compassionately to another human being while they tell their story (Baker & Diekelmann, 1994; Heinrich, 1992; Lindesmith & McWeeny, 1994; Roche, 1994). Simply put, this is caring enough about another person to listen to what they have to say (Kelly, 1995) and to listen with one's heart (Heiney, 1995).

Everyone complains about the lack of communication, of the failure to understand the what and the why and the how. To stretch and make room for the thoughts, ideas, or goals of others, all must learn to listen. It may be true that hearing is the one sense that becomes full-blown when life begins, and it can be the last to survive (Wilson, 1979).

4. *Spontaneity and creativity:* Storytelling requires no training or skill (Heiney, 1995). However, stories come alive when we let the story "lift and flow" and let the story "laugh and cry" (Wilson, 1979, p.3). Imagination, flexibility, and creativity flow forth naturally in storytelling (Kuhrik, 1995; Larkin & Zabourek, 1988; Wenckus, 1994), thereby allowing these traits to emerge.

5. *Presence:* To be present is to consciously stay in the moment. Change takes place in the present, not in the past or in the future. When one is present in the moment, a state of noninterfering attention that allows natural healing to flow is generated (Dossey, Keegan, & Guzzetta, 2000).

6. *Empathy and caring:* Storytelling increases empathy (Heinrich, 1992). Empathy is defined as "the action of understanding, being aware of, being sensitive to, and vicariously experiencing the feelings, thoughts, and experience of another . . . without having the feelings, thoughts, and experiences fully communicated in an objectively explicit manner" (Webster, 1984, p. 407).

According to Diekelmann (1994/1995), as the story unfolds the participants in the narrative travel together to the place of intertwining where "one
no longer knows who speaks and who listens" (p. 67). This sets up the possibility for one of us to dwell within the lived experience of another (Heinrich,
1992; Witherell & Noddings, 1991). Also, to listen is to display caring.
Caring is a factor Western society tends to neglect.

7. *Community:* In the process of storytelling, a feeling of community is
established (Bowman, 1995; Lindesmith & McWeeny, 1994). This feeling
creates bonding or strengthening of intimate relationships with others like
themselves and this in turn facilitates survival and well-being (Banks-Wallace,
1998). This sense of community decreases the invisibility and isolation of
people (Heinrich, 1992). Everyone desires to belong and be accepted in a
group environment. Community is a sense of this desire. According to Crain
(1995), people seem isolated, rootless, and disconnected. They desperately
seek love, and may even temporarily find it, but the emptiness and isolation
soon returns. A connection and belonging develops during the storytelling
process that not only connects us to other people (Kelly, 1995), but connects us to higher truths (Heiney, 1995). According to Levine (1995) truth
connects. This connection can provide a liberating experience (Baker &
Diekelmann, 1994).

8. *Learning and sharing*: Learning from one another when we share our
stories is automatic (Lindesmith & McWeeny, 1994) because storytelling
provides a vehicle to share knowledge and wisdom (Banks-Wallace, 1998).
According to Heiney (1995), part of this learning means we are able to see
things on many different levels and a prism may be provided through
which a single event may be viewed. New perspectives may emerge (Bowles,
1995) as stories are told. In the process of storytelling, validation (Heinrich,
1992; Wenckus, 1994), recognition and knowing self (Kelly, 1995), and
meaning for self evolve. It is in these acknowledgments that the spirit
evolves. According to Bondi (1993), the way of God and the way of knowing are one.

MEASUREMENT OF OUTCOMES

Storytelling is an encounter that can grant us positive advantageous effects
and outcomes that can facilitate a shift towards a balanced holistic health
status. Healing can occur when the above circumstances happen simultaneously. When we tell our stories, we release energy, which is healing for ourselves and others (Nagai-Jacobson & Burkhardt, 1996).

As demonstrated by the research studies that have used storytelling as a
therapeutic intervention, a variety of tools can be used to measure outcomes.

Depending on the purpose for which storytelling is used, instruments that measure anxiety, depression, social isolation, spirituality, caring, and sense of well-being may be appropriate.

PRECAUTIONS

Those using storytelling need to be prepared to deal with strong emotions the stories may evoke. Health professionals should be ready to assist and support the participants, as diverse reactions can occur. A list of available resources to make referrals for follow-up may be helpful after the session ends. Only persons trained in psychotherapy should utilize storytelling with people who have psychological problems.

USES

Nurses have used narrative storytelling in multiple situations across the life span for a variety of purposes. Uses of storytelling are identified in Table 12.1.

Many of the 12-step self-help programs, such as Alcoholics Anonymous (AA), are based on storytelling. Individuals qualify or tell of the development of their illnesses and subsequent recovery process. Reach for Recovery for mastectomy patients is also based on a similar premise (Larkin & Zabourek, 1988).

FUTURE RESEARCH

Nurses have always utilized stories in their practice. Clearly, much research needs to be conducted to document storytelling as a proven therapeutic modality. Even though many qualitative studies have been conducted that utilize storytelling to explore phenomena or to illuminate experiences in the discipline, storytelling must be viewed for its effect on patient outcomes. Examples of future research questions related to storytelling include the following:

1. What situations are appropriate for storytelling?
2. Which clients benefit from storytelling?
3. Which environments enhance storytelling?
4. What therapeutic skills are required when utilizing storytelling?
5. How can stories assist with teaching students, culture, health behavior, and health outcomes?
6. How does culture affect the art of storytelling?
7. What effects do talking circles have on spirituality?

TABLE 12.1   Uses of Narrative Storytelling

- To discover knowledge, uncover knowledge embedded in practice, recover the art of nursing, and rediscover the "every-dayness" of nursing practice (Sandelowski, 1994).
- To explain procedures, invoke hope, obtain information, resolve conflicts, teach students (Dicke, 1992).
- To honor one's experience and personal wisdom and assist with the teaching of health behaviors (Lawlis, 1995).
- To conduct qualitative research that allows access to the human experience of time, order, and change; and to format case studies (Sandelowski, 1991).
- To entertain, teach morals and values, promote critical thinking, relieve tension, and pass on traditions and preserve culture and history (Kirkpatrick et al., 1997).
- To facilitate self-awareness and search for personal truth (Bowles, 1995).
- To provide frameworks for healing encounters (Struthers, 1999).
- To enhance learning, professional development, and clinical practice among practicing nurses (Wadell, Durrant & Avery, 1999).
- To increase the quality of care in long-term care settings (Heliker, 1999).
- To conduct research (Diekelmann, 1994/1995; Kelly, 1995; Sandelowski, 1991).
- To relate culture and history and teach ethics and morals (Wenckus, 1994).

REFERENCES

Banks-Wallace, J. (1998). Emancipatory potential of storytelling in a group. *Image: Journal of Nursing Scholarship, 30*(1), 17–21.

Baker, C., & Diekelmann, N. (1994, March/April). Connecting conversations of caring: Recalling the narrative to clinical practice. *Nursing Outlook, 42*(2), 65–70.

Bondi, R. (1993). Spirituality and higher learning: Thinking and loving. *The Cressent, 6*(3), 5–12.

Bowles, R. (1995). Storytelling: A search for meaning within nursing practice. *Nursing Education Today, 15*(5), 365–369.

Bowman. A. (1995). Teaching ethics: Telling stories. *Nurse Education Today, 15*(1), 33–38.

Bramlett, M. H., & Gueldner, S. H. (1993). Reminiscence: A viable option to enhance power in elders. *Clinical Nurse Specialist, 7*(2), 68–74.

Collins, A. M. (1991). Perceived stress and stress projected into the spontaneous storytelling of two groups of fourth-grade children. *Journal of Child and Adolescent Psychiatric and Mental Health Nursing, 4*(3), 83–89.

Crain, W. (1995, Winter). Love of nature: Lessons from the Lakota. *Holistic Education Review, 8*(4), 27–36.

Crazy Bull, C. (1997). A Native conversation about research and scholarship. *Tribal College: Journal of American Indian Higher Education* , 9(1), 17–23.

Dicke, P. (1985). Storytelling. In M. Snyder (Ed.), *Independent Nursing Interventions.* Albany, NY: Delmar Publishers, Inc.

Diekelmann, N. (1994/1995, December/January). Sharing nursing work through stories. *Nursing New Zealand, 2*(11), 8.

Dossey, B. M., Keegan, L., & Guzetta. C. E. (2000). *Holistic nursing: A handbook for practice* (3rd ed.). Gaithersburg, MD: Aspen.

Heiney, S. P. (1995). The healing power of story. *Oncology Nursing Forum, 22*(6), 899–904.

Heinrich, K. L. (1992, March). Create a tradition: Teach nurses to share stories. *Journal of Nursing Education, 31*(3), 141–143.

Heliker, D. (1999). Transformation of story to practice: An innovative approach to long-term care. *Issues in Mental Health Nursing, 20,* 513–525.

Hodge, F. S., Fredericks, L., & Rodriguez, B. (1996). American Indian women's talking circle: A cervical cancer screening and prevention project. *Cancer Suppl., 78*(7), 1592–1597.

Hodge, F. S., Stubbs, H. A., Gurgin, V., & Fredericks, L. (1998). Cervical cancer screening: Knowledge, attitudes, and behavior of American Indian women. *Cancer Suppl., 83*(80), 1799–1802.

Howard, G. S. (1991). A narrative approach to thinking, cross-cultural psychology, and psychotherapy. *American Psychologist, 46*(3), 187–197.

Jones, D. (1995). The etymology of Anishinaabe. *Oshkaabewis Native Journal, 2*(1), 43–48.

Kelly, B. (1995, Winter). Storytelling: A way of connecting. *Nursing Connections, 8*(4), 5–11.

Kirkpatrick, M. K., Ford, S., & Castelloe, B. P. (1997). Storytelling: An approach to client-centered care. *Nurse Educator, 22*(2), 38–40.

Kuhrik, M. (1995). Telling stories in the classroom. *Nurse Educator, 20*(5), 4–5.

Larkin, D. M., & Zabourek, R. P. (1988). Therapeutic storytelling and metaphors. *Holistic Nursing Practice, 2*(3), 45–53.

Lawlis, G. F. (1995, May). Storytelling as therapy: Implications for medicine. *Alternative Therapies, 1*(2), 40–45.

Lee, S. C. (1995). The circle is sacred: A medicine book for women. Tulsa, OK: Council Oak Books.

Levine, P. M. (1995, Winter). Recovering the aesthetics of love: Teacher-as-loving-artist. *Holistic Education Review, 8*(4), 11–19.

Lindesmith, K. A., & McWeeny, M. (1994, July/August). The power of storytelling. *The Journal of Continuing Education in Nursing, 25*(4), 186–187.

Nagai-Jacobson, M., & Burkhardt, M.A. (1996, July). Viewing persons as stories: A perspective for holistic care. *Alternative Therapies, 2*(4), 54–58.

Newman, M. A. (1994). *Health as expanding consciousness.* New York: National League for Nursing.

Noddings, N. (1994). Learning to engage in moral dialogue. *Holistic Education Review*, 7(2), 5–11.

Roche, S. J. (1994). The story: A primary spiritual tool. *Health Progress*, 75(6), 60–63.

Sandelowski, M. (1991, Fall). Telling stories: Narrative approaches in qualitative research. *Image: Journal of Nursing Scholarship*, 23(3), 161–166.

Sandelowski, M. (1994). We are the stories we tell: Narrative knowing in nursing practice. *Journal of Holistic Nursing*, 12(1), 23–33.

Snyder, M. (1992). *Independent nursing interventions* (2nd ed.). Albany, NY: Delmar.

Strickland, C. J., Squeoch, M. D., & Chrisman, N. J. (1999). Health promotion in cervical cancer prevention among the Yakima Indian women of the Wa'Shat Longhouse. *Journal of transcultural Nursing*, 10(3), 190–196.

Struthers, R. (1999). *The lived experience of Ojibwa and Cree women healers*. Unpublished Dissertation, Minneapolis: University of Minnesota.

Thorne, S. (1993). Health belief systems in perspective. *Journal of Advanced Nursing*, 18, 1931–1941.

Waddell, J., Durrant, M., & Avery, S. (1999). The integration of research by nurse educators: Advancing practice through professional development programs. *The Journal of Continuing Education*, 30(6), 267–271.

Walker, C. L. (1988). Stress and coping in siblings of childhood cancer patients. *Nursing Research*, 37(4), 208–212.

Merriam-Webster's new collegiate dictionary (9th ed.), (1984). Springfield, MA: Merriam-Webster.

Wenckus. E. M. (1994). Storytelling: Using an ancient art to work with groups. *Journal of Psychosocial Nursing*, 32(7), 30–32.

Wilson, J. B. (1979). *The story experience*. Metuchen, NJ: The Scarecrow Press.

Witherell, C., & Noddings, N. (Eds.). (1991). *Stories lives tell: Narrative and dialogue in education*. New York: Teachers College Press.

The National Association for the Preservation and Perpetuation of Storytelling holds an annual convention each October in Jonesboro, Tennessee, (Larkin & Zabourek, 1988) for anyone who may be interested in exploring this ancient art further.

13

Journaling

Mariah Snyder

J ournal writing is one of a group of therapies that provide an opportunity for persons to reflect on and analyze their lives and the events and people surrounding them. Reminiscence, life review, and storytelling are other interventions that utilize a similar scientific basis. Journal writing (journaling) requires the active involvement of the person in reflecting and analyzing their experiences.

Since the beginning of written history, people have recorded the events of their lives. Libraries abound with volumes of personal journals, and countless journals are stashed away in closets and attics. *The Diary of Anne Frank* is an example of a journal that has had an impact on many lives. Journals provide a unique perspective on the thinking and struggles of individuals and on the *real* life in a particular era.

Although much anecdotal evidence exists about the beneficial effects of journaling, research on the use of journals is sparse. In nursing, research has related primarily to journaling as an educational tool (Fox & Fox, 1990; Gehrke, 1994). Research by J. W. Pennebaker, a psychologist, and his colleagues provides evidence of the positive effects of journaling (Booth, Petrie, & Pennebaker, 1997; Esterling, L'Abate, Murray, & Pennebaker, 1999; Pennebaker, 1997; Pennebaker & Seagal, 1999). Despite the lack of a large body of empirical data to support its use as a complementary therapy, the pervasive use of journaling across the centuries and anecdotal accounts point to its value in promoting positive health outcomes.

DEFINITION

The terms journal, diary, and writing are often used interchangeably. According to Baldwin (1977), a diary is a more formal pattern of entries in which observations and experiences are recorded. Diaries are more superficial than journals as the latter are a tool for recording the process of one's life (Baldwin, 1977). Events and experiences are noted in journals with emphasis placed on the person's reflections about these events and the personal meaning assigned to them. In journal writing, an interplay between the conscious and unconscious often occurs. Writing, another term, has been used when the focus has been on a theme or topic (Esterling et al., 1999). For example, people may be asked to record their thoughts and feelings about stressful events in their lives. Forms of expressive writing, such as poetry, are another form of writing. The term journaling will be used in this chapter and will encompass these three forms of written expression.

SCIENTIFIC BASIS

Journaling is a holistic therapy because it involves all aspects of a person: physical (muscular movements), mental (thought processes), emotional, and spiritual. Through journal recordings, people are able to connect with the continuity of their lives and thus enhance wholeness. Awareness of this is furthered as they reflect on specific events, thoughts, or feelings as they record them, link them with past feelings and meanings, and consider present and future implications.

Progoff (1975), a Jungian psychologist who developed a systematized method for journaling called the intensive journal, noted that this transpsychological approach provided "active techniques that enable the individual to draw upon his inherent resources for becoming a whole person" (p. 9). Through journaling, Progoff maintained, people become more self-reliant as they develop their inner strengths and can use these when faced with problems and challenges such as illness.

Journaling provides an opportunity for catharsis about highly emotional events (Pennebaker, 1997). Unlike merely venting feelings, journaling furnishes the avenue for a person to explore the causes and solutions and to gain insights. A participant in a study by Pennebaker noted,

> Although I have not talked with anyone about what I wrote, I was finally able to deal with it, work through the pain instead of trying to block it out. Now it doesn't hurt to think about it. (p. 38)

Inhibiting feelings about an event results in increased autonomic activity that often has long-lasting harmful effects on the body such as hypertension. Therapies that will assist the person in venting feelings may help to improve a person's health. In a study by Pennebaker and Beall (1986), students who wrote about their deepest feelings and emotions surrounding a traumatic event had fewer visits to the health center following the writing sessions than did those in the control group. The journaling resulted in better moods, a more optimistic outlook on life, and improved physical health. Further support for the efficacy of writing about traumatic events was documented in a second study in which students who journaled about a traumatic event had heightened immune function compared to the control group who wrote about superficial topics (Pennebaker, Kiecolt-Glaser, & Glaser, 1988). Spera, Buhrfeind, and Pennebaker (1994) found that 52% of persons in their study who had lost their jobs and engaged in journaling about the event had obtained employment after 8 months, compared to only 14% in the non-writing group and 24% in the group who wrote about superficial events.

Esterling and colleagues (1999) proposed three hypotheses for why journaling may be helpful in bringing about positive physical and emotional outcomes when someone writes about traumatic events:

1. Journaling allows the person to access multiple aspects of the event including its significance and meaning.

2. Journaling makes the event more readily accessible. People can recall more dimensions of the event and as they deal with it over time, the event becomes more automatic and thus less effort is needed to process events about the trauma.

3. Journaling transfers feelings into language. Applying a label to an emotion may help to reduce its intensity.

INTERVENTION

Many techniques for journaling exist: free flowing writing; intensive journaling (Progoff, 1975); and topical or focused journaling in which the writing relates to a specific topic such as an illness, transition, or traumatic event. The period of time for which journaling is carried out (weeks, months, or years) will depend on the purpose of the journaling. Sometimes people initially write during a specific time in their lives but become "hooked" and continue writing after the precipitating event or purpose has ended.

Some general guidelines or rules apply to all techniques. Journals are private; people may volunteer to share entries they have made, but this should never be an expectation when instructing a person about journaling. If a person has to share the entry, an internal monitor is put in place that often restricts what a person will write. Entries are made in a special notebook; this may be a fancy journal book or an inexpensive spiral notebook. Since pencil recordings fade over time, a pen should be used as it may be helpful to re-read past entries. Some may prefer to use word processing for journaling. If this type of recording is done, strategies are needed for keeping the contents secure and private. Establishing a specific time of day to make entries is helpful. Cameron (1992) suggested making entries in the early morning as it is easier to access the unconscious upon awakening. Many recommend making entries on a daily basis. However, Simons (1978) noted that journal writing needs to be the servant and not the master.

TECHNIQUES

Free Flow Journaling

This is the most common type of journaling. Cameron (1992) describes it as "the act of moving the hand across the page and writing down whatever comes to mind. Nothing is too petty, too silly, too stupid, or too weird to be included" (p. 10). No attention is given to grammar, punctuation, or spelling. The main goal is to put one's thoughts on paper, and Cameron suggests writing three pages a day. Persons using free flow journaling often do this every day for many years.

Topical Journaling

This type of journaling can take a number of forms. The focus can be the person's illness or that of a family member. The person writes about his or her feelings, how the illness will affect or has affected their lives, fears they have about the treatment or outcome. Pennebaker has focused his research on using journaling to assist persons dealing with trauma in their lives. They are instructed to consider multiple aspects of the event: who was involved, reasons they attribute for why the event occurred, how the event affected their lives, and the associated feelings. They just *write* with no attention to the structure of what is written. No constraints are imposed.

Intensive Journaling

Progoff (1975) developed the intensive journal method, a systematic way of making entries and dialoguing with and between topics. In addition to the book he authored, workshops on the intensive journaling method are held across the country. The structured process enables people to reflect upon their lives and to grow. Guidelines assist them in exploring specific areas of their lives. An entry relating to one area often evokes thoughts in another area; thus, they move between and among various areas.

Table 13.1 presents the 19 topics or sections contained in the intensive journal. These topics fit into three dimensions: life/time, dialogue, and depth.

TABLE 13.1 The "Intensive Journal" Method (Progoff, 1975)

Life/Time Dimension
  Life history log
  Stepping-stones
  Intersections
  Roads taken and not taken
  Now: The open moment

Dialogue Dimension
  Dialogue with persons
  Dialogue with work
  Dialogue with society
  Dialogue with events
  Dialogue with the body

Depth Dimension
  Dream log
  Dream enlargements
  Twilight imagery log
  Imagery extensions
  Inner wisdom dialogue

Period Log

Daily Log

Each has a specific role in helping people to explore their lives to become more self-reliant. In addition, a period log and a daily log are used.

The daily log section provides opportunities to record events and their reactions to these events as they happen, much as in free flowing journaling. Progoff (1975) noted that the focus should be on the essence of the experience and accompanying mental images and emotions. Writing thoughts and feelings may be therapeutic in and of itself.

Although Progoff saw the intensive journal method as a complete process, sections can be used separately. For example, the "Dialogue With Body" can be used by those diagnosed with a chronic illness or a serious health condition. Journaling may help them become more accepting of the illness and moving forward. "Roads taken and not taken" can be used when they are faced with decisions about their future, reviewing past choices and exploring what might have occurred if a different choice had actually been made. These reflections may provide insights about the current decision needed to be made.

MEASUREMENT OF OUTCOMES

Many of the outcomes of journal writing may not be immediately discernable. Some of the possible areas to measure are improvement in self-esteem, reduction in anxiety, and acceptance of a chronic condition. Because journaling is very personal, it may be difficult for the nurse to evaluate specific outcomes, but patients doing journaling can report changes that have occurred.

PRECAUTIONS

Fear that others will find and read journal entries is a common concern. This fear may prevent some persons from being completely open in expressing themselves. The heightened anxiety that the journal might be found may prevent unconscious thoughts from entering consciousness and thus decrease the efficacy of the intervention. Caution is needed in using journaling with those who are extremely introspective. However, Simons (1978) noted that journal writing may be useful in helping heal memories and become less introspective.

USES

Journaling has been used to achieve a variety of outcomes. Table 13.2 shows some of those uses.

One is with persons who are newly diagnosed with a chronic condition. Recording their perspectives may help them to uncover fears, which could then be discussed with a health professional. Some fears may be unfounded. Journaling also provides an avenue for persons to increase knowledge about themselves and to uncover hidden resources or strengths they possess that can be used in living with the chronic illness. Cameron (1992) urged people to provide positive affirmations to themselves. Writing positive statements and then reading these may help them gain confidence in their abilities. Johnson and Kelly (1990) had patients with breast cancer use journaling to help them gain insights about their lives.

Research and anecdotal evidence supports the use of journaling to improve well-being. Runions (1984) instructed the mother of a seriously ill adolescent to keep a journal. She found that journaling helped her in coping with the stressful situation. Hall (1990) found that journaling by high school students helped them to identify their potential and develop techniques for managing conflict.

TABLE 13.2 Uses of Journaling

Assisting with transitions (Spera, Buhrfeind, & Pennebaker, 1994)
Decreased anxiety (L'Abate & Baggett, 1997)
Decreased depression (L'Abate, Boyce, Fraizer, & Russ, 1992)
Increased creativity (Cameron, 1992)
Improved critical thinking (Hahnemann, 1986)
Improved well-being (Booth et al., 1997)
Personal growth (Johnson & Kelly, 1990; Patton, Woods, Agarenzo, Brubaker, Metcalf, & Sherrer, 1997)

FUTURE RESEARCH

Research on the efficacy of journaling is only beginning to be conducted and few findings exist to guide clinicians in its use with patients. There are some areas in which research is needed:

1. Studies to identify persons who will most benefit from journaling. McKinney (1982) reported that 43% of the students in his study were enthusiastic about keeping a journal. Although journaling may appear to have a more feminine appeal, history abounds with examples of males who have kept journals. However, little is known about the overall appeal of journaling or the specific technique that might be helpful.

2. Initial studies have been conducted on the impact that journaling has on the psychoneuroimmunological system (Booth et al., 1997; Pennebaker et al., 1988). Additional studies with various populations are needed to validate and extend these findings.

3. Studies using qualitative methodologies will help to identify the processes people use in journaling. This information can then be used by health professionals to assist patients to use journaling.

REFERENCES

Baldwin, C. (1977). *One to one.* New York: M. Evans.
Cameron, J. (1992). *The artist's way.* New York: G. P. Putnam's Sons.
Booth, R. J., Petrie, K. J., & Pennebaker, J. W. (1997). Changes in circulating lymphocyte numbers following emotional disclosure: Evidence of buffering? *Stress Medicine, 13,* 23–29.

Esterling, B. A., L'Abate, L., Murray, E. J., & Pennebaker, J. W. (1999). Empirical foundations for writing in prevention and psychotherapy: Mental and physical health outcomes. *Clinical Psychology Review, 19,* 79–96.

Fox, E., & Fox, D. L. (1990). Journal writing in health education: An introduction to purposes and methods. *Health Education, 21*(3), 53–54.

Gehrke, P. (1994). Finding voices through writing. *Nurse Educator, 19*(2), 28–30.

Hahnemann, B. K. (1986). Journal writing: A key to promoting critical thinking in nursing students. *Journal of Nursing Education, 25*(5), 213–215.

Hall, E. G. (1990). Strategies for using journal writing in counseling gifted students. *The Gifted Child Today, 13*(4), 2–6.

Johnson, J. B., & Kelly, A. W. (1990). A multifaceted rehabilitation program for women with cancer. *Oncology Nursing Forum, 17,* 691–695.

L'Abate, L., & Baggett, M. S. (1997). *Manual: Distance writing and computer assisted training mental health.* Atlanta, GA: Institute for Life and Empowerment.

L'Abate, L., Boyce, J., Frazier, R., & Russ, D. (1992). Programmed writing: Research in progress. *Comprehensive Mental Health Care, 2,* 45–62.

McKinney, F. (1982). Free writing as therapy. In E. Nickerson & K. O'Laughlin (Eds.), *Helping through action: Action-oriented therapies* (pp. 60–65). Amherst, MA: Human Resources Development Press.

Patton, J. G., Woods, S. J., Agarenzo, T., Brubaker, C. M., Metcalf, T., & Sherrer, L. (1997). Enhancing the clinical practicum through journal writing. *Journal of Nursing Education, 36,* 238–240.

Pennebaker, J. W. (1997). *Opening up: The healing power of expressing emotions.* New York: Guilford Press.

Pennebaker, J. W., & Beal, S. K. (1986). Confronting a traumatic event: Toward an understanding of inhibition and disease. *Journal of Abnormal Psychology, 95,* 274–281.

Pennebaker, J. W., Kiecolt-Glaser, J. K., & Glaser, R. (1988). Disclosure of traumas and immune function. *Journal of Consulting Clinical Psychology, 56,* 239–245.

Pennebaker, J. W., & Seagal, J. D. (1999). Forming a story: The health benefits of a narrative. *Journal of Clinical Psychology, 55,* 1243–1254.

Progoff, I. (1975). *At a journal workshop.* New York: Dialogue House Library.

Runions, J. (1984). The diary: A self-directed approach to coping with stress. *Canadian Nurse, 80*(5), 24–28.

Simons, G. (1978). *Keeping your personal journal.* New York: Paulist Press.

Spera, S. P., Buhrfeind, E. D., & Pennebaker, J. W. (1994). Expressive writing and coping with job loss. *Academy of Management Journal, 37,* 722–733.

14

Reminiscence

Mariah Snyder

A reflective process characterizes several therapies: reminiscence, life review, story telling, and journal writing. The techniques used in these therapies help people to connect with their mind, body, and spirit. Thus, reminiscence is a mind-body therapy. Although reminiscence has been primarily used with older adults, the universality of reminiscing makes it an appropriate planned therapy for all age groups across health care settings (Comana, Brown, & Thomas, 1998; Jones, 1995; Nugent, 1995; Sellers & Stork, 1997).

DEFINITION

Reminiscence and life review have many commonalities and numerous authors fail to distinguish between the these two therapies. This has contributed to difficulties in interpreting and comparing results of research on reminiscence. Reflection on one's past life through memory and recall is common in the two interventions. However, differences do exist.

Life review, according to Haight and Burnside (1993), is a critical analysis of one's past life. The goal of life review is to facilitate the achievement of integrity. Life review follows a very specific format, with a person reflecting on the various stages of life. In contrast, reminiscence focuses more on an event or topic and not the entire life sequence.

Reminiscence has been defined in numerous ways. King (1982) says it is "memory that has been filtered through time and altered by the person's other life experiences" (p. 22). In this definition, memories do not necessarily have to match life facts. According to Kovach (1991) reminiscence is "a cognitive process of recalling events from the past that are personally significant and perceived as reality based" (p. 14). Although persons reminisce sponta-neously, the discussion in this chapter will focus on the use of reminiscence as a planned strategy in which persons are assisted to recall past events, inter-actions, experiences, and feelings.

Several types of reminiscence have been identified. Kovach (1991) iden-tified two types of reminiscence: validating and lamenting. In validating reminiscence, the memories confirm or validate that the person's life has been fruitful and enriching. Lamenting reminiscences, in contrast, focus on negative life events or experiences and difficulties that a person has encoun-tered. Merriman (1989) classifies reminiscence as either recreational or ther-apeutic. Recreational reminiscence is a spontaneous recall of the past that occurs when people sit around and talk about "the good old days." Therapeutic reminiscence is used by health professionals to help people achieve a spe-cific outcome; these explorations may focus on pleasant or negative feelings or experiences.

SCIENTIFIC BASIS

Erikson's developmental stages (1950) have been proposed as a possible basis for using reminiscence. It has been hypothesized that reminiscence assists older adults in achieving ego integrity rather than despairing. Reminiscence allows them to let go, realizing that the past is past and that what happened during that part of life was alright. According to Kovach (1993), data have not supported the hypothesis that reminiscence promotes ego-integrity; however, findings from a study by Newbern (1992) document that reminiscence pro-vided people with an opportunity to improve their self-esteem.

Parker (1995) proposed the continuity theory as a theoretical perspective that accounts for the therapeutic effects of reminiscence. Reminiscence provides a sustaining sense of self and a mechanism for connecting across the many developmental stages through which they have progressed. Recalling the past helps one adapt to life's changes and thus provide a sense of continuity. Parker contends that individuals reminisce more dur-ing times of personal transitions than during more stable periods. Within the continuity perspective, reminiscence would be an appropriate inter-vention to use with persons of any age group who are experiencing a tran-sition in their lives. While the continuity theory appears to provide a logi-cal basis for the efficacy of reminiscence, research is needed to validate this relationship.

INTERVENTION

TECHNIQUE

Many different techniques have been used to assist people in reminiscing. In many instances it is done in groups, but can be done on an individual basis (Burnside & Haight, 1994). The degree to which sessions are structured has differed greatly in the articles describing the use of reminiscence. An important component of the use of reminiscence is for the nurse to assess the health status and needs of each patient and determine which format would have the potential of bringing about the best outcomes. Two techniques that are described in the literature will be presented.

Individual Unstructured Sessions

After discussing the intervention with the patient and gaining the patient's consent, the nurse ensures that the patient is comfortable. In unstructured reminiscing, the patient is invited to talk about past experiences or feelings; no specific topic for reflection is proposed by the nurse. Good listening skills on the part of the nurse are essential. The nurse assists the patient by providing comments that are supportive of the ideas or feelings being expressed. When a patient repeats an idea or returns to one that has been previously expressed, the nurse may suggest that this topic seems to be important to the person and encourages the expression of associated memories or feelings. Both positive and negative feelings are acknowledged. If a nurse does not feel competent in dealing with strong negative feelings, a referral to a psychiatric clinical nurse specialist can be offered to the patient. The patient may wish to audiotape the memories recalled and share these with his or her family, to whom these memories can serve as a legacy.

The number of reminiscence sessions with each patient will vary and many times this number cannot be predicted when initiating the intervention. Sessions may be held several times a week or on a weekly basis. The specific length of sessions has not been established; the frailty of the patient and the nature of the reminiscing are factors to consider in determining the length of sessions. Whenever a patient appears to be tiring, the nurse should offer to terminate the session and return at a later time.

Individual reminiscence sessions have a number of advantages. One-to-one sessions facilitate establishing a good relationship between the patient and the nurse. Unstructured individual sessions require less planning and coordination than do group sessions. One-on-one sessions tend to be best for persons who have moderate to severe cognitive deficits or who are shy. However, individual reminiscence sessions are time consuming and may not be feasible in busy nursing homes or acute care settings.

Group Structured Sessions

Because of time constraints, group structured sessions are used more frequently than individual sessions. Guidelines for group size have varied in the studies; hence, no set size for groups appears to be the ideal. If older adults who are confused or cognitively impaired will be included, the size of the group should be smaller. Whether the group will be open (anyone can join at any session) or closed (only those present at the first session can attend subsequent sessions) needs to be discussed and a group consensus reached. A deciding factor may be whether subsequent sessions will build on the content presented at previous sessions or whether each session will be free-standing.

Conducting a reminiscence group requires that the nurse be skillful in group techniques. It is important that everyone in the group has an opportunity to share their reminiscences if they so desire. However, no one should feel pressured to share memories. Some group participants may need encouragement to share their reminiscences. Several meetings of the group may be needed before all of the members feel comfortable in sharing their memories. The leader needs to be aware that despite the seeming pleasantness of the suggested topic, such as a holiday, some participants may have sad or negative memories associated with it. Attentiveness to non-verbal behaviors is needed. When sadness or withdrawal is noted, the leader should seek out the person at the end of the session and ask if they would like to talk about their feelings apart from the group.

For a structured reminiscence group, a special topic or theme is chosen. Props are often used to provide an atmosphere that helps the group recall memories related to the theme. For example, if the theme is holidays, decorations and foods for a particular holiday will help members get in the mood. Flags, patriotic music, and watermelon could be used if the Fourth of July is the theme. Table 14.1 provides guidelines for structured reminiscence with a group.

MEASUREMENT OF OUTCOME

The outcome measures chosen will be determined by the purpose for which reminiscence is being used. The most commonly measured outcome has been mood state; depression and overall well-being were explored in a number of studies (Ha, 1993; Stevens-Ratchford, 1993), and self-esteem has also been studied (Stevens-Ratchford). A qualitative approach to examining patients' perspectives about reminiscence was used in some studies (Kovach, 1993; Sellers & Stork, 1997). Because reminiscence may stimulate the patient to continue to think about the past, family members can be encouraged to report positive or negative reactions. Also, nurses may want to record their perspectives about a session and patients' reactions.

TABLE 14.1   Technique for Group Structured Reminiscence

1. Contact potential participants; decide on size of group; determine length of session (45–60 minutes), date, and time; establish whether it will be an open or closed group; select number of weekly sessions to hold.

2. Select meeting place; arrange the room: comfortable chairs, quiet space, pleasant environment.

3. Remind participants about session and arrange for participants to attend.

4. At first session, introduce your self and have participants introduce themselves; take time for persons to get to know one another. Describe the purpose of reminiscence and format of sessions. Have group establish ground rules regarding sharing reminiscences.

5. Introduce the theme for the session, such as grade school. (This would be an appropriate topic if the group is beginning in September. Show pictures of old-fashioned schools and school buses or children walking to school. Ask participants to share memories of their first day of school or early school days.) Allow sufficient time for participants to reflect and respond. Let them ask questions about experiences related by other members. If group members are hesitant to initiate sharing of memories, the leader can share his or her memories or ask probing questions to elicit memories.

6. When 10 minutes remain, provide an opportunity for those who have not spoken to share their memories if they wish to do so.

7. Summarize the general memories that have been shared; thank the members for their contributions and inform them about the next meeting time and the topic.

PRECAUTIONS

Assessment of individuals prior to initiating reminiscence will help to avoid its use with individuals for whom it may produce negative effects. Awareness that outcomes of reminiscence may not always be pleasant and positive should alert nurses to be attentive to possible negative outcomes. Reminiscing may result in the recall of painful memories. Lashley (1993) noted that nurses need to be attentive to possible signs of grief or guilt, such as problems with sleeping, eating, or concentrating, that may occur during the days following reminiscence session. Thus, follow-up evaluation is an important component of the intervention. Also, some persons may use reminiscence as an escape from the present situation and not problem-solve about current issues.

USES

As noted earlier, reminiscence has traditionally been thought of as a therapy for older adults. However, more reports support its use with many populations. Table 14.2 identifies conditions or purposes for which reminiscence has been used.

OLDER ADULTS

Reminiscence has been used extensively with this population. The majority of the outcomes that were explored relate to improved mood state. Some of the specific outcomes tested include improvement of self-esteem (Nugent, 1995), lessening of depression (Ha, 1993); improving life satisfaction (Ha, 1993; Sherman, 1987); and decreasing stress/anxiety (Rybarczyk & Auerbach, 1990). Because of the multiplicity of techniques used, including life review, it is difficult to determine which technique or techniques would be the most beneficial. Overall, evidence has documented that reminiscence does produce beneficial effects in older adults.

FAMILIES/STAFF

A growing body of literature documents the use of reminiscence with families (Comana et al., 1998) and nursing staff (Hammer et al., 1992; Puentes, 1999). Comana and colleagues used reminiscence with patients who had chronic renal failure and their family members. This therapy assisted families in increasing their coping skills. Remembrance groups, similar to reminiscence, were used by Hammer and colleagues to help staff resolve their grief associated with the death of patients. Puentes found that a continuing education offering using reminiscence improved nurses' attitudes about aging elders.

THE ACUTELY ILL

Because of the short stays of most patients in acute care settings, reminiscence may not appear a realistic therapy. However, studies have reported its use in critical care settings. Jones (1995) used reminiscence in a critical care unit to encourage communication between the nurse and the patient, to provide a relief from stressful situations, and to promote interaction between the family and the patient. Nugent (1995) provided case studies to illustrate the use of reminiscence with patients who had cancer. According to Beadleston-Baird and Lara (1988), reminiscing by acutely ill older patients resulted in

TABLE 14.2   Uses of Reminiscence

Older Adults
  Acutely ill (Beadleson-Baird & Lara, 1988)
  Depressed (Ha, 1993)
  Improved life satisfaction and well-being (Cook, 1998)
  Coping with medical procedures (Rybarczyk & Auerbach, 1990)

Nurses
  Increase knowledge about older adults (Puentes, 1999)
  Reduce grief (Sellers & Stork, 1997)

Families
  Assist with grieving (Hammer, Nichols, & Armstrong, 1992)
  Improve coping (Comana et al., 1998)

Intensive Care
  Critically ill patients (Jones, 1995)

the patients' being less anxious, frightened, and depressed. They noted that older adults who are faced with life-threatening conditions indicated a strong desire to reminisce.

FUTURE RESEARCH

A number of authors (Kovach, 1990; Merriman, 1989) have done critical reviews of the research on reminiscence. The Cochrane Database of Systematic Reviews includes a review on the use of reminiscence for persons with dementia. A major problem in the research is the lack of specificity in describing the technique used and the mixing of components of reminiscence and life review. Merriman noted that the lack of consistency in findings may be the result of the various techniques that have been used. The following are areas in which further research is needed:

1. Numerous techniques have been used in reminiscence research. Testing one technique with multiple samples would provide guidance about the efficacy of specific techniques. Furthermore, careful descriptions of the techniques used would allow readers to know specifically what was done.
2. Studies on the use of reminiscence with persons of various age groups will add to the scientific knowledge base. The small sample sizes and its limited reported use with younger populations provides little guidance for the use of reminiscence in practice settings with younger persons.

3. More explorations on the use of reminiscence for the resolution of guilt and negative feelings are needed. Qualitative studies may help in identifying how reminiscence is used in these situations.

REFERENCES

Beadleson-Baird, M., & Lara, L. L. (1988). Reminiscing: Nursing actions for acutely ill geriatric patients. *Issues in Mental Health Nursing, 9,* 83–94.

Burnside, I., & Haight, B. (1994). Reminiscence and life review: Therapeutic interventions for older people. *Nurse Practitioner, 19,* 55–61.

Comana, M. T., Brown, V. M., & Thomas, J. D. (1998). The effect of reminiscence on family coping. *Journal of Family Nursing, 4,* 182–197.

Cook, E. A. (1998). Effects of reminiscence on life satisfaction of elderly female nursing home residents. *Health Care of Women International, 19,* 109–118.

Erikson, E. (1950). *Childhood and society.* New York: Norton.

Ha, Y. S. (1993). The effect of group reminiscence on the psychological well-being of the elderly. *The Seoul Journal of Nursing, 7*(1), 35–60.

Haight, B., & Burnside, I. (1993). Reminiscence and life review: Explaining the differences. *Archives of Psychiatric Nursing, 7*(2), 91–98.

Hammer, M., Nichols, D. J., & Armstrong, L. (1992). A ritual of remembrance. *Maternal Child Nursing, 17,* 310–313.

Jones, C. (1995). "Take me away from all of this" . . . Can reminiscence be therapeutic in an intensive care unit? *Intensive and Critical Care Nursing, 1,* 341–343.

King, K. (1982). Reminiscing psychotherapy with aging people. *Journal Psychiatric Nursing and Mental Health Services, 20*(2), 20–25.

Kovach, C. R. (1990). Promise and problems in reminiscence research. *Journal of Gerontological Nursing, 16*(4), 10–14.

Kovach, C. (1991). Reminiscence: Exploring the origins, processes, and consequences. *Nursing Forum, 26*(3), 14–20.

Kovach, C. (1993). Understanding autobiographical memories. *Journal of Holistic Nursing, 11,* 149–163.

Lashley, M. E. (1993). The painful side of reminiscence. *Geriatric Nursing, 14,* 138–141.

Merriman, S. B. (1989). The structure of simple reminiscence. *The Gerontologist, 29,* 761–767.

Newbern, V. B. (1992). Sharing the memories: The value of reminiscence as a research tool. *Journal of Gerontological Nursing, 18*(5), 13–18.

Nugent, E. (1995). Try to remember . . . reminiscence as a nursing intervention. *Journal of Psychosocial Nursing, 33*(11), 7–11.

Parker, R. G. (1995). Reminiscence: A continuity theory framework. *The Gerontologist, 35,* 515–525.

Puentes, W. J. (1999). Effect of reminiscence on nurses' attitudes and empathy with older adults. *Image: The Journal of Nursing Scholarship, 31,* 94–96.

Rybarczyk, B. D., & Auerbach, S. M. (1990). Reminiscence interviews as stress management interventions for older patients undergoing surgery. *The Gerontologist, 30,* 522–528.

Sellers, S. C., & Stork, P. B. (1997). Reminiscence as an intervention: Rediscovering the essence of nursing. *Nursing Forum, 32,* 17–23.

Sherman, E. (1987). Reminiscence groups for community elderly. *The Gerontologist, 27,* 569–572.

Spector, A., Orrell, M., Davies, S., & Woods, R. T. (2001). Reminiscence therapy for dementia. *Cochrane Database of Systematic Reviews, 1.* On-line.

Stevens-Ratchford, R. G. (1993). The effect of life review reminiscence activities on depression and self-esteem in older adults. *American Journal of Occupational Therapy, 47,* 413–420.

15

Animal-Assisted Therapy

Jennifer Jorgenson

A nimal-assisted therapy (AAT) is grounded in research on the human-animal bond. Until recently this body of knowledge has been largely anecdotal, based on pet ownership and casual interactions between people and animals. Since the 1970s, research has begun to establish a link between animal companionship and improved health and well-being. The evolution of this research has promoted AAT as a therapeutic healing modality that can help promote physical, social, and psychological benefits. Today AAT has been implemented as an adjunctive therapy by nurses across the health care continuum in outpatient, acute care, and extended care facilities, as well as in all patient populations from pediatrics to geriatrics (Cole, 1999). It is important that nurses as advocates in the promotion of optimal holistic healthcare are aware of the role animals can play.

Throughout history animals have played a significant role in our customs, legends, and religions. Primitive people found that human-animal relationships were important to their very survival, and keeping pets was common in hunter-gatherer societies (National Institutes of Health [NIH], 1987). The process of domestication, which began more than 12,000 years ago, continues today as humans and domestic animals coexist, interact, and profoundly influence the shape of each other's social space (Young, 1985). The most recent data on pet ownership indicates that approximately 58.9% of all U.S. households contained a companion animal (American Veterinary Medical Association, 1997).

The first recorded setting in which animals were used therapeutically was the York Retreat in England (Netting, Wilson, & New, 1987). Founded in 1792, the retreat kept small animals such as rabbits and poultry, which were cared for by psychiatric patients. The nursing establishment recognized the benefits of AAT early on. In 1860, Florence Nightingale observed that "a small pet is often an excellent companion for the sick, for long chronic cases especially" (Nightingale, 1860/1969, p. 103). She suggested the use of a caged bird as the only pleasure an invalid confined for years to the same room might enjoy. The use of animals in a therapeutic setting began in the U.S. in 1944 at the Army Air Corps Convalescent Hospital at Pawling, New York. Patients recovering from war experiences were encouraged to work at the hospital's farm with hogs, cattle, horses, and poultry (NIH, 1987).

DEFINITION

AAT has had many names including pet-facilitated therapy, pet-assisted therapy, pet therapy, pet-oriented child psychotherapy, animal-facilitated therapy, animal-assisted activity, and animal visitation. These generic terms allude to programs that include visitation, attempts at milieu therapy, and animal-assisted psychotherapy (Berrisford, 1995). Today the terminology tends to differentiate between two distinct types of interventions, pet visitation and AAT.

The most simple use of animals in health care is pet visitation. This intervention is intended to foster rapport and initiate communication between therapists and patients. It is often effective in increasing patient responsiveness, giving patients a pleasurable experience, enhancing the treatment milieu, and helping to keep patients in touch with reality (Barba, 1995a). The animal initiates contact with patients, and the direction of the visit is determined by patients' needs at that particular time. Social interaction is often increased using the animal as a springboard for conversation. This therapeutic modality has demonstrated success in psychological counseling, as well as in long-term care facilities. Visitation may be provided by one or more animal and volunteer teams and may occur in individual or group settings. A variety of animals have been used favorably in this intervention including cats, rabbits, birds, and dogs.

By contrast, AAT is a goal-directed intervention in which an animal, usually a dog, that meets specific criteria is an integral part of the treatment process. This intervention, directed by a health or human-services provider, is designed to promote improvement in human physical, social, emotional, and cognitive functioning. AAT can be utilized in a variety of group or individual settings, often in acute care facilities, and is documented and evaluated (Delta Society, 1991). AAT exercises are purposeful, individually goal-oriented, and can provide multiple benefits that include but are not limited to improvement in fine and gross motor skills; verbal, tactile, and auditory stimulation; verbalization skills; ambulating and equilibrium; following instructions and decision-making; memory recall; and increased concentration and extended attention span. Often AAT interventions may occur during a visitation program and the two terms are frequently used interchangeably.

SCIENTIFIC BASIS

There are many theoretical frameworks to support the use of AAT in healthcare. The most commonly cited is the social support theory (Barba, 1995b). The social support theory recognizes that buffers against stress are developed in relationships in which people gain a sense of security and a feeling of being needed. Using this framework, studies conducted with companion animals have demonstrated that animals promote well-being, health, and longevity and provide a source of relief, love, and companionship (Carmack, 1998). Willis (1997) applied Roy's Adaptation model to the extent that animals in the environment are factors which can influence adaptation and interdependence as a response. Studies by Calvert (1988) and Friedmann, Katcher, Lynch, and Thomas (1980) have supported the hypothesis that interaction between people and companion animals has a positive influence on loneliness. As early as 1965, family systems therapist Murray Bowen recognized the influence of animals in the dynamic family. Cain (1991) validated the notion that companion animals are often given "people-status," that pets can provide the emotional devotion that persons may be seeking from others, and that many family members believe that their pets are "tuned in" to the members' feelings.

The idea that human interactions with companion animals can result in physiological and psychological benefits is gradually gaining acceptance. Many research studies have indicated that people's health and well-being benefit from AAT. Table 15.1 lists research studies that support these conclusions in a variety of populations in a range of settings with many different types of interventions.

One of the first nursing studies to associate health benefits from animal contact was performed by Baun, Bergstrom, Langston, and Thoma (1983). Their study revealed a decrease in subjects' heart rate, respiratory rate, and blood pressure while petting a companion animal with which they had a bond.

Research conducted by Siegel (1990) suggested that pet ownership could influence physician utilization in older adults. Ownership of pets appeared to help individuals in times of stress. The accumulation of stressful events was associated with increased physician contacts for respondents without pets; however, this association did not emerge for pet owners. Data revealed that owning a dog provided a stress buffer, whereas owning other types of pets

TABLE 15.1   Populations in Which Animals and Animal-Assisted Therapy Have Been Studied (Cole & Gawlinski, 1995)

Adolescents with special education needs (Cawley, Cawley, & Retter, 1994)

Adults in the community (Raina, 1999; Sebkova, 1977)

Adult pet owners (Anderson, Reid, & Jennings, 1992; Serpell, 1991)

College students (Wilson, 1991)

Older persons in elder residences (Mugford & M'Comsky, 1975);

Older adults apartment residents (Riddick, 1985)

Heart patients (Friedmann et al., 1980; Friedmann et al., 1983; Friedmann & Thomas, 1995)

Hospice patients (Chinner & Dalziel, 1991)

Hospitalized psychiatric patients (Barker & Dawson, 1998)

Persons with Alzheimer's disease (Batson, McCabe, Baun, & Wilson, 1995; Kongable, Stolley, & Buckwalter, 1990)

Persons requiring wheelchair use (Allen & Blaskovich, 1966)

Pet-owning children (Triebenbacher, 1998)

Physically challenged school-aged children (Madder, Hart, & Bergin, 1989)

Women in prison (Walsh, 1994)

Cole & Gawlinski, 1995

did not. The advantages associated with dog ownership included the companionship functions of talking and spending more time outdoors and an increased sense of security.

More recently Cole and Gawlinski (2000) explored the value of aquariums in promoting relaxation in patients awaiting heart transplants. Benefits included humanizing the hospital environment and patients reported a sense of control in choosing feeding schedules and in performing the feeding ritual. Many patients described the fish as soothing and comforting at night. The aquariums also provided cognitive stimulation and became a bridge for communication among patients.

INTERVENTION

One of the newer and more exciting ways AAT has been utilized is in critical care settings. Several successful programs have been documented in the literature. Connor and Miller (2000) have implemented an extensive program at Trinity Mother Frances Health System in Tyler, Texas, as well as

Giuliano, Bloniasz and Bell (1999) at Baystate Medical Center in Springfield, Massachusetts.

The author is involved in expanding an existing pet visitation program in pediatrics and rehabilitation at WakeMed Hospital to include the surgical intensive care unit (SICU). WakeMed is a 650-bed level-II trauma center with a nine-bed SICU located in Raleigh, North Carolina. The program was implemented in order to reduce patients' anxiety and stress, improve communication, aid in reality orientation, and to provide a more humanistic environment.

The preparation for obtaining approval was fairly rigorous and involved many disciplines. Physicians were surveyed about their support for the program, staff in the SICU was educated, and the volunteer department was involved to refine the existing policies and protocols. An extensive literature search was performed, highlighting other successful programs around the country, and a final proposal was prepared and presented to the hospital's infection control committee. Approval was obtained for a 6-month pilot program. Next the actual volunteers and dog teams were oriented to the unit to ensure that the dog and the volunteer would be comfortable in the ICU setting. Issues addressed were sights, smells, equipment, appearances of patients, and guidelines for prevention of disease transmission. The program was well received by patients and families as well as staff and physicians. During the first 6 months approximately 25 visits were provided, there were no untoward events, and the positive feedback was phenomenal.

GUIDELINES

Policies and procedures were developed for pet visitation in the SICU at WakeMed. Visits in the unit were conducted twice a week, and each visit lasted approximately 20 minutes. These policies are unique to the facility, but may be viewed as general guidelines (Table 15.2).

MEASUREMENT OF OUTCOMES

In the evaluation of AAT, there are frequent methodological limitations often caused by the complexity of the subject area. Small sample sizes, failure to randomize subjects, and poor design are cited most often as the shortcomings to fully appreciating the results of many AAT studies (Brodie & Biley, 1999). Failure to correct and design appropriate studies will only slow the acceptance of AAT as a legitimate, research-based intervention.

Outcome measurements are assessed relative to the various types of interventions and their intended effects. To date, published material on AAT suggests that the human-animal bond could have positive effects on human

TABLE 15.2   Guidelines for Pet Visitation

Inclusion criteria for potential patients to receive pet visitation:
- Length of stay > 72 hours
- Patient is awake and alert
- Patient is hemodynamically stable
- Patient meets the screening for exclusion criteria

Exclusion criteria: Any patients with the following diagnoses or conditions would be excluded from participating in a pet visitation:
- Fear of animals
- Any patient in the SICU with a documented allergy to dogs
- Pet visitation not supported by the attending physician
- Patient is diagnosed with any of the following:
  - Methicillin-resistant *staphylococcus*
  - Tuberculosis
  - Group A *streptococcus*
  - Hepatitis
  - *Salmonella*
  - *Staphylococcus aureus*
  - Ringworm
  - *Shigella*
  - Fever of unknown origin

- All patients in the SICU, who have been medically cleared and have guardian or patient permission, may participate in a pet visitation, unless otherwise ordered by the physician.
- Staff RNs in the SICU will be responsible to ask if patient/family members would like a pet visit. If they are agreeable, a note confirming verbal consent will be placed in the nursing notes.
- The charge RN will evaluate the unit acuity and level of activity to determine if a pet visitation is appropriate.
- Volunteer team will contact the charge RN for a list of appropriate patients prior to entering the unit.
- Prior to the visit, linen or bedding will be placed on the patient's bed as a barrier.
- Dog and volunteer team will go directly to the appropriate room; once inside, the door is closed with a sign posted outside to indicate pet visitation is in progress.

physical, social, and psychological health. Brodie and Biley (1999) performed a review of the literature on animal-induced health benefits and concluded that evidence exists to promote the use of AAT as a therapeutic intervention by nurses. Improvements in physical health including reduced risk of cardiac problems, lowered blood pressure, and increased overall health. When AAT is employed, increased social interaction, happiness, and harmony appear elevated in the general population and in specified groups such as children, older adults, and those with disabilities. Decreased loneliness, improved morale, and increased levels of relaxation appear to be some of the psychological benefits.

PRECAUTIONS

The strongest opposition to using AAT is found in acute care facilities. The major concern is the potential for transmitting disease. For this reason dogs are the most frequently used species since specific guidelines have been well established to ensure that the risk of disease transmission is minimized. The Delta Society (1991) and Therapet (Bernard, 1998) are two well-known programs that have developed standards for policy, protocol, and procedures that clearly outline the criteria for AAT visits. Protocols for the health and grooming of dogs are addressed, along with policies for patient selection and handler responsibilities. Dogs in the program are carefully screened by a veterinarian for any physical or behavioral problems. A primary concern is patient exposure to animal feces, saliva, blood, or parasites. Stool samples to screen for any enteric pathogens and parasites are taken from the dogs on entry to the program and on an ongoing basis thereafter. Patients and staff members must wash their hands after petting the dogs. In addition, the dogs never ride the elevators, thus avoiding encounters with people who may be allergic or phobic.

Dr. Sandra Wallace, an infectious-disease specialist and chairwoman of the infection control committee at Huntington Memorial Hospital, Pasadena, California, reports that thoroughly screened dogs in controlled programs can interact with hospital patients without transmitting zoonotic infections or serving as transient carriers of nosocomial pathogens. Huntington Memorial Hospital has been host to 3,281 dog visits to 1,690 patients over 5 years. In that time no zoonotic infections have been reported (Huntington Memorial Hospital, 1992).

Yamauchi and Olmsted (1996) have developed specific guidelines for AAT, which are presented in *APIC-Infection Control and Applied Epidemiology.* This comprehensive overview is an invaluable tool for creating policies for new or existing programs. It is noted that while the transmission of nosocomial infection associated with AAT programs is theoretically possible, there are no documented cases.

USES

In addition to the types of interventions already mentioned, the variety of ways and settings in which AAT can be used is almost limitless. One only has to be creative when designing this intervention. The following is a partial list of additional ways AAT can be utilized.

- "Hippotherapy," or horseback riding is used in a variety of ways to influence the physical and psychological well-being of a person with movement disorders. Specially trained physical and occupational therapists prescribe therapeutic riding to improve a patient's posture, balance, mobility, and function (NIH, 1987).
- Porpoises and dolphins have helped autistic children become more responsive. A 1989 study demonstrated that dolphins, used as both stimulus and reinforcement, were 2 to 10 times more effective at increasing attention and language skills among children with mental disabilities than were other stimuli and reinforcements used in land-based classrooms (Nathanson & de Faria, 1993).
- Psychotherapy has utilized animals in an effort to decrease anxiety and open up the lines of communication. Often patients will more readily talk about painful experiences in their lives when they are petting a dog (Connor & Miller, 2000).
- Companion dogs have been used with great success for people who are blind and in recent years by those or are hearing impaired or using a wheelchair. Not only do service dogs provide for more independence and greater mobility, but the presence of a companion dog also creates a "magnet" effect that serves to increase the quantity and quality of attention directed toward those who are handicapped (Edney, 1992).
- Rehabilitation units in acute care facilities have begun to utilize AAT to increase motor skills through activities that challenge balance, fine and gross motor skills, and endurance; improve stress management and coping skills; improve cognitive function; and assist with adjusting to life changes (Jorgenson, 1997).
- Several prisons have recently begun limited trials in which inmates are given animals to raise for service programs or local shelters. These programs are carefully supervised. Pet visitation to inmates is also being used as a form of behavior modification (Connor & Miller, 2000).

FUTURE RESEARCH

Because the interventions available to AAT are virtually limitless, so too are the areas for further research. In critical care the effect of therapy dogs on ventilatory weaning, pain medication requirements, length of stay, and body image are interesting areas for further research. Determining the most effective delivery aspects of AAT (i.e., timing and frequency of visits) and comparing AAT outcomes to other types of therapy should also be investigated. Finally, studies to determine the cost effectiveness of AAT in improving recovery rates and long-term health benefits would substantially increase the acceptance of AAT.

ACKNOWLEDGMENT

The author is grateful to Angie Bullock, RN, MSN, Nurse Manager, SICU, WakeMed for her support in initiating the AAT program in the SICU. I am also grateful to Elizabeth VanHorn, RN, MSN, for her editorial help and encouragement throughout the project.

REFERENCES

Allen, K. M., & Blaskovich, J. (1996). The value of service dogs for people with severe ambulatory disabilities. *Journal of the American Medical Association, 275,* 1001–1006.

American Veterinary Medical Association. (1997). *U.S. pet ownership & demographics sourcebook, 1997.* Schaumburg, IL: Center for Information Management.

Anderson, W. P., Reid, C. M., & Jennings, G. L. (1992). Pet ownership and risk factors for cardiovascular disease. *Medical Journal of Australia, 157,* 298–301.

Barba, B. (1995b). A critical review of research on the human-companion animal relationship 1988–1993. *Antrozoos, 8*(1), 9–15.

Barba, B. (1995a). The positive influence of animals: Animal-assisted therapy in acute care. *Clinical Nurse Specialist, 9*(4), 199–202.

Barker, S. B., & Dawson, K. S. (1998). The effects of animal-assisted therapy on anxiety ratings of hospitalized psychiatric patients. *Psychiatric Service, 49,* 797–801.

Batson, K., McCabe, W., Baun, M. M., & Wilson, C. (1995). The effect of a therapy dog on socialization and physiologic indicators of stress in persons diagnosed with Alzheimer's disease. In C. C. Wilson & C. C. Turner (Eds.), *Companion animals in human health* (pp. 203–215). Thousand Oaks, CA: Sage.

Baun, M. M., Bergstrom, N., Langston, N. F., & Thoma, L. (1983). Physiological effects of human/companion animal bonding. *Nursing Research, 33*(3), 126–130.

Bernard, S. (1998). *Animal assisted therapy: A guide for health care professionals and volunteers.* Whitehouse, TX: Therapet. [on-line]. Available: www.therapet.com

Berrisford, J. A. (1995). Implications of pet-facilitated therapy in palliative nursing. *International Journal of Palliative Nursing, 1,* 86–89.

Brodie, S. J., & Biley, F. C. (1999). An exploration of the potential benefits of pet-facilitated therapy. *Journal of Clinical Nursing, 8,* 329–337.

Cain, A .D. (1991). Pets and the family. *Holistic Nurse Practice, 5*(2), 58–63.

Calvert, M. (1988). Human-pet interaction and loneliness: A test of concepts from Roy's adaptation model. *Nursing Science Quarterly, 2*(4), 194–202.

Carmack, B. J. (1998). Companion animals: Social support for orthopedic clients. *Orthopedic Nursing, 33*(4), 701–711.

Cawley, R., Cawley, M. S., & Retter, M. (1994). Therapeutic horseback riding and self-concept in adolescents with special educational needs. *Anthrozoos, 7,* 129–134.

Chinner, T. L., & Dalziel, F. R. (1991). An exploratory study on the viability and efficacy on a pet-facilitated therapy project with a hospice. *Journal of Palliative Care, 7,* 13–20.

Cole, K. (1999). Animal-assisted therapy. In G. M. Bulechek & J. C. McCloskey (Eds.), *Nursing interventions: Effective nursing treatments* (3rd ed., pp. 508–519). Philadelphia: WB Saunders.

Cole, K. M., & Gawlinski, A. (1995). Animal-assisted therapy in the intensive care unit. *Nursing Clinics of North America, 30*(3), 529–537.

Cole, K. M. & Gawlinski A. (2000). Animal-assisted therapy: The human-animal bond. *AACN Clinical Issues, 11*(1), 139–149.

Conner, K., & Miller, J. (2000). Animal-assisted therapy: An in-depth look. *Dimensions of Critical Care Nursing, 19*(3), 20–26.

Delta Society. (1991, February) *Task force meeting of the standards committee.* Rowley Educational Consulting: Author.

Edney, A. T. B. (1992). Companion animals and human health. *Veterinary Record, 130*(4), 285–287.

Friedmann, E., Katcher, A. H., Lynch, J. J., & Thomas, S. A. (1980). Animal companions and one-year survival of patients after discharge from a coronary care unit. *Public Health Reports, 95*(4), 307–312.

Friedmann, E., Katcher, A. H., Lynch, J. J., Thomas, S. A., & Messent, P. (1983). Social interaction and blood pressure: Influence of animal companions. *Journal of Mental Disorders, 171,* 461–465.

Friedmann, E., & Thomas, S. A. (1995). Pet ownership, social support, and one-year survival after acute myocardial infarction in the cardiac arrhythmia suppression trial (CAST). *American Journal of Cardiology, 76,* 1213–1217.

Giuliano, K. K., Bloniasz, E., & Bell, J. (1999). Implementation of a pet visitation program in critical care. *Critical Care Nurse, 19*(3), 43–50.

Huntington Memorial Hospital. (1992, December). Patients best friend? Hospital dogs raise spirits, not infection rates. *Hospital Infection Control.* Interagency Communication: author.

Jorgenson, J. (1997). Therapeutic use of companion animals in health care. *Image: Journal of Nursing Scholarship, 29*(3), 249–254.

Kongable, L. G., Stolley, J. M., & Buckwalter, K. C. (1990). Pet therapy for Alzheimer's patient: A survey. *Journal of Long-term Care Administration, 18*(3), 17–21.

Madder, B., Hart, L. A., & Bergin, B. (1989). Social acknowledgements for children with disabilities: Effects of service dogs. *Child Development, 60*(6), 1529–1534.

Mugford, R., & M'Comsky, J. (1975). Some recent work on the psychotherapeutic value of caged birds with old people. In R. Anderson (Ed.), *Pet animals and society* (pp. 54–65). London: Balliere Tindall.

Nathanson, D. E., & de Faria, S. (1993). Cognitive improvements to children in water with and without dolphins. *Anthrozoos* 6(1), 17–27.

National Institutes of Health. (1987). *The health benefits of pets* (1988-216-107). Washington, DC: U.S. Government Printing Office.

Netting, F. E., Wilson, C. C., & New, J. C. (1987). The human-animal bond: Implications for practice. *Social Work, 12*(1), 60–64.

Nightingale, F. (1860/1969). *Notes on nursing.* New York: Dover.

Raina, P., Waltner-Toews, D., Bonnett, B., Woodward, C., Abernathy, T. (1999). Influence of companion animals on the physical and psychological health of older people: An analyses of a one-year longitudinal study. *American Geriatric Society, 47,* 323–329.

Riddick, C. C. (1985). Health aquariums and the non-institutionalized elderly. In M. B. Sussman (Ed.), *Pets and the family* (pp. 163–172). New York: Haworth Press.

Sebkova, J. (1977). *Anxiety levels as affected by the presence of a dog.* Unpublished thesis, University of Lancaster.

Serpell, J. (1991). Beneficial effects of pet ownership on some aspects of human health and behavior. *Journal of Royal Society of Medicine, 84,* 717–720.

Siegel, J. M. (1990). Stressful life events and use of physician services among the elderly: The moderating role of pet ownership. *Journal of Personality and Social Psychology, 58*(6), 1081–1086.

Triebenbacher, S. L. (1998). The relationship between attachment of companion animals and self-esteem: A developmental perspective. In C. C. Wilson & D. C. Turner (Eds.), *Companion animals in human health* (pp. 135–148). Thousand Oaks, CA: Sage.

Walsh, P. G., & Mertin, P. G. (1994). The training of pets as therapy dogs in a women's prison: A pilot study. *Anthrozoos, 7,* 124–128.

Willis, D. A. (1997). Animal therapy. *Rehabilitation Nursing, 22*(2), 78–81.

Wilson, C. C. (1991). The pet as an anxiolytic intervention. *Journal of Nervous Disorders, 179,* 482–489.

Yamauchi, T., & Olmsted, R. N. (1996). Animal assisted therapy. In R. N. Olmsted (Ed.), *APIC infection control and applied epidemiology: principles and practice* (pp. 1–5). St. Louis, MO: Mosby-Year Book.

Young, M. S. (1985). The evolution of domestic pets and companion animals. *The Veterinary Clinics of North America, 15*(2), 297–310.

PART III

Energy Therapies

OVERVIEW

In a recent classification of complementary/alternative therapies, the National Center for Complementary/Alternative Medicine combined biofield therapies and bioelectromagnetics into one category: energy therapies. These therapies focus on energy originating in or near the body and energy coming from other sources. The concept of energy and its use in healing is universal. Most cultures have a word to describe energy. *Qi*, (pronounced *chee*) is a basic element of Traditional Chinese Medicine. The Japanese word is *ki*, while in India energy is *prana* and in ancient Egypt it was called *ankh*. The Dakota Indians' word for energy is *ton*, and the Lakota Indians call it *wakan* (Hover-Kramer, Mentgen, & Scandrett, 1996).

Nurses have used energy therapies for many years. The most familiar is therapeutic touch that Krieger described in the 1970s. Therapeutic touch is part of the larger group of therapies included under the umbrella of healing touch. The "touch" noted in these therapies may or may not involve actual physical touching of the body. Rather the nurse or therapist seeks to bring energy into the patient or to balance the energy within the patient. As noted in the chapter on healing touch, nurses can use many techniques for administering energy therapies. Educational programs that prepare nurses to become certified healing-touch practitioners are offered at many sites across the United States and in other countries.

Other energy therapies are less well known but are increasing in popularity. Many nurses have taken education offerings to become competent in the administration of qi gong, a Traditional Chinese Medicine that used meditation and breathing to enhance and balance qi to promote health. *Reiki*, an energy therapy originating in Japan, is another therapy that nurses are using to promote healing; energy is channeled through the practitioner to achieve healing of the total person.

163

Content on bioelectromagnetics is not included in this book. A variety of techniques are based on the use of electromagnetic fields: pulsed fields, transcutaneous electrical nerve stimulation, low-energy emission therapy, and magnets. Bioelectromagnetic therapies are used more extensively in Japanese health care than in the United States. Although questions about the efficacy of bioelectromagnetic therapies have been raised, particularly about the use of magnets, there is an increasing body of research and much anecdotal evidence to support the use of these therapies in conditions such as arthritis, bone repair, wound healing, and stimulation of the immune system (Fontaine, 2000).

Establishing a scientific base to support the use of energy therapies has been challenging because many of the measurements and designs typically used in Western clinical trials are sometimes difficult to apply when studying the effectiveness of energy therapies. It is difficult to observe energy, and some have questioned whether the effects are real or merely a placebo effect. Strides have been made in developing techniques to measure energy. Nurse researchers can play a critical role in the ongoing research to document the efficacy of complementary therapies.

REFERENCES

Fontaine, K. L. (2000). *Healing practices.* Upper Saddle River, NJ: Prentice Hall.
Hover-Kramer, D., Mentgen, J., & Scandrett-Hibdon, S. (Eds.). *Healing touch: A resource for health care professionals.* Albany, NY: Delmar.

16

Healing Touch

Alexa W. Umbreit

ll cultures, both ancient and modern, have developed some form of touch therapy as part of their desire to heal and care for one another. The oldest written evidence of the use of touch to enhance healing comes from China more than 5,000 years ago (Dossey , Keegan, Guzzetta, & Kolkmeier, 1995; Hover-Kramer et al., 1996; Krieger, 1979). This therapeutic use of the hands has been passed on from generation to generation as a tool for healing. However, there have been philosophical and cultural differences that have influenced how touch has been used throughout the world. The Eastern viewpoint has based its touch healing practices on energy channels (called meridians), energy fields (auras), and energy centers (chakras). Expert practitioners in energetic touch therapies use their hands to influence this flow of energy to promote balance and healing. The Western viewpoint focuses on physiological changes that occur at the cellular level from touch therapies that are believed to influence healing. A blending of both Eastern and Western techniques has led to an explosion of a wide variety of touch therapies that are being used (Dossey et al., 1995). Nursing has used touch throughout its history and today's nurses are integrating many touch techniques into their practice. Hands-on touch modalities are used by more than 30,000 nurses in hospitals each year (Healing Touch International, Inc., 1998). One of these therapies is healing touch, which now has more than 56,000 participants who have been trained during the past 10 years.

DEFINITION

Healing touch (HT) is a type of complementary therapy that uses energy-based techniques to balance and align the human energy field. Based on a holistic view of health and illness, HT focuses on creating an energetic balance of the whole body at the physical, emotional, mental, and spiritual levels rather than on a dysfunctioning part. Through this process of balancing the energy field and therefore opening up energy blockages, an environment is created that is conducive to self healing. Through the interaction of the energy fields between the practitioner and client, the use of the HT practitioner's hands, an intention focusing on the client's highest good, and a centering process, HT techniques specific for the client's needs are used to create this energetic balance (Umbreit, 2000). Krieger (1979) describes the centering process as a meditation in which one eliminates all distractions and concentrates on that place of quietude within where one can feel truly integrated, unified, and focused. Finding this "place of quietude within" is achieved by many through deep belly breathing, prayer, meditation, or any other technique that slows one down, calms the mind, and accesses a deeper spirit of compassion and strength. To be centered is to be fully present with another person or situation, with both heart and mind, deeper feelings, and thoughts. The centered state of mind is maintained throughout the healing touch treatment.

Umbreit (2000) describes the role of the HT practitioner as observation, assessment, and repatterning of the client's energy field because, the pattern and organization of the energy field is disrupted when there is disease, illness, psychological stressors, and pain. Practitioners describe these disruptions in the energy field as blockages, leaks, imbalances, or congestion. The goal of the HT practitioner is to open up these blockages, seal the leaks, rebalance the energy field to symmetry, and release congestion.

The healing touch program, started in 1989 and endorsed by the American Holistic Nurses' Association, involves a formal educational program that teaches techniques including therapeutic touch (TT) developed by Dolores Krieger (1979), interventions described by Brugh Joy (1979), concepts presented by Rosalyn Bruyere (1989) and Barbara Brennan (1986), and original techniques developed by the founder of the healing touch program, Janet Mentgen, and her students (Scandrett-Hibdon, 1996). The multilevel HT educational program in energy-based practice moves from beginning to advanced practice and certification. Advanced practice requires at least 90 hours of workshop instruction plus at least 2 years of study, practice, and working as an apprentice with mentors in the field (Umbreit, 2000). The HT course work is open to nurses, physicians, body therapists, counselors, psychotherapists, other health care professionals, and individuals desiring an in-depth understanding and practice of healing work using energy based concepts and principles (Mentgen & Bulbrook, 1995).

SCIENTIFIC BASIS

Nursing has long described the profession as one dedicated to the art and science of human caring. Rogers (1990) and Watson (1985) have written extensively about caring as a central quality of the nursing profession, along with nursing's concern for the promotion of health and well-being, taking into account the individual's constant interaction with their environment. It was this concern that led nurse theorist Rogers to develop her concepts of the nature of individuals as energy fields in constant interplay with the surrounding environment (Hover-Kramer et al., 1995). The most concentrated part of the energy field is the physical body, but the energy field also extends beyond the level of the skin, imperceptible to the untrained senses (Wright, 1987). Simply stated, Rogers' theoretical framework emphasizes that every living thing is composed of energy, that living things are continually, simultaneously, and mutually exchanging energy with each other, striving toward the goal of balance and universal order (Sayre-Adams, 1994). Using the hands, intention, and centering, the HT practitioner assesses the client's energy field and helps direct the field to a more open, symmetrical pattern that enhances the client's ability to self-heal. Scientific studies on healing energy have suggested that healers can interact with energy fields even without actually touching the client (Fedoruk, 1984; Keller & Bzdek, 1986; Quinn, 1984; Wirth, Richardson, Eidelman, & O'Malley, 1993). These findings support Rogers' concept that humans and environment are energy fields constantly interacting (Miller, 1979). However, it still is not clear how the energy of a practitioner balances the energy patterns of a recipient or how recipients utilize the energy to enhance their self-healing processes (Egan, 1998). The fields of physics, engineering, biology, and physiology continue to research this area of energy exchange in an attempt to explain what occurs during an energetic interaction (Oshman, 2000; Stouffer, Kaiser, Pitman, & Rolf, 1998). Oshman (2000) reports that various energy therapies (including complementary therapies and those approved by current medical practice) actually stimulate tissue healing by the production of pulsating magnetic fields that induce currents to flow within the body's tissue. A superconducting quantum interference device (SQUID) has actually been used for more than 20 years to measure these biomagnetic fields emanating from the hands of energy field practitioners who use therapeutic touch, qi gong, yoga, and meditation. Infrared energy (heat) and other forms of energy yet unnamed from the interaction of energy fields between practitioner and client may also affect the healing process.

This concept of energy field as part of the human interactive environment and healing has been part of many cultures for centuries. Ancient Indian traditions, speak of a universal energy *(prana)* that flows and activates the life force *(kundalini)* (Hover-Kramer et al., 1995). In China, Japan, and Thailand, the basic life energy is called *chi* or *qi*. The Egyptians called it *ka* and the Hawaiians refer to it as *mana* (Umbreit, 2000). The belief is that an imbalance in this energy force could result in illness.

It is unknown precisely how symptoms are managed by HT interventions. What has been observed are changes in outcomes being measured in the nursing research. It may be postulated that because energy fields are in constant interaction within and outside the physical body, internal mechanisms are stimulated by this movement of energy (Umbreit, 2000). Over the past 25 years, published studies on therapeutic touch (TT)—a foundational technique used in HT—have supported observed changes in some of these internal mechanisms. Krieger, Peper, and Ancoli (1979) demonstrated a high abundance of large amplitude alpha brain activity through electroencephalography monitoring in subjects receiving TT. These results demonstrated that a state of deep relaxation occurred in the subjects. Several TT studies have shown positive changes in hematologic measures of blood samples (Krieger, 1976; Olson et al., 1997; Quinn & Strelkauskas, 1993; Wirth, Change, Eidelman, & Paxton, 1996) and dermal wound healing (Wirth, Richardson, Eidelman, & O'Malley, 1993) indicating that physiologic changes at the cellular level can be affected by working with the body's energy fields. Published studies specific to other HT interventions and physiological changes are currently in process (Healing Touch Research Survey, 2000).

What has been reported repeatedly in the HT literature is managing the symptoms of pain and anxiety, decreasing the side effects of cancer treatments, promoting faster postoperative recovery, improving depression, increasing relaxation, and promoting a sense of well being (Bulbrook, 2000; Healing Touch Research Survey, 2000; Hover-Kramer et al., 1996; Hutchison, 1999; Scandrett-Hibdon, Hardy, & Mentgen, 1999; Silva, 1996; Umbreit, 1997, 2000). Since the HT program was started in late 1989, research that incorporates some of the other HT techniques (other than TT) began in the mid 1990s. As of January 2000, there are 29 completed HT studies and 23 in progress (Healing Touch International, 2000).

Umbreit (2000) proposed a model of how HT may promote positive changes in symptoms (Figure 16.1). A trained HT practitioner moves and repatterns a client's energy field, promoting a more open and symmetric pattern to enhance the client's perceived sense of well-being. This movement of energy may stimulate physiological, neurochemical, and psychological changes that promote positive impacts on pain, anxiety, wound healing, immune system function, depression, and sense of well-being.

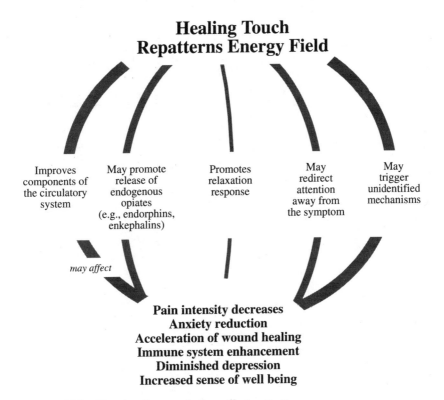

Healing Touch
Repatterns Energy Field

| Improves components of the circulatory system | May promote release of endogenous opiates (e.g., endorphins, enkephalins) | Promotes relaxation response | May redirect attention away from the symptom | May trigger unidentified mechanisms |

may affect

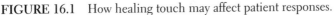

Pain intensity decreases
Anxiety reduction
Acceleration of wound healing
Immune system enhancement
Diminished depression
Increased sense of well being

FIGURE 16.1   How healing touch may affect patient responses.

Note: From "Healing Touch: Applications in the Acute Care Setting," by A. Umbreit, 2000, *AACN Clinical Issues, 11*(1), p. 107. Copyright 2000 by A. Umbreit. Reprinted with permission.

INTERVENTION

TECHNIQUES

More than 25 HT techniques are taught in the HT program from the simple to the complex. The HT practitioner determines which techniques to use after an assessment of the client's expressed needs, symptoms presented, and results of an energy-field hand scan. Techniques range from localized techniques to full-body techniques. Table 16.1 lists several basic techniques, including indications and a brief description of the procedures. These techniques treat a wide range of client symptoms, and it is recommended that they be practiced in a supervised setting with an instructor before working with a client.

TABLE 16.1 Basic Healing Touch Techniques (Hover-Kramer et al., 1996; Mentgen & Bulbrook, 1994, 1995)

	Indications	Brief Description of Procedure
Full-Body Techniques		
Therapeutic touch	Promote relaxation Relieve pain Lower anxiety, tension, stress Accelerate wound healing Promote restoration of the body Promote a sense of well-being	1. Center oneself physically and psychologically 2. Assess the client's energy field with a hand scan over the body. 3. Unruffle clear the energy field. 4. Direct and modulate the energy (i.e., hold the hand over the areas where blockages or congestion were detected). 5. Stop when the energy field feels symmetrical.
Magnetic unruffle	Clear the body's energy field of congested energy and emotional debris Used for history of drug use, post-anesthesia, chronic pain, trauma, systemic disease, breathing polluted air, history of smoking, environmental sensitivities, release of emotional debris and unresolved feelings (e.g., anger, fear, worry, tension, anxiety)	1. Center oneself physically and psychologically. 2. Place hands 12 inches above the client's head with fingers spread, relaxed, and curled, thumbs touching or close together. 3. Move hands very slowly in long continuous raking motions over the body from above the head to the toes. 4. Repeat procedure (should be repeated 30 times and take about 15 minutes).
Chakra connection	Connect, open, and balance the energy centers (chakras), enhancing the flow of energy throughout the body	1. Center oneself physically and psychologically. 2. Place hands on or over the minor energy centers (chakras) on the extremities and the major energy centers (chakras) on the trunk in a defined sequential manner, holding each area for a least one minute.

Chakra spread

Opens the energy centers (chakras), producing a deep clearing of energy blocks

Used for those in severe pain, pre- and postoperatively, severe stress reactions with the terminally ill, and assisting a client who has chosen to enter a profound spiritual state

1. Center oneself physically and psychologically.
2. Hold the client's feet, then hands, one by one in a gentle embrace.
3. Place the hands (palms facing) above each energy center (chakra), moving the hands slowly downward toward the chakra, then spreading the hands outward as far as possible; motion is repeated 3 times for each energy center, moving from the upper to the lower chakras.
4. Repeat the entire sequence two more times.
5. End the treatment with the practitioner holding the client's hand and heart center.
6. This procedure is generally gone in silence and takes about 10 minutes. It is used very carefully by experienced practitioners for special needs and sacred moments in healing.

Localized Techniques

Ultrasound

Break up congestion, energy patterns, and blockages

Relieve pain

Assist in stopping internal bleeding, sealing laceration, healing fractures, and joint injuries

1. Center oneself physically and psychologically.
2. Hold the thumb, first and second fingers together, directing energy from the palm to the fingers.
3. Imagine a beam of light coming from the fingers into the body.
4. Move the whole hand in any direction over the affected part continuously for 3–5 minutes.

(continued)

TABLE 16.1 Basic Healing Touch Techniques (Hover-Kramer et al., 1996; Mentgen & Bulbrook, 1994, 1995) (Continued)

	Indications	Brief Description of Procedure
Laser	Cuts, seals, and breaks up congestion in the energy field Relieves pain	1. Center oneself physically and psychologically. 2. Hold the fingers still and pointed toward the problem area. 3. Sense an intermittent pulsing light penetrating the problem area. 4. Use for a few seconds to 1 minute.
Mind clearing	Promotes relaxation and focusing of the mind	1. Center oneself physically and psychologically. 2. Hold fingertips or palms on designated parts of the neck and head holding each part about 1 minute. 3. Gently massage the mandibular joint. 4. End with light sweeping touches 3 times across the brow and cheeks.
Pain drain	Eases pain or energy congestion	1. Center oneself physically and psychologically. 2. Place the practitioner's left hand on the area of pain and hold the right hand downward away from the body.

3. The client's congested energy from the painful area is siphoned off through the practitioner's left hand and travels out the right hand.
4. Next the practitioner moves the right hand on the painful area and places the left hand upward in the air to bring in healing energy from the universal energy field.
5. Each position is generally held for 3–5 minutes.

Wound sealing — Repairs energy field leaks that occur as a result of the physical body's experiencing trauma, incisions, or childbirth

1. Center oneself physically and psychologically.
2. Hand scans over the body above a scar or injury to determine if any leaks of energy are coming from the site (this may feel like a column of cool air).
3. Move the hands over the area gathering energy.
4. Bring down the gathered energy to the client's skin over the injury and hold for a minute with the hands.
5. Re-scan the area to determine that the energy field feels symmetrical over the entire body.

From "Healing Touch: Applications in the Acute Care Setting," by A. Umbreit, 2000, AACN *Clinical Issues*, *11*(1), pp. 109–110. Copyright 2000 by A. *Umbreit*. Reprinted with permission.

Most of the HT techniques involve two basic types of hand gestures that are described in terms of movement or stillness (Hutchison, 1999). In the movement gestures, the hands make gentle brushing or combing motions (called *unruffling* or *clearing*), usually downward and outward, in order to remove congested energy from the field. The hands remain relaxed, palms facing downward toward the patient, between 2 and 12 inches from the skin. The hand strokes may be slow and sweeping or short and rapid. In the stillness hand position, the practitioner holds his or her hands over a specific part of the client's body for one to several minutes (called *directing, modulating,* or *sending* energy), either lightly touching or just above the skin. The practitioner uses intent to facilitate a transfer of energy to the specific body part of the client from a "universal source" of energy, the practitioner being the conduit of this energy.

Although several of the HT techniques can be done in a seated position, most techniques are done while the client is lying down so that the client can be in the most relaxed state possible in order to promote a more profound effect. When working with a client, the practitioner briefly describes HT and what the practitioner plans to do, invites the client to ask any questions at any time, and receives the client's permission to do the treatment and to touch the client.

MEASUREMENT OF OUTCOMES

Measurement of HT outcomes have included patient satisfaction, anxiety and stress reduction, pain reduction, improved sense of well-being, decrease in depression, changes in blood pressure, accelerated wound healing, diminished agitation levels in dementia patients, and immunological changes. Studies currently in progress are also examining cost effectiveness outcomes like length of procedure and length of stay in the hospital. Until a tool is developed to measure changes in the energy system, objective measuring of changes in the flow of an energy field is not possible. Practitioners do report a change in the client's energy field that they perceive through the use of their senses, most commonly through the sense of touch.

Outcomes measured must reflect the specific client need and presenting symptoms and the particular HT technique used to treat the need or symptoms. Tools that have been used to measure client outcomes have included measuring patient satisfaction and well-being using Likert-type scale responses; the Spielberger State/Trait Anxiety Inventory, Profile of Moods State, or an Anxiety Visual Analog Scale; a Pain Visual Analog Scale, the McGill-Melzack Pain Questionnaire, or the Chronic Pain Experience

Instrument; Beck's Depression Inventory; cardiovascular variables (heart rate, systolic/diastolic blood pressure, and mean arterial blood pressure); oxygenation variables (pH, CO_2, PO_2, and HCO_3); accelerated healing (rate of epithelialization); Recovery Index; the Cohen-Mansfield Agitation Inventory; and immunoglobulin concentrations pre- and posttreatments.

It is difficult to determine whether the outcome of the HT intervention is solely from the treatment or due to another factor. The effect of the practitioner's presence has always been considered a confounding variable affecting client outcome, but this is true in many nursing interventions.

PRECAUTIONS

Precautions to be aware of when using HT techniques include the following:

- The energy field of infants, children, older people, the extremely ill, and the dying are sensitive to energy work so treatments should be gentle and time limited.
- Gentle energy treatments are also required for pregnant women since the energy field also includes the fetus.
- Energy work with a cancer patient should be focused on balancing the whole field rather than concentrating on a particular area.
- The effect of medications and chemicals in the body may be enhanced with energy work so one must be alert to the possibility of side effects and sensitivity reactions to these substances.

It is recommended that experienced practitioners work with clients in the above situations. However, an apprentice in HT can provide treatments in these situations if supervised by a mentor to help develop a knowledgeable practice (Umbreit, 2000).

Healing touch is not considered a curative treatment and must always be used in conjunction with conventional medical care. However, practitioners and clients have reported that clients have experienced a sense of healing at a more holistic level of mind, body, and spirit, even if a cure is not possible. Umbreit (2000) reports anecdotal comments from clients that include: "I feel wonderful," "relaxed," "peaceful," "in a meditative state," "warm," "soothed," "safe," "reassured," "more balanced," "mellow," "happier with life," "as if all my tension was melting," and a "sense of inner peace." Since HT is a noninvasive intervention, these client responses have enormous implications for improving a client's quality of life in their striving toward wellness.

USES

Healing touch interventions have been supported by several research studies (mostly on therapeutic touch), but the majority of the time support comes through anecdotal stories in a variety of clinical situations in all age groups and states of illness or wellness (Bulbrook, 2000; Hover-Kramer et al.,1996; Scandrett-Hibdon et al., 1999, Umbreit, 1997, 2000). Healing touch has been used in the following clinical situations:

- Reduction of anxiety and stress
- Promotion of relaxation
- Reduction in acute and chronic pain
- Acceleration of wound healing, bone healing, and recovery level
- Aid in preparation for medical treatments and procedures
- Immune system enhancement
- Reducing symptoms of depression
- Promoting a sense of well-being
- Reduction in agitation levels
- Support for the dying process
- Opening up a blocked energy field
- Enhancement of spiritual development

Table 16.2 lists several research studies that have supported the use of healing touch interventions in some of these clinical situations over the past 10 years. Many of these studies are not yet published in medical, nursing, or psychology journals, but information can be accessed through Healing Touch International's research department. The research continues to be controversial because the exact mechanism of action cannot be seen or easily explained in our Western view of what constitutes sound scientific research, and few double-blind studies have ever been done in this area.

FUTURE RESEARCH

Research studies and anecdotal cases in healing touch offer promising, yet certainly not conclusive, data on the positive outcomes from this complementary therapy. Qualitative responses from clients have been especially important in helping guide the direction of the research and may provide insight into the phenomenon of energy exchange in the future. Some of the problems encountered in nursing research include insufficient funding to support the work, multiple variables that are hard to control in a clinical

TABLE 16.2   Research Studies Using Healing Touch Interventions
            1992–2000

Uses	Selected sources
Anxiety/stress relief	Dubrey (1997); Olson, Sneed, Bonadonna, Ratliff, & Dias (1992); Olson & Sneed (1995); Samarel, Fawcett, Davis, & Ryan (1998); Simington & Laing, (1993); Turner, Clark, Gauthier, & Williams (1998)
Relaxation response initiated	Snyder, Egan, & Burns (1995); Vaughn (1995)
Pain relief	Barrington (1994); Biley (1996); Darbonne & Fontenot (1997); Gordon (1997); Meehan (1993); Peck (1997); Turner et al. (1998)
Wound healing/postoperative recovery	Silva (1996); Wirth et al., (1993)
Aid in medical procedures/treatments	Norris (2000)
Immune system enhancement	Quinn & Strelkauskas (1993); Olson et al., (1997)
Diminished depression	Bradway (1998)
Enhancement of well-being	Giasson & Bouchard (1998); Semple (2000)
Agitation levels	Snyder et al., (1995); Wang & Hermann (1999); Woods, Craven, & Whitney (1996)
Enhancement of spiritual development	Geddes (1999); Wardell (1999)

setting versus a laboratory setting, and the use of small sample sizes that can be easily affected by highly variable data and sampling error. Added to this is the difficulty of testing the efficacy of an energy-based therapy, in which the energy exchange between practitioner and client cannot be seen by most but is only observed as subjective responses from clients. The whole conceptual framework of energy fields and energy exchange does not fit the cause-effect model that Western science is focused on. Rogers' theory (1990) speaks about energy changing, exchanging, and patterning, one moment in time never replicating itself to another. The focus is on nature's restoring universal order and balance, and restoring energy balance is the goal of HT. This is a huge area of research that obviously will require a multidisciplinary effort by Western and Eastern medicine, quantum physics, biology, psychology, philosophy, spirituality, and nursing. Outcome studies, as well as studies of mechanism, will help support the development and understanding of the phenomenon of energy exchange. As postulated in Figure 16.1, there are many mediating factors that may contribute to decreases in pain intensity, anxiety reduction, acceleration of wound healing, immune system enhancement, diminished depression, and increased sense of well-being. More studies that measure some of these mediating mechanisms are recommended.

The choice of a valid instrument in measuring outcomes is critical in HT studies. Results of studies can be skewed in either direction if the instrument is not reliable. However, in order to get subject cooperation when working with persons who are ill, the measuring instrument must be simple to use and not burdensome to some one who is already facing difficulties.

Other challenges to be controlled in conducting a HT research study include the experience of the HT practitioner, the presence phenomenon of the caregiver, the type of HT treatment modality chosen, the length and number of treatments, when the treatment is done, and when measurements are done. There are a wide range of skill levels of HT practitioners from novice to certified practitioner and like skill level would be important in planning a research study. The phenomenon of presence of the HT practitioner may also affect the outcome of the research and needs to be controlled in the research design. Since there are many HT interventions that can be used, a research study would need to be consistent in the type of chosen therapy. The challenge with length and number of treatments is that under normal circumstances, a HT intervention is not used for a prescribed length of time or number of treatments. The practitioner does the work until she or he senses and intuits that it is time to stop or that more treatments are needed. Research could restrict this professional decision-making process in a false manner. Choosing when to give a HT treatment and when to measure outcomes and how long the outcome may last continues to be a challenge. Experienced HT practitioners must have input into determining these time lines by observing patterns they may typically see in their own professional practice.

The next steps for research must build upon the small studies already completed. Replication of studies would help strengthen the validity of HT. The following are specific areas to build upon:

1. Is HT equally effective in acute versus chronic pain? How long and how often do treatments need to be for the client to report a decrease in pain? How long does this last?

2. How is postoperative recovery affected by administering HT (pain relief, wound healing, restoring of bowel function, ease of physical activity, length of stay in the hospital)?
3. Does HT have a positive effect on degenerative diseases such as arthritis, multiple sclerosis, fibromyalgia, stroke, immune deficiency disorders, chronic lung conditions?
4. Does HT assist in managing the side effects of treatments in the patient with cancer?
5. What are the psychological and spiritual benefits reported by HT recipients?
6. What tools are effective in measuring a change in energy in the recipient before and after HT or an exchange of energy between practitioner and recipient?

In the quest to examine the impact of HT scientifically, we must not be too quick to dismiss the overwhelming positive client feedback from its clinical application. Creativity is necessary in conducting research of this phenomenon that cannot be seen by the naked eye, but is so often felt by the human spirit.

FOR MORE INFORMATION ON HEALING TOUCH:

Healing Touch International
12477 W. Cedar Drive, Suite 202
Lakewood, CO 80228
(303)989-7982
E-mail HTIheal@aol.com
Available on line at http://healingtouch.net

Colorado Center for Healing Touch
12477 West Cedar Drive, Suite 206
Lakewood, CO 80228
(303)989-0581
E-mail: ccheal@aol.com
Available on line at http://www.healingtouch.net

American Holistic Nurses Association (AHNA)
P.O. Box 2130
Flagstaff, AZ 86003-2130
(800)278-AHNA
Available on line at http://www.ahna.org

REFERENCES

Barrington, R. (1994). A naturalistic inquiry of post-operative pain after therapeutic touch. In D. Gaut & A. Boykin (Eds.), *Caring as healing: Renewal through hope* (pp. 199–213). New York: National League for Nursing Press.

Biley, F. (1996). Rogerian science, phantoms, and therapeutic touch: Exploring potentials. *Nursing Science Quarterly, 9*(4), 165–169.

Bradway, C. (1998). The effects of healing touch on depression. *Healing Touch Newsletter, 8*(3), 2.

Brennan, B. (1986). *Hands of light.* New York: Bantam.

Bruyere, R. L. (1989). Wheels of light. New York: Simon & Schuster.

Bulbrook, M. J. T. (2000). *Healing stories to inspire, teach and heal.* Carrboro, NC: North Carolina Center for Healing Touch.

Darbonne, M. & Fontenot, T. (1997). The effects of healing touch modalities on patients with chronic pain. *Healing Touch Research Survey January 2000.* Lakewood, CO: Healing Touch International.

Dossey, B. M., Keegan, L., Guzzetta, C. E., & Kolkmeier, L. H. (1995). *Holistic nursing: A handbook for practice.* Gaithersburg, MD: Aspen.

Dubrey, R. (1997). Perceived effectiveness of healing touch treatments by healees. *Healing Touch Research Survey January 2000.* Lakewood, CO: Healing Touch International.

Egan, E. C. (1998). Therapeutic touch. In M. Snyder & R. Lindquist, *Complementary/alternative therapies in nursing* (3rd ed., pp. 49–62). New York: Springer.

Fedoruk, R. B. (1984). Transfer of the relaxation response: Therapeutic touch as a method of reduction of stress in premature neonates. Unpublished doctoral dissertation, University of Maryland.

Geddes, N. (1999). The experience of personal transformation in healing touch practitioners: A heuristic inquiry. *Healing Touch Newsletter, 9*(3), 5.

Giasson, M. & Bouchard, L. (1998). Effect of therapeutic touch on the well-being of persons with terminal cancer. *Journal of Holistic Nursing, 16*(3), 383–398.

Gordon, A. (1997, September). *Therapeutic touch in the treatment of osteoarthritis.* Research report presented at the Complementary and Alternative Health Care conference, Minneapolis, MN.

Healing Touch International, Inc. (1998). *Did you know?* [On-line]. Available: www.healingtouch.net/index.shtml

Healing Touch International, Inc. (2000). *Healing Touch Research Survey.* Lakewood, CO: Author.

Hover-Kramer, D., Mentgen, J., & Scandrett-Hibdon, S. (1996). *Healing touch: A resource for health care professionals.* Albany, NY: Delmar.

Hutchison, C. P. (1999). Healing touch: An energetic approach. *American Journal of Nursing, 99*(4), 43–48.

Joy, B. (1979). *Joy's way.* New York: G. P. Putnam's Sons.

Keller, E., & Bzdek, V. (1986). Effects of therapeutic touch on tension headache pain. *Nursing Research, 13*(2), 101–106.

Krieger, D. (1976). Healing by the laying on of hands as facilitator of bioenergetic change: The response of in-vivo hemoglobin. *Psychoenergetic Systems, 1*, 121–129.

Krieger, D. (1979). *The therapeutic touch: How to use your hands to help or to heal.* New York: Simon & Schuster.

Krieger, D., Peper, E., & Ancoli, A. (1979). Therapeutic touch: Searching for evidence of physiological change. *American Journal of Nursing, 79*, 660–662.

Meehan, T. (1993). Therapeutic touch and post-operative pain: A Rogerian research study. *Nursing Science Quarterly, 6*(2), 69–78.

Mentgen, J., & Bulbrook, M. (1995). *Healing touch level I notebook.* Carrboro, NC: North Carolina Center for Healing Touch.

Miller, L. A. (1979). An explanation of therapeutic touch using the science of unitary man. *Nursing Forum, 18*(3), 278–287.

Norris, R. (2000, January). *Evaluation of energy-based relaxation techniques as nursing interventions to improve outcomes in patients undergoing nurse-performed screening flexible sigmoidoscopy.* Research report presented at the 2000 Healing Touch International Conference, Kauai, HI.

Olson, M., & Sneed, N. (1995). Anxiety and therapeutic touch. *Issues in Mental Health Nursing, 16*, 97–108.

Olson, M., Sneed, N., Bonadonna, R., Ratliff, J., & Dias, J. (1992). Therapeutic touch and post-Hurricane Hugo stress. *Journal of Holistic Nursing, 10*, 120–136.

Olson, M., Sneed, N., LaVia, M., Virella, G., Bonodonna, R., & Michel, Y.(1997). Stress-induced immunosuppression and therapeutic touch. *Alternative Therapies, 3*, 13–26.

Oschman, J. L. (2000). *Energy medicine: The scientific basis.* Dover, NH: Churchill Livingston.

Peck, S. (1997). The effectiveness of therapeutic touch for decreasing pain in elders with degenerative arthritis. *Journal of Holistic Nursing, 15*(2), 13–26.

Quinn, J. (1984). Therapeutic touch as energy exchange: Testing the theory. *Advances in Nursing Science, 6*(2), 42–49.

Quinn, J., & Strelkauskas, A. (1993). Psychoimmunologic effect of therapeutic touch on practitioners and recently bereaved recipients: A pilot study. *Advances in Nursing Science, 15*(4), 13–26.

Rogers, M. (1990). Nursing: Science of unitary, irreducible, human beings: Update 1990. In E. A. M. Barrett (Ed.), *Vision of Rogers' science-based nursing* (pp. 5–11). New York: National League for Nursing.

Samarel N., Fawcett, J., Davis, M. M., & Ryan, F. M. (1998, September). Effects of dialogue and therapeutic touch on preoperative and postoperative experiences of breast cancer surgery: An exploratory study. *Oncology Nursing Forum, 25*(8), 1369–1376.

Sayre-Adams, J. (1994). Therapeutic touch: A nursing function. *Nursing Standard, 8*(17), 25–28.

Scandrett-Hibdon, S. (1996). Research foundations. *In healing touch: A resource for health care professionals* (pp. 27–42). Albany, NY: Delmar.

Scandrett-Hibdon, S., Hardy, C., & Mentgen, J. (1999). *Energetic patterns: Healing touch case studies Vol. 1.* Lakewood, CO: Colorado Center for Healing Touch.

Semple, S. (2000). The psychosocial benefits of therapeutic touch as an adjunct to cancer treatments. *In Touch*, 12(1), 5.

Silva, C. (1996). The effects of relaxation touch on the recovery level of postanesthesia abdominal hysterectomy patients. *Alternative Therapies*, 2(4), 94.

Simington, J., & Laing, G. (1993). Effects of therapeutic touch on anxiety in institutionalized elderly. *Clinical Nursing Research*, 2(4), 438–450.

Snyder, M., Egan, E., & Burns, K. (1995). Interventions for decreasing agitation behaviors in persons with dementia. *Journal of Gerontological Nursing*, 21(7), 34–40.

Stouffer, D., Kaiser, D., Pitman, G., & Rolf, W. (1998, January). *Electrodermal testing to measure the effect of a healing touch treatment*. Paper presented at the Healing Touch Research Symposium, Denver, CO.

Turner, J., Clark, A., Gauthier, D., & Williams, M. (1998). The effect of therapeutic touch on pain and anxiety in burn patients. *Journal of Advanced Nursing*, 28(1), 10–20.

Umbreit, A. (1997). Therapeutic touch: Energy-based healing. *Creative Nursing*, 3, 6–7.

Umbreit, A. (2000). Healing touch: Applications in the acute care setting. *AACN Clinical Issues*, 11(1), 105–119.

Vaughn, S. (1995). The gentle touch. *Journal of Clinical Nursing*, 4, 359–368.

Wang, K., & Hermann, C. (1999). Healing touch on agitation levels related to dementia. *Healing Touch Newsletter*, 9(3), 3.

Wardell, D. (1999). Spirituality in healing touch practice. *Healing Touch Newsletter*, 9(3), 4.

Watson, J. (1985). *Nursing: The philosophy and science of caring*. Boulder: Colorado Associated University Press.

Wirth, D., Richardson, W., Eidelman, W., & O'Malley, A. (1993). Full thickness dermal wounds treated with non-contact therapeutic touch: A replication and extension. *Complementary Therapies in Medicine*, 1, 127–132.

Wirth, D., Chang, R., Eidelman, W., & Paxton, J. (1996). Haematological indicators of complementary healing intervention. *Complementary Therapies in Medicine*, 4(1), 14–20.

Woods, D., Craven, R., & Whitney, J. (1996). The effect of therapeutic touch on disruptive behaviours of individuals with dementia of the Alzheimer type. *Alternative Therapies*, 2(4), 95.

Wright, S. M. (1987). The use of therapeutic touch in the management of pain. *Nursing Clinics of North America*, 22, 705–714.

17

Therapeutic Touch

Janet F. Quinn

Therapeutic touch was developed from the laying-on of hands by Dora Kunz, a gifted healer, and Dolores Krieger, PhD, RN. In 1979 Krieger outlined the steps of the practice in her first book (Krieger, 1979). She introduced the method to students in the graduate nursing program at New York University in the early 1970s in a course called "Frontiers of Nursing," which continues today. Krieger estimates that as of 1990, "therapeutic touch has also been taught in more than 80 colleges and universities in the United States as well as in innumerable hospital and health facility in-service and continuing-education programs. In addition, therapeutic touch has been taught in 68 countries" (Krieger, 1993).

DEFINITION

Therapeutic touch (TT) is the use of the hands on or near the body with the intention to help or to heal. It is a contemporary intervention that is different from the laying-on of hands in several key ways. Perhaps most notable of these differences is that therapeutic touch need not take place within a religious or spiritual framework. It is seen as a natural human potential that can be actualized by anyone who has the intention to heal and makes the commitment to learning and practicing. Therapeutic touch has as its focus the facilitation and acceleration of the natural healing potential within all living systems.

SCIENTIFIC BASIS

Therapeutic touch is founded on three basic assumptions:

183

1. Human beings are energy fields and open systems.
2. Illness is an imbalance in energy flow or pattern.
3. Trained practitioners can perceive and intervene in the recipient's energy field to stimulate the recipient's own natural healing potential.

1. *Human beings are energy fields.* When Kunz and Krieger developed therapeutic touch, they called on understandings gained from Eastern thought to explain both the method and its effects. *Prana*, the vital life force energy identified in Indian philosophy and healing systems, is posited to be the energy that surrounds and pervades every living system. According to Krieger, *prana* is directed and modulated *by* the one in the role of healer *for* the one being healed (Krieger, 1973, 1979, 1993). Other theorists have developed Krieger's original hypothesis further by applying the theoretical framework postulated by Rogers. In *Science of Unitary Human Beings*, Rogers defines people as irreducible, indivisible, multidimensional energy fields integral with the environmental energy field (Rogers, 1990). In earlier conceptualizations of TT within this framework, the theory that there was an "energy transfer or exchange" between the practitioner and the recipient was a primary explanatory model (Heidt, 1981; Keller & Bzdek, 1986; Quinn, 1984); it was derived from Rogers' conceptual system and is consistent with theoretical explanations offered by earlier researchers (Grad, Cadoret, & Paul, 1961; Grad, 1963, 1964, 1965; Smith, 1972). More recently, it has been postulated that the therapeutic touch practitioner, knowingly participating in the mutual human/environment process by shifting consciousness into a state that may be thought of as a "healing meditation" (Krieger, Peper, & Ancoli, 1979), facilitates repatterning of the recipient's energy field through a process of resonance rather than "energy exchange or transfer" (Cowling, 1990; Quinn, 1992).

Because therapeutic touch practitioners believe that human beings are energy fields, they also believe that people are open systems. Neither the practitioner nor the recipient stops at their skin, so the therapeutic touch exchange may occur with no physical contact at all, or with a mix of physical contact and no physical contact. This becomes most relevant when actual physical contact between practitioner and recipient is undesirable for medical or sociocultural reasons.

2. *Illness is an imbalance in energy flow or pattern.* When there is illness or other dysfunction in the body-mind-spirit, there is a corresponding imbalance in the energy field. In the case of disease, the assumption made in this system is that a shift in the energy field probably preceded the onset of physical symptoms and clinical evidence of the disease. This assumption is consistent with current scientific theories concerning the relationship

between the state of the resistance of the host when exposed to pathogens and the onset of disease. In an energetic framework, one assumes that there are patterns or flows of energy that are more or less consistent with health and therefore provide greater or less resistance to disease.

3. *Trained practitioners can perceive and intervene in the recipient's energy field to stimulate the recipient's own natural healing potential.* Through the process of turning one's attention inward and becoming quiet, relaxed, and focused, one can begin to get a sense of the human energy field of another. The energy field is always there, but we are not always quiet enough and paying close enough attention to notice it. Through practice, TT practitioners can become extremely sensitive to even subtle changes in the field, and through gentle movements of the hands coupled with a very focused intention, they can assist in repatterning the field in a direction that is more conducive to health.

Tests of human beings' ability to perceive the energy of other human beings are described in the paper by Schwartz, Russek, and Beltran (1995). These authors report the results of several experiments in which blindfolded, randomly assigned subjects were able to correctly guess when another person's hand, palm open and facing, was held 3 to 4 inches above their own open palm. They guessed correctly at a rate statistically greater than chance would allow.

At this time there is not conclusive evidence acceptable in the Western scientific tradition that a human energy field exists. Therapeutic touch practitioners and practitioners of all so-called energy medicines like acupuncture, homeopathy, and qi gong, are well within the bounds of responsible scientific practice as long as they acknowledge this and continue to treat the theory of energy exchange as a working hypotheses. Theories, rather than confirmed facts, regarding the mechanisms by which interventions have effects are the rule, not the exception, across modern medical, pharmaceutical and nursing practice. The scientific evidence for the efficacy of TT will be discussed in the section on uses.

INTERVENTION

TECHNIQUE (TABLE 17.1)

Centering

The TT assessment of the human energy field is uncomplicated and simple, but developing a deep sensitivity to subtle cues and differences in the field will take practice. To facilitate this sensitivity and to create the most healing

TABLE 17.1   The Therapeutic Touch Process

The Steps of the Therapeutic Touch Process Are

- Centering
- Assessing the energy field
- Clearing and mobilizing the energy field
- Directing energy for healing
- Balancing the energy field

environment for both practitioner and recipient, the therapeutic touch practitioner prepares for the assessment and treatment by *centering*. Centering involves a shift from our ordinary state of being into a calm, relaxed, and focused healing presence; it is the turning inward of attention and the making of an intention to help or to heal. The mind is quieted, extraneous thoughts from the past or about the future are temporarily set aside, and the full awareness of the practitioner is brought into the present moment in the intention to heal. For this reason, therapeutic touch has been called a "healing meditation" (Krieger et al., 1979).

This intention to heal is believed to be the key variable in the efficacy of the treatment. In a randomized, placebo-controlled study, cardiac patients were given a TT treatment by nurses who were very experienced with therapeutic touch, and a control group received a mimic sham treatment by nurses with no training in TT. The nurses who were doing the real treatments centered themselves in the moment and made the intention to heal before beginning and during the movement of their hands. The nurses in the sham condition were taught how to mimic the hand movements exactly but were doing mental arithmetic while they simply went through the motions, rather than holding the intent to heal. Both groups of nurses were videotaped and the tapes were reviewed by naïve observers. No one could tell the difference in the treatments by looking at them. In the experimental group receiving therapeutic touch, there was a highly significant decrease in anxiety on posttest; anxiety didn't change in the mimic group (Quinn, 1984). This type of control has been used in other therapeutic touch research and demonstrates the same phenomenon; namely, that the intention of the practitioner not the hand movements, seems to be the critical variable. This is why centering is the most important step of the process. All the movements of the TT process are done within this context of the intention for healing, wholeness, and balance.

Assessing

The goal of the assessment is to gain information about the pattern and flow of energy in the field. During the entire TT session the patient can be seated sideways in an armless chair, so that his or her back is unobstructed. To complete an assessment, the practitioner stands behind the clothed patient, extends the hands over the top of the patient's head with palms turned toward the patient, and holds them about 2 to 4 inches away from the body. Maintaining this distance, the hands are held somewhat parallel to each other and palms parallel to the patient's body, and are moved gently from the top of the head to the level of the hips, while the practitioner mentally notes any areas in which the energy field feels different from the rest of the field. Next, the practitioner moves in front of the patient and repeats the assessment process from head to toe, again noting areas where the field feels different. Alternatively, the practitioner can assess front and back at the same time and compare them, by using one hand behind the patient and one hand in front and moving both hands from head to foot simultaneously. Patients can also be assessed while lying in bed or on an exam table.

In the healthy person, the energy field should feel essentially symmetrical from left to right and from top to bottom. There should be a sense of smoothness or evenness and there should not be areas where there is a sharp difference in temperature or rhythm or flow. When there is illness, there are often areas of the field in which the smoothness is broken, or where there is a sharp change in perceived temperature over the area. In the person with serious systemic illness or depression, the assessment may reveal a generalized disturbance over the entire field, such as a weakness, a thickness, a dullness or a sense of decreased flow or increased temperature. For an excellent discussion of the various perceptions and their meanings as developed by one expert therapeutic touch practitioner see Macrae's primer (1988).

Clearing and Mobilizing the Energy Field

Krieger refers to this step as *unruffling* while Macrae uses the language used here. The unruffling or clearing process prepares the field for further treatment and is also an extremely effective method for inducing a profound relaxation response. The practitioner again begins by holding the hands 2 to 4 inches away from the body at the top of the head and moves the hands, palms toward the patient, the length of the body from head to foot in a gently sweeping motion. The intention of the practitioner remains focused on wholeness and balance, imagining that the patient is becoming more and more relaxed and that the energy is flowing easily and freely, from head to toe, in a balanced and harmonious way. This process is repeated over the front of the patient's body, ending with the feet. When the practitioner is at the feet, it is useful to gently massage the bottoms of the feet to assist in the outward flow of energy.

Directing Energy for Healing

Using the assessment data as a guide, the practitioner now begins to direct energy with the intention of restoring imbalances in the field to order and harmony. The direction of energy is accomplished by placing the hands on or over the area of imbalance and allowing a sense of the healing energy to flow out through the practitioner and toward the patient. If it is useful, the practitioner may hold an image of the desired outcome in mind while directing this energy.

Balancing

The practitioner systematically treats each area of imbalance detected during assessment, as well as new areas uncovered through the clearing process. When the practitioner perceives that the imbalances have been eliminated or that the patient's system has taken as much energy as it can, the treatment ends with a general *balancing* and grounding process. The balancing consists of an additional head-to-toe clearing as before, but with the intention of smoothing and balancing the whole field. This process ends with the practitioner's touching the feet and imagining the patient as being whole, balanced and grounded or rooted—steady and strong like a tree with roots deep into the earth.

MEASUREMENT OF OUTCOMES

Because the focus of therapeutic touch is broader than curing physical disease, outcomes of the process are not uniformly predictable. In general, most patients experience therapeutic touch as calming, integrating, and balancing. A strong relaxation response, characterized by the usual indicators of this response, is usually seen, within minutes of the start of the treatment and deepens over its full course.

The therapeutic touch practitioner will be assessing the patient's energy field throughout the treatment, looking for changes in the pattern of the energy field compared to the initial assessment. These changes may be great or small and may or may not be perceived by the patient. There are also times when the practitioner may assess that although the pattern of imbalance has not shifted, the treatment is nevertheless over; the patient has gotten all that he or she can in this session. The intuitive capacity of the therapeutic touch practitioner helps to guide this process.

In addition to the energetic assessment, the therapeutic touch practitioner carefully monitors the patient's response throughout, and at the end of the treatment asks for feedback. Patients describe changes in their energetic, physical, emotional, and spiritual being. Some patients cannot report their perceptions—like the neonate in the NICU who promptly falls asleep during the treatment after crying for an extended period of time or the combative patient with Alzheimer's disease who becomes quiet and restful—but the practitioner can observe them. Sometimes there is no immediate response, but the patient will experience a decrease in physical symptoms in the 15 to 20 minutes following treatment. Sometimes the change will manifest as a good night's sleep.

When therapeutic touch is used over time as a course of therapy, these kinds of changes can be monitored by having the patient keep a treatment journal and review it with the practitioner before each session. Cumulative effects on the physical, emotional, or spiritual may become more obvious in this manner. Again, because the focus in therapeutic touch goes beyond yet includes the physical, changes in attitude, philosophy, and general well-being are all part of the process. These changes can be assessed best in dialogue with the patient over time.

PRECAUTIONS

The safety of therapeutic touch is borne out in clinical practice. Since its introduction by nurses into mainstream health-care institutions there have been no reported incidents of harm to a patient related to therapeutic touch. However, because we do not know the effects of energetic forms of healing on unborn children, therapeutic touch practitioners recommend that it not be used by inexperienced practitioners on pregnant women. Caution when treating the very old or the very young is also appropriate, and treatments with people in these age groups should be shorter and carefully modulated. Some people find direct treatment of the head uncomfortable, so the hands should be kept moving when working around the head.

USES

There is no way of knowing at the outset how any given person will respond to TT. What we do know is that therapeutic touch is a treatment for the whole person, not just for illness or disease, and so it is appropriate for use on virtually everyone. Therapeutic touch is almost always best when used as a complement to standard medical and nursing care, where it has been found clinically to be very useful in musculoskeletal conditions such as sprains, strains, muscle spasms, and fractures. Practitioners report that the sooner treatment is given in these cases the more effective TT seems to be. Research data supporting efficacy remains preliminary. Peters (1999) reports in a meta-analytic review of TT studies that "it is impossible to make any substantive claims [about the efficacy of therapeutic touch] at this time because there is limited published research and because many of the studies had significant methodological issues that could seriously bias the reported results" (p. 52). Nevertheless, observed effects have been demonstrated through well-designed, placebo-controlled research and clinical practice that suggest uses for TT. Table 17.2 indicates some of those uses.

A forthcoming meta-analysis of TT anxiety studies concludes that therapeutic touch is more effective than mock therapeutic touch or routine clinical touch in reducing anxiety symptoms (Warber, Gillespie, Kile, Gorenflo, & Bolling, in press). A pilot study where the immune systems of practitioners and recipients were examined before and after a course of therapeutic touch treatments suggests that TT may have an immunoenhancing effect in bereaved adults (Quinn & Strelkauskas, 1993) while Turner, Clark, Gauthier, and Williams (1998) found a similar effect in burn patients.

FUTURE RESEARCH

In 1989, three critical directions were proposed for future research efforts in TT that are still relevant and appropriate as guidelines (Quinn, 1989): new outcome/efficacy studies, replication of existing studies, and theory development studies. Although a small cadre of researchers has begun the rigorous work of explicating framework and outcomes of TT, much remains to be done. TT researchers must continue to explore the effects of TT in controlled outcome studies, by testing competing theoretical explanations for the outcomes observed, and participating in interdisciplinary efforts related to basic research about the human energy field. Because there are so few clinical situations in which TT outcomes have actually been researched, we should also expect that a significant amount of work will be done using simple descriptive designs, the most appropriate starting point when attempting to study a new area.

TABLE 17.2 Selected Therapeutic Touch Research, 1980–2000

Author/Yr.	Design	N	Variables/Population	Intervention	Control	Result
Heidt, 1981	Experimental pre-posttest	90	Anxiety (STAI)/ cardiac patients	TT	Casual touch; presence	Significant decrease in TT group
Keller & Bzdek, 1986	Experimental pre-posttest	60	Tension headache pain/college students	Non-contact TT (NCTT)	Mimic TT	Significant decrease in TT group immediately after treatment
Quinn, 1984	Experimental pre-posttest	60	Anxiety (STAI)/ cardiac patients	NCTT	Mimic NCTT	Significant decrease in TT group
Quinn & Strelkauskas, 1993	Descriptive pre-posttest; pilot	6	Immune status; anxiety (STAI); positive and negative affect (ABS)/ recently bereaved patients and TT nurses	TT	none	20% mean decreased suppressor T-cells; 29% decreased anxiety; increased positive affect, decreased negative affect in bereaved (not statistically analyzed)
Meehan et al., 1990	Experimental pre-posttest	159	Post-op pain (VAS); analgesia consumption	NCTT with narcotic	Mimic NCTT; standard care	TT group waited significantly longer time before requesting re-medication

(continued)

TABLE 17.2   Selected Therapeutic Touch Research, 1980–2000 (Continued)

Author/Yr.	Design	N	Variables/Population	Intervention	Control	Result
Meehan, 1993	Experimental pre-posttest	108	Post-op pain (VAS)	NCTT with narcotic	Mimic NCTT; standard care	Nonsignificant in pain (p. < .06); TT group waited significantly longer time before requesting re-medication
Simington & Laing, 1993	Experimental posttest only	105	Anxiety (STAI)/ institutionalized older adults	TT with back rub	back rub without TT; mimic TT with back rub	Significant decreases in TT with back-rub group compared to back rub without TT group
Gagne & Toye, 1994	Experimental pre-posttest	31	Anxiety (STAI)/ inpatient psychiatric patients	TT; relaxation therapy	Mimic TT	Significant decreases in anxiety in both TT and relaxation therapy
Peck, 1997	Experimental repeated measures	2	Pain and distress (VAS/older arthritis patients)	TT; progressive muscle relaxation (PMR)	Subjects served as own controls: routine care for baseline	Significant decreases in pain and distress with both TT and PMR
Olson et al., 1997	Experimental pre-posttest	20	T-lymphocyte function (CD25); immuno-globulin level/stressed college students	TT	No treatment	Significant differences in IgA and IgM (immunoglobulins); between groups differences in CD25 non-significant

Study	Design	N	Variables/Population	Intervention	Control	Results
Gordon et al., 1998	Experimental	25	Pain (West Haven-Yale Multidimensional Pain Inventory; VAS); level of functioning (Stanford Health Assessment Questionnaire) general well being (VAS)/ patients with osteoarthritis of knee	TT	Mimic TT; standard care	Significant decrease in pain and increase in functional ability in TT group compared to controls
Lin & Taylor, 1998	Experimental pre-posttest	95	Chronic musculo-skeletal pain (numeric rating scale) anxiety (STAI), salivary cortisol/older adults	TT	Mimic TT; standard care	Significant decrease in pain and anxiety in TT group compared to controls; no differences in cortisol
Peck, 1998	Experimental repeated measures	82	Functional ability (VAS)/older arthritis patients	TT; progressive muscle relaxation (PMR)	Subjects served as own controls: routine care for baseline	Significantly increased functional ability after TT and PMR; significantly better functional ability in TT group

(continued)

TABLE 17.2   Selected Therapeutic Touch Research, 1980–2000 (*Continued*)

Author/Yr.	Design	N	Variables/Population	Intervention	Control	Result
Turner, et al, 1998	Experimental pre-posttest	99	Pain (McGill pain questionnaire); anxiety (VAS); lymphocytes subsets for 11 patients/burn patients	TT	Mimic TT	Significant decrease in pain and anxiety in TT group; decrease in CD8 (suppressor T-cells) and lymphocyte concentration in TT group
Lafreniere, et al, 1999	Experimental pre-posttest	41	Biochemical and mood indicators (multiple measures)/ healthy women	TT	No treatment	Significant decrease in mood disturbance, levels of nitric oxide in TT group

REFERENCES

Cowling, R. W. (1990). A template for unitary pattern-based nursing practice. In E. A. M. Barters (Ed.), *Visions of Rogers' science-based nursing*. New York: National League for Nursing.

Gagne, D., & Toye, R. C. (1994). The effects of therapeutic touch and relaxation therapy in reducing anxiety. *Archives of Psychiatric Nursing, 8*(3), 184–189.

Gordon, A., Merenstein, J. H., D'Amico, F., & Hudgens, D. (1998). The effects of therapeutic touch on patients with osteoarthritis of the knee. *Journal of Family Practice, 47*(4), 271–277.

Grad, B. (1963) A telekinetic effect on plant growth. *International Journal of Parapsychology* , 5, 117–133.

Grad, B. (1964). A telekinetic effect of plant growth II. *International Journal of Parapsychology* , 6, 473–485.

Grad, B. (1965). Some biological effects of the laying-on of hands: Review of experiments with animals and plants. *Journal of the American Society for Psychical Research, 59*, 95–127.

Grad, B., Cadoret, R. J., & Paul, G. I. (1961). An unorthodox method of wound healing in mice. *International Journal of Parapsychology, 3*, 5–24.

Heidt, P. (1981). Effect of therapeutic touch on anxiety level of hospitalized patients. *Nursing Research, 30*, 32–37.

Keller, E., & Bzdek, V. M. (1986). Effects of therapeutic touch on tension headache pain. *Nursing Research, 35*(2), 101–106.

Krieger, D., Peper, E., & Ancoli, S. (1979). Physiologic indices of therapeutic touch. *American Journal of Nursing, 4*, 660–662.

Krieger, D. (1973). The relationship of touch, with intent to help or heal, to subjects' in-vivo hemoglobin values: A study in personalized interaction. *Proceedings, Ninth American Nurses Association Nursing Research Conference, San Antonio, TX*, 39–58.

Krieger, D. (1979). *The therapeutic touch: How to use your hands to help or to heal.* Englewood Cliffs, NJ: Prentice-Hall.

Krieger, D. (1993). *Accepting your power to heal: The personal practice of therapeutic touch.* Santa Fe, NM: Bear.

Lafreniere, K. D., Mutus, B., Cameron, S., Tannous, M., Giannotti, M., Abu-Zahra, H., & Laukkanen, E. (1999). Effects of therapeutic touch on biochemical and mood indicators in women. *Journal of Alternative and Complementary Medicine, 5*(4), 367–70.

Lin, Y., & Taylor, A. G. (1998). Effects of therapeutic touch in reducing pain and anxiety in an elderly population. *Integrative Medicine, 1*(4), 155–62.

Macrae, J. (1988). *Therapeutic touch, a practical guide.* New York: Alfred Knopf.

Meehan, T. C. (1993). Therapeutic touch and postoperative pain: A Rogerian research study. *Nursing Science Quarterly, 6*(2), 69–78.

Meehan, T. C., Mersmann, C. A., Wiseman, M., Wolff, B. B., & Malgady, R. (1990). The effect of therapeutic touch on postoperative pain [Abstract]. *Pain* (Suppl. 5), 149.

Olson, M., Sneed, N., LaVia, M., Virella, G., Bonadonna, R., & Michel, Y. (1997). Stress-induced immunosuppression and therapeutic touch. *Alternative Therapies in Health and Medicine, 3*(2), 68–74.

Peck, S. D. (1997). The effectiveness of therapeutic touch for decreasing pain in elders with degenerative arthritis. *Journal of Holistic Nursing, 15*(2), 176–198.

Peck, S. D. (1998). The efficacy of therapeutic touch for improving functional ability in elders with degenerative arthritis. *Nursing Science Quarterly, 11*(3), 123–132.

Peters, R. M. (1999). The effectiveness of therapeutic touch: A meta-analytic review. *Nursing Science Quarterly, 12*(1), 52–61.

Quinn, J. F: (1984). Therapeutic touch as energy exchange: Testing the theory. *Advances in Nursing Science, 6,* 42–49.

Quinn, J. (1989). Future directions for therapeutic touch research. *Journal of Holistic Nursing, 7*(1), 19–25.

Quinn, J. F. (1992). Holding sacred space: The nurse as healing environment. *Holistic Nursing Practice, 6*(4), 26–35.

Quinn, J. F. (1996). *Therapeutic touch: Healing through human energy fields: A 3-tape video course for health care professionals.* New York: National League for Nursing. [Distributed by HaelanWorks, Boulder, CO.]

Quinn, J. F., & Strelkauskas, A. J. (1993). Psychoneuroimmunological effects of therapeutic touch on practitioners and recently bereaved recipients: A pilot study. *Advances in Nursing Science, 15*(4), 13–26.

Rogers, M. E. (1990). Nursing: Science of unitary, irreducible human beings: Update 1990. In: E. A. M. Barrett, Ed., *Visions of Rogers science-based nursing.* New York: National League for Nursing.

Schwartz, G. E., Russek, L. G., & Beltran, J. (1995). Interpersonal hand-energy registration: Evidence for implicit performance and perception. *Subtle Energies, 6*(3), 183–200.

Simington, J. A., & Laing, G. P. (1993). Effects of therapeutic touch in the institutionalized elderly. *Clinical Nursing Research, 2*(4), 438–450.

Smith, M. J. (1972). Paranormal effects on enzyme activity. *Human Dimensions, 1,* 12–15.

Turner, J. G., Clark, A. J., Gauthier, D. K., & Williams, M. (1998). The effect of therapeutic touch on pain and anxiety in burn patients. *Journal of Advanced Nursing, 28*(1), 10–20.

Warber, S. L., Gillespie, B. W., Kile, G. L., Gorenflo, D., & Bolling, S. F. (in press). Meta-analysis of the effects of therapeutic touch on anxiety symptoms. *Focus on Alternative and Complementary Therapies.*

18

Reiki

Linda L. Halcón

*R*eiki is an energy healing method that can be used as an alternative or complementary therapy for a broad range of acute and chronic health problems. Although anyone can benefit from Reiki, a Canadian study comparing the social characteristics of users of five modes of treatment for various conditions found that persons who used Reiki had higher education levels and were more likely to be employed as professionals or managers than those seeking treatment from medical doctors, chiropractors, acupuncturists, or naturopaths.

Its origins are unclear, but Reiki historians generally agree that this therapy may have its roots in hands-on healing techniques that were used in Tibet or India more than 2,000 years ago. Reiki emerged in modern times around 1900 through the work of a Japanese scholar and businessman, Mikao Usui. According to William Lee Rand, founder of the International Center for Reiki Training (1999), Usui searched many years for knowledge of healing methods that do not deplete the practitioner's personal energy. Finally, after a period of fasting and meditation, he had a profound, transformative experience and received direct revelation of what became known as Reiki. Following this experience, Usui worked with the poor in Kyoto and Tokyo teaching classes and giving treatments in what he called "the Usui system of Reiki healing." One of Dr. Usui's students, Chujiro Hayashi, wrote down the hand positions and suggested ways of using them for various ailments. Hawayo Takata is credited with the spread of Reiki in the Americas and Europe; in 1975, she began to train other Reiki teachers in Hawaii. Although 22 master teachers trained with her, the widespread practice of Reiki was limited until the 1980s, in part because of the high price of training. This situation changed in recent years as Reiki masters made this therapy more accessible to the general public and the healing community.

Reiki is not only a healing technique, but also a philosophy of living that acknowledges mind-body-spirit unity and human connectedness to all things. This philosophy is reflected in the Reiki ethical principles for living:

Just for today I will give thanks for my many blessings.
Just for today I will not worry.
Just for today I will not be angry.
Just for today I will do my work honestly.
Just for today I will be kind to my neighbor and every living thing.
                                                              —(Stein, 1996)

DEFINITION

The word Reiki is composed of two Japanese words—*rei* and *ki. Rei* is usually translated as "universal," although some authors suggest that it also has a deeper connotation of all-knowing spiritual consciousness. *Ki* refers to life force energy, known in certain other parts of the world as *Chi* (qi), *prana*, or *mana*, "the biomagnetic energy of the aura". This life force flows through all living things. When *ki* energy is unrestricted, there is thought to be less susceptibility to illness or imbalances of mind, body or spirit. In its combined form, Reiki is taken to mean spiritually guided life-force energy or universal life-force energy.

The ability to practice using Reiki is transmitted in stages directly from teacher to student via initiations called attunements. The one-on-one attunement process differentiates Reiki from other hands-on healing methods. During attunements, teachers transmit to students specific visual symbols that were revealed to Dr. Usui. These symbols support expansion of the flow of *ki* in the student and allow the student to be a more effective channel for transmitting *ki* to others in treatment sessions. The levels or degrees of attunement allow gradual adjustment to the increased flow of *ki*. The attunements do not give the recipient anything new; rather, they might be compared to gradually increasing the flow of water from a trickle to full flow through a faucet. The water was always flowing, but at a lesser force. In the Usui Reiki tradition, there are generally three degrees of attunement in order to achieve the status of master teacher, at which stage the practitioner is considered fully open to the flow of universal life-force energy. Some teachers may require a period of apprenticeship and integration before students are authorized to practice independently or initiate others. In recent years, additional branches of Reiki with further degrees of attunement have developed; two of these are Karuna Reiki and Reiki Seichim.

SCIENTIFIC BASIS

An emerging body of evidence confirms the existence of energy fields and suggests new ways of measuring energy, although they are not specific to Reiki. Traditional electrical measurements such as electrocardiograms and electroencephalograms can now be supplemented by biomagnetic field mapping to obtain more accurate information about the human condition. Superconducting quantum interference devices have been used to show the effect of disease on the magnetic field of the body, and pulsating magnetic fields have been used to improve healing. In a small experimental study concerning the effects of one type of energy therapy, researchers found consistent, marked decreases in gamma rays measured at several sites within intervention subjects' electromagnetic fields during treatment. To a lesser extent, the findings indicated a decrease also during sham treatment, but not among control subjects. The authors hypothesized that the effect among sham treatment recipients resulted from human touch. Brewitt, Vittetoe, and Hartwell (1997) studied electrical skin resistance at selected body points to measure the effects of Reiki treatments. Charman's research (2000) suggests that intention to heal transmits measurable wave patterns to recipients. Taken together, these studies suggest that in the future it may be possible to directly measure subtle elements of the human energy field in order to elucidate mechanisms by which Reiki and other energy healing techniques lead to changes in health outcomes.

INTERVENTION

The Reiki practitioner acts as a conduit for this healing-intended energy to self or others. During treatments, a practitioner may use various Reiki symbols to focus the *ki* energy. By tradition, the Usui Reiki symbols and their Japanese names are kept confidential. This seems to arise from a sense of their sacred nature rather than proprietary motives, as the symbols are not held to carry power if used by non-initiates. In the second-degree attunement, students are imbued with conscious access to three symbols that can further focus *ki* energy for specific purposes. These are the power symbol, which can increase desirable energy or disperse unwanted energies; the mental-emotional symbol; and the distance-healing symbol. The third degree attunement adds the Reiki master symbol. These symbols are not unique to Reiki and there is some variation in their written form.

VARIOUS TECHNIQUES

Practitioners can apply Reiki with or without direct contact, and they can also use Reiki for distance healing. If touch is contraindicated for any reason, the hands can be held 1 to 4 inches above the body. A full Reiki session usually lasts 60 to 90 minutes. Reiki practitioners, especially if they are nurses working in a clinical setting, often do not have the luxury of providing a full session. At such times, shorter treatments may be offered for specific purposes. Recommendations exist for the use of particular hand positions to address specific health problems. For example, holding the hands over the thymus area has been recommended to stimulate production of T cells.

GUIDELINES FOR FULL HANDS-ON REIKI SESSION

The recipient may sit or lie down, but since Reiki tends to be very relaxing, it is often preferable to lie down. Patients should be advised to wear comfortable clothing for the session. A calm space with soft lighting can aid relaxation, but this is not necessary for the treatment to be effective. After practitioners center themselves and establish intent to heal with Reiki, the energy flows automatically from their hands without cognitive effort. The hands rest gently on the person's body, with the fingers straight and touching so that each hand functions as a unit. Both hands are used, held parallel or one in front of the other. Starting at the head, the practitioner gradually moves down the front of the body and then the back. The sequence of hand positions may vary, but will generally include all seven major chakras and the endocrine glands. The length of time for each hand position is determined by the subjective sensations of the healer. Sensations may include "heat, cold, water flowing, vibrating, trembling, magnetism, static electricity, tingling, color, sound, or (extremely rare) pain" (Stein, 1996). These sensations crescendo and subside generally in 3 to 5 minutes, after which the practitioner moves to the next position.

MEASUREMENT OF OUTCOMES

Recipients' subjective feelings during a Reiki session are not considered indications of effectiveness. Patients may feel sensations similar to those of the practitioner, but they may feel nothing. Physiologic outcome measures examined in other healing touch studies are also appropriate for Reiki, such as hematologic tests, blood pressure and heart rate, bioelectric measures, wound healing rate, inhibition of harmful microorganisms, and body temperature changes. Psychological measures are equally important, including perceived pain, cognitive function, memory and levels of anxiety, depression, anxiety, or hostility.

PRECAUTIONS

No serious adverse effects of Reiki treatments have been published. Some patients, however, may experience emotional release that can feel uncomfortable or even frightening. Therefore, practitioners must be prepared to provide assistance and appropriate referrals if emotional distress persists. Moreover, some individuals may dislike being touched. Practitioners can avoid this discomfort by assessing the person's comfort level with touch and by taking into account gender and cultural considerations. One way to do this is to describe the hand placements beforehand and alter or omit those that might cause discomfort or distress. The success of a Reiki treatment does not depend on the use of certain hand positions, for the *ki* energy goes where it is needed. Few patients who are fully informed object, and even among vulnerable populations such as adolescent psychiatric patients, responses to hands-on energy healing methods have been found to be very favorable..

USES

Increasingly, nurses are using Reiki in their practice. It can be employed in any practice setting to enhance healing and wellness. Besides offering treatment sessions to patients, nurses can use Reiki for self-care and to avoid burnout, to increase touch sensitivity, and to increase perception and assessment skills. The range of potential practical applications with patients is broad and depends on the setting. Table 18.1 provides a list of populations and settings in which Reiki has been used. In a biomedical treatment setting, Reiki is best seen as a complementary healing modality, whereas in other circumstances it can either be used alone or with other approaches.

FUTURE RESEARCH

Most published research on Reiki has been conducted with small, non-controlled, convenience samples, raising questions about the validity of findings and whether they can be generalized. Such studies have measured the effects of Reiki on hematocrit and hemoglobin levels, as well as blood urea nitrogen and glucose levels (Wirth, Chang, Eidelman, & Paxton, 1996) and the

TABLE 18.1   Suggested Applications for Reiki in Clinical Settings

Application	Reference
Promoting relaxation in labor and delivery	Buenting, 1993
Enhancing the effectiveness of dialysis	Tattum, 1994
Supporting pre- and post-operative surgical patients	Alandydy & Alandydy, 1999
	Swayer, 1998
Palliative care for cancer patients	Starn, 1998
	Bullock, 1997
Pain management	Dressen & Singg, 2000
	Olson & Hanson, 1997
Decreasing anxiety and stress levels	Dressen & Singg, 2000
	Neklason, 1987
	Thornton, 1996
Enhancing immune function	Brewitt et al., 1997
	Van Sell, 1996
Promoting wound healing	Papantonio, 1998
Respiratory problems	Chan, 1999
Addiction and chemical dependency treatment	Burkert, 1999
Improving hematologic measures	Wetzel, 1989; Wirth et al., 1996

results are positive and intriguing despite methodological limitations. In the area of mental health there have been small studies of Reiki's effects on anxiety, depression, and hostility, and one larger experimental study of effects on mood level and personality characteristics. This study, as well as others, have investigated the impact of Reiki treatments on pain and the course of chronic illnesses such as fibromyalgia.

The growing body of experimental evidence on therapeutic touch and other energy healing methods suggests that similar research on Reiki is possible. Mansour, Beuche, Lang, Leis, & Nurse (1999) published methods for conducting randomized controlled trials of Reiki outcomes that can be used to plan other experiments. Combining subjective and physiological measures in such research studies will allow a broad assessment of the Reiki's effects. Because the goals of Reiki may be broader than symptom relief and include concepts of physiologic and psychological balance, qualitative studies that can address values and meaning are also important. Suggested questions for future research include the following:

- What are the physiologic and psychological effects of Reiki treatments for specific conditions, either used alone or with other measures?
- Are there differences in selected outcome measures between Reiki and other forms of treatment?
- What groups of people are more likely to experience positive effects from Reiki treatments?
- What are the mechanisms of action underlying Reiki?

REFERENCES

Alandydy, P., & Alandydy, K. (1999). Performance brief: Using Reiki to support surgical patients. *Journal of Nursing Care Quality, 13*(4), 89–91.

Benford, M. S., Talnagai, J., Doss, D. B., Boosey, S., & Arnold, L. E. (1999). Gamma radiation fluctuations during alternative healing therapy. *Alternative Therapies,* 5(4), 51–56.

Brewitt, B., Vittetoe, T., & Hartwell, B. (1997). The efficacy of Reiki hands-on healing: Improvements in spleen and nervous system function as quantified by electrodermal screening. *Alternative Therapies, 3*(4), 89.

Brown, C. K. (2000). Methodological problems of clinical research into spiritual healing: The healer's perspective. *Journal of Alternative and Complementary Medicine, 6*(2), 171–176.

Buenting, J. A. (1993). Human energy fields and birth: Implications for research and practice. *Advances in Nursing Science, 15*(4), 53–59.

Bullock, M. (1997). Reiki: A complementary therapy for life. *American Journal of Hospice and Palliative Care, 14*(1), 31–33.

Burkert, L. (1999). *Reiki for the recovering alcoholic and addict.* International Center for Reiki Training. [on-line] [2000, August 22]. Available: http://www.reiki. org/reikinews/reikin20.html.

Chan, P. (1999). *Reiki and the conventional health care provider: Recommendations and potholes.* International Center for Reiki Training. [on-line] [2000, August 22]. Available: http://www.reiki.org/reikiews/reikin10.html.

Charman, R. A. (2000). Placing healers, healees, and healing into a wider research context. *Journal of Alternative and Complementary Medicine, 6*(2), 177–180.

Dressen, L. J., & Singg, S. (2000). Effects of Reiki on pain and selected affective and personality variables of chronically ill patients. *Subtle Energies and Energy Medicine, 9*(1), 51–82.

Herron, D. (2000). *History of Reiki* [on-line] [2000, August 22]. Available: http://reiki.7gen.com/history.html.

Hughes, P. P., Meize-Grochowski, R., & Harris, C. N. D. (1996). Therapeutic touch with adolescent psychiatric patients. *Journal of Holistic Nursing, 14*(1), 6–23.

Kelner, M., & Wellman, B. (1997). Who seeks alternative health care? A profile of the users of five modes of treatment. *Journal of Alternative and Complementary Therapies, 3*(2), 127–140.

Lipinski, K. (1999). *Enhancing nursing practice with Reiki.* International Center for Reiki Training. [on-line] [2000, August 22]. Available: http://www.reiki.org/reikinews/Nursingand Reiki.html.

Liverani, A., Minelli, E., & Ricciuti, A. (2000). Subjective scales for the evaluation of therapeutic effects and their use in complementary medicine. *Journal of Alternative and Complementary Medicine, 6*(3), 257–264.

Mansour, A. A., Beuche, M., Laing, G., Leis, A., & Nurse, J. (1999). A study to test the effectiveness of placebo Reiki standardization procedures developed for a planned Reiki efficacy study. *Journal of Alternative and Complementary medicine, 5*(2), 153–164.

Mitchell, A. (2000). Researching healing: A psychologist's perspective. *Journal of Alternative and Complementary Medicine, 6*(2), 181–186.

Neklason, Z. T. (1987). *The effects of Reiki treatment on telepathy and personality traits.* Unpublished master's thesis. California State University, Hayward.

Olson, K., & Hanson, J. (1997). The effect of Reiki in the management of pain: A preliminary report. *Cancer Prevention Control, 1,* 108–113.

Oschman, J. L., & Oschman, N. H. (1999). *Science measures the human energy field.* International Center for Reiki Training. [on-line] [2000, August 22]. Available: http://www.reiki.org/reikinews/ScienceMeasures.thm.

Papantonio, C. (1998). Alternative medicine and wound healing. *Ostomy/Wound Management, 44*(4), 44–55.

Rand, W. L. (1991). *Reiki: The healing touch: First and second degree manuals* (Rev. ed.). Southfield, MI: Vision.

Rand, W. L. (1999). *Usui Reiki symbols.* International Center for Reiki Training. [on-line] [2000, August 28]. Available: http://www.reiki.org/reikinews/usuisym.html.

Rand, W. L. (2000). *What is the history of Reiki?* International Center for Reiki Training. [on-line] [2000, August 8] Available: http://www.reiki.org/FAQ/HistoryOfReiki.html.

Rand, W. L., & Gifford, L. E. (1999). *Discovering the roots of Reiki.* International Center for Reiki Training. [on-line] [2000, August 22]. Available: http://www.reiki.org/reikinews/roots/rootsreiki.html.

Sawyer, J. (1998). The first Reiki practitioner in our OR. *AORN Journal, 67*(3), 674–676.

Starn, J. R. (1998). Energy healing with women and children. *JOGNN, 27*(5), 576–584.

Stein, D. (1996). *Essential Reiki: A complete guide to an ancient healing art.* Freedom, CA: The Crossing Press.

Tattum, A. (1994). Reiki: Healing and dealing. *Australian Nursing Journal, 2*(2), 3, 52.

Thornton, L. M. (1996). A study of Reiki, an energy treatment, using Roger's science. *Rogerian Nursing Science News, 8,* 14–15.

Van Sell, S. L. (1996). Reiki: An ancient touch therapy, *RN, 59*(2), 57–59.

Wetzel, W. S. (1989). Reiki healing: A physiologic perspective. *Journal of Holistic Nursing, 7*(1), 47–54.

Wirth, D. P., Chang, R. J., Eidelman, W. S., & Paxton, J. B. (1996). Hematological indicators of complementary healing intervention. *Complementary Therapies in Medicine, 4,* 4–20.

19

Acupressure

Pamela Weiss

Touch has been central to the practice of nursing since its inception. This chapter will discuss a traditional Chinese medicine form of touch known as acupressure and its application in nursing care. This method of treatment is common in many cultures. As Dossey, Keegan, and Guzzetta (2000) note, "All cultures have demonstrated that some form of rubbing, pressing, massaging or holding are natural manifestations of the desire to heal and care for one another" (p. 615). Acupressure is also integral to the practice of *shiatsu, tui na, tsubo,* and *jin si ju jitsyu.*

DEFINITIONS

Acupressure is defined by Gach (1990) as "an ancient healing art that uses the fingers to press certain points on the body to stimulate the body's self-curative abilities" (p. 3). To assist the reader, the following other definitions are provided.

Acupuncture: One of the treatment modalities of traditional Chinese medicine in which fine sterile needles are inserted into specific points on the body. It is a treatment of greater intensity than acupressure.
Auriculotherapy: Needling or pressure to ear points.
Jin Shin Jyutsu: A gentle acupressure type of massage for self-care.
Meridians: A traditional Chinese medicine term for the pathways throughout the body for the flow of *qi*, or vital energy, accessed through acupuncture points.

Moxibustion: The method of burning mugwort (an herb) directly on the
skin, on the needle, or in a tool to stimulate acupuncture points.

Qi: Pronounced "chee," the life force or vital force.

Shiatsu: Finger pressure stimulation of acupuncture points and meridians to stimulate the movement of qi.

TRADITIONAL CHINESE MEDICINE

Traditional Chinese Medicine (TCM) is an ancient system of health developed more than 3,000 years ago in Asia. This system is based on the concept
that *qi* that flows throughout the body and that balance of yin and yang forces
represents health and well being. As Kaptchuk (1983) describes it,

> This system of care is based on ancient texts and is the result of a continuous
> process of critical thinking, as well as extensive clinical observation and test-
> ing. It represents a thorough formulation and reformulation of material by
> respected clinicians and theoreticians. It is also, however, rooted in the phi-
> losophy, logic and sensibility, and habits of a civilization entirely foreign to our
> own. It has therefore developed its own perception of the body and health and
> disease. (p. 2)

The focus of care within this system is to restore balance in the body. To
do so, yin and yang must be balanced. Yin aspects are associated with cold,
passivity, interiority, and decreases. Yang aspects are associated with warmth,
activity, external forces, and increases. Yin and yang are always in relation to
each other (Kaptchuk, 1983). According to this conceptualization, yin and
yang are in continuous flux and there is always yin within yang and yang
within yin.

Unschuld (1999) reflects that TCM theory is a mixture of beliefs that
pathogenic influences from the outside combine with the lack of balance or
harmony within the person and result in illness. TCM is also concerned with
the concept of *qi* . Qi flows in the body through specific pathways identified
as meridians or channels. If the *qi* is blocked or diminished, a person experiences pain or illness.

There are 12 bilateral meridians and 8 extra meridians. All meridians have
an exterior and an interior pathway and are named according to the organ
system. Located on the meridians are specific points. In the 12 major meridians, the points are bilateral and in the West called acupuncture points. This
nomenclature implies that the points are designated for needle insertion and
does not fully reflect the TCM concept of the point.

Acupuncture points are used for acupressure. The points do not have a
corresponding anatomic structure but are described by their location relative

to other anatomical landmarks. This contributes to the skepticism of many Western-trained scientists about their existence. In Chinese, the name of the point usually is descriptive of its function or location. Mistranslation over the years has often limited the substantial amount of anatomical basis for the nomenclature of points and the apparent knowledge of anatomy of Chinese scholars (Schnorrenberger, 1996).

There are 365 (Kaptchuk, 1983) to 700 (Jwing-Ming, 1992) major points on the meridians. Jwing-Ming stated that 108 could be stimulated using the fingers. In a traditionally formulated TCM treatment plan, whether the modality is needles or pressure, the points are combined to achieve maximum benefit for the patient. Rarely is only one point used. There are points that should not be stimulated, especially during pregnancy, and are referred to as "forbidden points."

SCIENTIFIC BASIS

"Western" medicine is the dominant system of health care in the United States. It is characterized by hospitals, clinics, pharmaceutical resources and by a work force of physicians, nurses, specialized therapists, and various support service personnel. There are many differences between Western medicine and TCM, which become more evident as nurses seek to add TCM modalities to their practice. Western medicine emphasizes disease, causal agents, and treatments that are designed to control or destroy the cause of disease (Kaptchuk, 1983). Once a causal agent or mechanism is identified, treatment plans are developed that focus on the agent or mechanism as a consistent factor in all human manifestations of the disease. In Western journals, almost all studies using the modality of acupuncture and acupressure emphasize the specific effects of needling one point known to address a specific symptom; medical researchers are eager to find the mechanism by which acupuncture alleviates the symptoms and some of the mechanisms have been suggested in Western medical research (National Institutes of Health [NIH]), NCCAM, 2000). Stimulation of the points with needles or with pressure may produce a therapeutic effect due to the following:

1. Conduction of electromagnetic signals that may start the flow of pain-killing biochemicals, such as endorphins, and of immune system cells to specific sites in the body that are injured or vulnerable to disease (Dale, 1997; Takeshige, 1989)
2. Activation of opioid systems thereby reducing pain (Han, 1997)

3. Changes in brain chemistry, sensation, and involuntary responses by changing the release of neurotransmitters and neurohormones in a health promoting way (Wu, Zhou, & Zhou, 1994; Wu, 1995).

The scientific research into an underlying mechanism demonstrates one of the differences between Western medicine and the TCM system. The focus in TCM is the imbalance in the patient, and the causality of is always multifactorial. The function of the points is described in terms of TCM diagnosis. For example, Western medicine research has focused on pericardium 6, or *nei guan*, for the treatment of nausea. In English its name means inner border gate. Lade (1986) describes the point:

> The name refers to the point's role as the gateway or connecting point of the triple burner channel and the yin linking vessel. Inner refers to the palmar aspect of the forearm and to the point's location on the yin channel. The actions of this point are: to regulate and tonify the heart, transform heart phlegm, facilitate *qi* flow, regulate the yin-linking vessel and clear heart fire, redirect rebellious *qi* downward, expand and relax the chest and benefit the diaphragm (p. 196). The indications for use of the point are: asthma, bronchitis, pertussis, hiccups, vomiting, diaphragmatic spasms, intercostal neuralgia, chest fullness, and pain and dyspnea. (p. 197)

While Western medicine focuses on the treatment of nausea for this point, the TCM paradigm suggests multiple uses. In TCM theory, nausea is considered rebellious *qi* (*qi* that flows in the wrong direction). Nausea and vomiting are examples of this. *Nei guan* (pericardium 6) is used as one of the points in the treatment of a patient who presents with nausea. In TCM theory, nausea is considered one of the external manifestations of the imbalance, but in an authentic TCM treatment, a TCM practitioner would evaluate the imbalances that set up the manifestation and would treat the underlying condition. Therefore, a combination of points to treat nausea would be used, possibly including other primary points for antiemesis (Hoo, 1997): S 36 on the stomach meridian located on the knee; ren 12 on the ren/conceptional meridian located on the upper abdomen; or the Sp 4 on the spleen meridian located on the foot. Application of multiple acupoints may be more effective for the treatment of nausea; however, in Western medicine, the focus of finding the single active point or the mechanism creates an almost insurmountable challenge to the fullest application of the therapy.

In 1997, the National Institutes of Health held the first consensus conference on acupuncture. The conference concluded that

Acupuncture is effective in the treatment of adult nausea and vomiting in chemotherapy and probably pregnancy and in postoperative dental pain. The conference members stated there is an indication that acupuncture may be helpful in the treatment of addiction, stroke rehabilitation, headache, menstrual cramps, tennis elbow, fibromyalgia, myofascial pain, osteoarthritis, low back pain, carpal tunnel syndrome, and asthma, in which acupuncture may be useful as an adjunct treatment or an acceptable alternative or be included in a comprehensive management program. (NIH, 1997).

Research evidence underlying the use of the point called *nei guan* (pericardium 6) for nausea is reviewed below. Table 19.1 indicates just a few studies of the effect of this point on nausea.

There are many limitations to the research done in acupuncture and therefore acupressure. Harris (1997) states that

The scientific quality of most of the published studies examining the effectiveness of multipoint acupressure, predominantly auriculotherapy, has been poor, without adequate control groups, randomization, placebos, blinding, and statistical analyses. There seems to be a cultural divide between theory and methodological rigor. The scientifically rigorous studies have tended to be atheoretical in selecting the acupoint for treatment and in explaining how the points may work. (p. 157)

Table 19.2 presents a brief overview of recent studies examining the use of acupuncture and acupressure in a variety of populations

INTERVENTION

A diagnostic process is used to choose the correct points to stimulate. In TCM, the process includes an extensive history, observing the patient's appearance and demeanor, noticing the patient's odor, checking the tongue, palpating the abdomen, points on the body, and palpating the pulses at the radial location on the wrists. A diagnosis is developed and a treatment plan is implemented and may use a variety of techniques. Nurses will not follow this process and will therefore be using a Western symptom-based system of determining the correct treatment plan.

GUIDELINES FOR USE

Nurses can incorporate acupressure into the care of patients by using some common points that have specific actions to relieve common symptoms. The

TABLE 19.1   Sample of Studies Using P 6 for Treating Nausea

Condition Causing the Nausea	Modality: Acupressure/ Acupuncture	Author/Date	Conclusion
Morning sickness	Acupressure	Bayreuther, Lewith, & Pickering (1994)	Acupressure reduced nausea of participants.
Dental procedures	Acupressure	Chate, 1998	Of the 13 patients who completed the study, acupressure on P 6 did not relieve the nausea better than sham point.
Nausea of chemotherapy	Acupressure on P 6 and ST 36	Dibble, Chapman, Mack, & Shih (2000)	During the first 10 days of the chemotherapy cycle, women with breast cancer who were taught and practiced acupressure of P 6 experienced a decreased intensity and frequency of nausea.
Postoperative nausea	Acupressure	McConaghy, Bland, & Swales (1996)	Patients treated with P 6 acupressure had a greater mean improvement in their visual analog score for nausea.
All nausea studies (review)	Acupuncture/ acupressure	Jewell & Young (2000); Cochrane Collaborative (2000)	The studies on nausea are limited and the results are equivocal.

TABLE 19.2   Review of Effective Uses of Acupuncture/Acupressure

Condition	Modality: Acupressure/ Acupuncture	Author/Date	Conclusion
Wandering behaviors in Alzheimer's	Acupressure	Sutherland, Reakes, & Bridges (1999)	Foot acupressure may have produced a decrease in wandering, pulse and respirations, and an increase in quiet time.
Angina	Acupuncture as an addition to pharmacological intervention to reduce costs	Ballegaard, Johannessen, Karpatschof, & Nyboe, (1999)	The addition of acupuncture and self-care education was found to be cost beneficial in patients with advanced angina pectoris.
Effect on cardiovascular system	Active stimulation consisting of pressure on acupoints (P); active stimulation consisting of stroking along the meridians (S); or a control stimulation	Felhendler & Lisander (1999)	The acupressure group differed significantly from the control group and the stroking-only group demonstrating a decrease in systolic and diastolic arterial pressure, mean arterial pressure, heart rate, and skin blood flow. Pressure on acupoints can significantly influence the cardiovascular system.
Constipation	Pressing of a stimulating seed at appropriate acupressure points	Ma (1999), (Case study reports only; no controls or rigorous design)	Of 123 patients all but 6 had improvement.
Postoperative pain/knee arthroscopy	Stimulated 15 classical acupoints in the active stimulation group, on the side	Felhendler & Lisander (1996)	The results indicate that pressure on acupoints can decrease postoperative pain.

(continued)

TABLE 19.2   Review of Effective Uses of Acupuncture/Acupressure (*Continued*)

Condition	Modality: Acupressure/ Acupuncture	Author/Date	Conclusion
(cont.)	contralateral to surgery, with a firm pressure and a gliding movement across the acupoint		
Posttraumatic somatic pain	Auricular acupressure	Tekeoglu, Adak, & Ercan (1996)	The auriculopressure group increase in pain threshold was statistically significant. These results suggest that auriculopressure could be a useful method for suppression of posttraumatic somatic pain.
Patello-femoral pain syndrome	Acupuncture	Jensen, Gothesen, Liseth, & Baerheim (1999)	Acupuncture may be an alternative treatment for patello-femoral pain syndrome.
Rheumatoid arthritis	Acupuncture	David, Townsend, Sathanathan, Kriss, & Dore (1999)	Acupuncture cannot be considered a useful adjunct to therapy in patients with RA.
Osteoarthritis of the knee	Acupuncture	Berman et al. (1999)	Acupuncture is an effective and safe adjunctive therapy to conventional care for patients with OA of the knee.
Frozen shoulder	Acupuncture	Tukmachi (1999)	No control group, but treatment group had a high level of improvement.

TABLE 19.2 *(Continued)*

Condition	Modality: Acupressure/ Acupuncture	Author/Date	Conclusion
Pain in labor	Acupuncture	Kvorning, Buchhave, Svensson, & Akeson (1998)	Acupuncture reduces the use of other methods of labor analgesia with no major side effects in mothers or infants.
Breech presentation	Moxibustion	Berman, Singh, Lao, Langenberg, et al. (1998)	Among prima-gravidas with breech presentation during the 33rd week of gestation, moxibustion for 1 to 2 weeks increased fetal activity during the treatment period and cephalic presentation after the treatment period.

nurse can treat the patient with acupressure or teach the patient or family members how to use acupressure as part of a care plan.

Prior to touching any patient, the nurse must assess the readiness of the client. Shames and Keegan (2000) recommend the following assessment of clients:

- perception of mind-body situation
- pathophysiological problems that may require referral
- history of psychological disorders
- cultural beliefs about touch
- previous experience with body therapies (p. 624)

Each point is a located using an anatomical marker. There are many books describing point location. The standard measure is the *cun*, which is different for each individual. One *cun* for a particular patient is defined as the "width of the interphalangeal joint of the patient's thumb or as the distance between the two radial ends of the flexor creases of a flexed middle finger of the patient. Two *cun* is the width of the index finger, the middle finger and the ring finger (Ho, 1997).

Stimulating the Point

There are several different types of techniques to stimulate the points according to Gach (1990):

- *Firm pressure* using the thumbs, fingers, palms, the sides of hands, or knuckles using a firm stationary pressure
- *Slow motion kneading* using the thumbs and fingers along with the heels of the hands to squeeze large muscle groups
- *Brisk rubbing* using friction to stimulate the blood and lymph
- *Quick tapping* with the fingertips stimulates muscles on unprotected areas of the body such as the face (p. 9)

EVALUATING ACUPRESSURE'S EFFECT

Gach (1990) has developed guidelines for the assessing results. The elements of the assessment include:

- Identifying the problems being addressed with acupressure
- Identifying the points being used for the treatment
- The length of time for the acupressure
- Identifying what makes the condition worse (e.g., standing, cold weather, menstruation, constipation, lack of exercise, stress, traveling, and other)
- Describing the changes experienced by the patient after 3 days and after one full week of treatment
- Describing the changes in the condition and overall feeling of well-being (p. 13)

USES

There are many uses for acupressure. Some conditions for which it has been used are shown in Table 19-2. The use of acupuncture for nausea, pain, and gastrointestinal disorders is described below.

NAUSEA

Point: Pericardium 6 (nei guan, "inner gate")

Location: Pericardium 6 is located on the inner aspect of the wrist 2 *cun* (units) proximal to the transverse crease of the wrist between the tendons of the palmaris longus and flexor carpi radialis muscles (Lade, 1986). Have the patient place the middle three fingers (index, middle, and ring fingers) on the opposite hand that is palm upward. The point under the ring finger between the two tendons is pericardium 6 (see Figure 19.1).

Functions: Its functions were outlined previously in the discussion on the research on this point.

Method of stimulation: The point can be stimulated using firm pressure either with a rotating pattern with the thumb or the static pressure of a Sea Band (elastic bands with a small imbedded plastic button that can be applied to the wrist).

Indications in nursing: This point can be used for the treatment of nausea in many situations, but research as cited previously has focused on postoperative nausea, the nausea of pregnancy, and the nausea accompanying chemotherapy.

PAIN AND GASTROINTESTINAL DISORDERS

Point: Large intestine 4 (LI 4) (hoku, "joining the valley")

Location: This point is on the back of the hand halfway between the junction between the first and second metacarpal bones, which form a depression or valley when the thumb is abducted (Lade, 1986). There are two ways to easily locate this point. Have the patient hold the hand with the thumb touching the index finger; hold the hand at eye level and the highest mound at the base of the thumb and index finger is the location of LI 4. Or instruct the patient to place the thumb of one hand in the web between the thumb and index finger of the opposite hand. The patient should match the first crease on the thumb of one hand to the web of the other and then rotate the thumb to touch the fleshy area between the index finger and thumb. The point is where the tip of the thumb touches the area between the thumb and the index finger.

Functions: This point has multiple functions and is one of the most important points of the body. It alleviates pain, tones *qi*, and protective *qi* (in Western medicine this would be considered an immune system building function); moistens the large intestine and in so doing relieves diarrhea or constipation; clears the nose, regulates the lungs in asthma, bronchitis, or the common cold; and expedites labor. This point is contraindicated in early pregnancy because of this function (Lade, 1986, pp. 40–41).

Indications in nursing: This point will relieve any pain in the body. In addition, persons with diarrhea or constipation may receive relief because

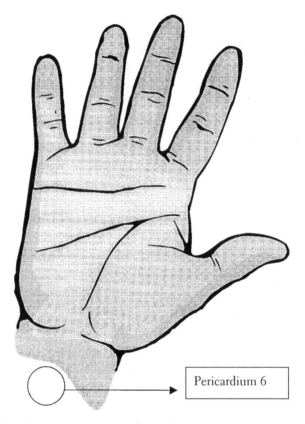

FIGURE 19.1 Pressure point pericardium 6.

stimulating the point balances the gastrointestinal functions. This point can be used to induce labor and coupled with its pain relieving effect may be useful.

Method of stimulation: Firm pressure can be applied on this point with a rotating thumb massage technique. This point is often sensitive and the patient will report the feeling of discomfort. This is normal and not indicative of a problem.

PRECAUTIONS

There are overall guidelines and precautions carefully outlined by Michael Reed Gach (1990) in his book, *Acupressure Potent Points.*

- Never press any area in an abrupt, forceful or jarring way.
- Use abdominal points cautiously especially if you are ill. Avoid the abdominal area altogether if patient has a life-threatening disease, especially intestinal cancer, tuberculosis, or leukemia. Avoid the abdominal area during pregnancy.
- During pregnancy, strong stimulation of certain points should be avoided: LI 4 (four point on the large intestine meridian), K 3 (third point on the kidney meridian), and SP 6 (sixth point on the spleen meridian). Each of these points may have an effect on the pregnancy (p. 192).
- Lymph areas such as the groin, the area of the throat just below the ears, and the outer breast near the armpits are very sensitive. Touch these areas lightly.
- Do not work directly on a serious burn or ulcer or area of infection.
- Do not work directly on a newly formed scar. New surgical or other wounds should not be touched directly. Continuous holding on the periphery of the injury will stimulate the injury to heal.
- After an acupressure treatment, tolerance to cold is lowered and the energy of the body is focused on healing, so advise the patient to wear warm clothes and keep out of drafts (p. 193).
- Apply finger pressure in a slow, rhythmic manner to enable the layers of tissue and the internal organs to respond.
- Use cautiously in persons with a new acute or serious illness.
- Acupressure is not a sole treatment for cancer, contagious skin disease, or sexually transmitted disease (Gach, 1990, pp. 11–12).
- Brisk rubbing, deep pressure, or kneading should not be used for persons with heart disease, cancer, or high blood pressure (Gach, 1990, p. 9).

FUTURE RESEARCH

There are many areas of future research in which the methods of traditional Chinese medicine and the underlying theory can be tested using Western medical research techniques. Research questions about the usefulness of acupressure techniques can be posed in many areas of nursing including the use of acupressure for palliative care, rehabilitation nursing, support of women in labor, and health promotion and disease prevention.

Acupressure is used by millions of persons around the world. Incorporating this technique into nursing care plans will unite us in the commonality we share—the desire to relieve human suffering (Serizawa, 1976).

REFERENCES

Ballegaard, S., Johannessen, A., Karpatschof, B., & Nyboe, J., (1999). Addition of acupuncture and self-care education in the treatment of patients with severe angina pectoris may be cost beneficial: An open, prospective study. *Journal of Alternative and Complementary Medicine, 5*, 405–413.

Bayreuther, J., Lewith, G. T., & Pickering, R. (1994). A double blind crossover study to evaluate the effectiveness of acupressure at pericardium 6 (P 6) in the treatment of early morning sickness (EMS). *Complementary Therapies in Medicine 2*, 70–76.

Berman, B. M., Singh, B. B., Lao. L., Langenberg, P., Li, H., Hadhazy, V., Bareta, J., Cardini, F., & Weixin, H. (1998). Moxibustion for correction of breech presentation: A randomized controlled trial. *Journal of the American Medical Association, 280*(18), 1580–1584.

Chate, R. A. (1998). PC.6 Acupressure for dental nausea: A prospective randomized double blind clinical trial with crossover (Pt. 2). *Acupuncture in Medicine,16*(2), 69–72.

Cho, Z. H., Chung, S. C., Jones, J. P., Park, J. B., Park, H. J., Lee, H. J., Wong, E. K., & Min, B. I. (1998). New findings of the correlation between acupoints and corresponding brain cortices using functional MRI. *Proceedings of the National Academy of Science, U.S.A. 95*, 2670–2673.

Cochrane Collaborative. (2000). Overview of Cochrane Collaborative [on-line]. Available: http://www.cochrane.de/cochrane/cc-broch.htm#CC

Dale, R. A. (1997). Demythologizing acupuncture, part 1: The scientific mechanisms and the clinical uses. *Alternative and Complementary Therapies Journal, 3*(2), 125–131.

David, J., Townsend, S., Sathanathan, R., Kriss, S., & Dore, C. J. (1999). The effect of acupuncture in patients with rheumatoid arthritis. A randomized placebo-controlled cross-over study. *Rheumatology (Oxford), 38*, 864–869.

Dibble, S. L., Chapman, J., Mack, K. A., & Shih, A. S. (2000). Acupressure for nausea: Results of a pilot study. *Oncology Nursing Forum, 27*(1), 41–47.

Dossey, B. M., Keegan, L., & Guzzetta, C. E. (2000). *Holistic nursing: A handbook for practice.* Gaithersburg, MD: Aspen.

Felhendler, D., & Lisander, B. (1996). Pressure on acupoints decreases postoperative pain. *Clinical Journal of Pain, 12*(4), 326–329.

Felhendler, D., & Lisander, B. (1999). Effects of non-invasive stimulation of acupoints on the cardiovascular system. *Complementary Therapies in Medicine, 7*(4), 231–234.

Gach, M. (1990). *Acupressure potent points.* New York: Bantam Books

Han, J. S. (1997). Acupuncture activates endogenous systems of analgesia. *National Institutes of Health Consensus Conference on Acupuncture: Program and Abstracts.* Bethesda, MD: National Institutes of Health

Harris, P. E. (1997). Acupressure: A review of the literature. *Complementary Therapies in Medicine, 5*(3), 156–161.

Hochberg, M. (1999). A randomized trial of acupuncture as an adjunctive therapy in osteoarthritis of the knee. *Rheumatology* 3(4), 346–354.

Hoo, J. J. (1997). Acupressure for hyperemesis gravidarum. *American Journal of Obstetrics and Gynecology, 176*(6), 1395–1396.

Jewell, D., & Young G. (2001). *Interventions for nausea and vomiting in early pregnancy.* The Cochrane Library (Oxford).

Jensen, R., Gothesen, O., Liseth, K., & Baerheim, A. (1999). Acupuncture treatment of patellofemoral pain syndrome. *Journal of Alternative and Complementary Medicine, 5*(6), 521–527.

Jwing-Ming, Y. (1992). *Chinese qigong massage.* Jamaica Plain, MA: Yangs' Martial Arts Association.

Kaptchuk, T. J. (1983). *The web that has no weaver.* New York: Congdon & Weed.

Kvorning, T. N., Buchhave, P., Svensson, G., & Akeson, J. (1998). Acupuncture during childbirth reduces use of conventional analgesia without major adverse effects: A retrospective study. *American Journal of Acupuncture, 26*(4), 233–239.

Lade, A. (1986) *Images and functions.* Seattle, WA: Eastland Press.

Ma, J. (1999). Ear point pressing in treatment of constipation: Clinical observation of 123 cases. *International Journal of Clinical Acupuncture,10*(1), 69–72.

McConaghy, P., Bland, D., & Swales, H. (1996). Acupuncture in the management of postoperative nausea and vomiting in patients receiving morphine via a patient-controlled analgesia system. *Acupuncture in Medicine, 14*(1), 2–5.

National Center for Complementary/Alternative Medicines. (2000). Acupuncture information and resources [on-line] http://nccam.nih.gov/fcp/factsheets/acupuncture/acupuncture.htm

National Institutes of Health. (1997). NIH Consensus Development conferencs Statement. Acupuncture. [on-line] http://odp.od.nih.gov/consensus/cons/107/107_statement.htm.

Schnorrenberger, C. C. (1996). Morphological foundations of acupuncture: An anatomical nomenclature of acupuncture structures. *Acupuncture in Medicine, 14*(2), 89–103.

Shames, K. H., & Keegan, L. (2000). Touch: Connecting with the healing power in 2000. In B. Dossey, L. Keegan, & C. E. Guzzetta (Eds.), *Holistic nursing* (3rd ed., pp 613–635). Gaithersberg, MD: Aspen.

Serizawa, K. (1976). *Tsubo.* Tokyo: Japan Publications.

Sutherland, J. A., Reakes, J., & Bridges, C. (1999). Foot acupressure and massage for patients with Alzheimer's disease and related dementias. *Image: The Journal of Nursing Scholarship, 31*(4), 347–348.

Takeshige, C. (1989). *Mechanism of acupuncture analgesia based on animal experiments: Scientific bases of acupuncture.* Berlin, Germany: Springer-Verlag.

Tekeoglu, I., Adak, B., & Ercan, M. (1996). Suppression of experimental pain by auriculopressure. *Acupuncture in Medicine, 14*(1), 16–18.

Tukmachi, E. S. (1999). Frozen shoulder: A comparison of western and traditional Chinese approaches and a clinical study of its acupuncture treatment. *Acupuncture in Medicine, 17*(1), 9–21.

Unschuld, P. (1999). The past 1,000 years of Chinese medicine. *Lancet*, *354*(Suppl.), SIV9.

Wu, B., Zhou, R. X., & Zhou, M. S. (1994). Effect of acupuncture on interleukin-2 level and NK cell immunoactivity of peripheral blood of malignant tumor patients. *Chung Kuo Chung Hsi I Chieh Ho Tsa Chich*, *14*(9), 537–539.

Wu, B. (1995). Effect of acupuncture on the regulation of cell-mediated immunity in patients with malignant tumors. *Chen Tzu Yen Chiu Acupuncture Research*, *20*(3), 67–71.

PART IV

Manipulative and Body-Based Therapies

OVERVIEW

This category of the National Center for Complementary/Alternative Medicine (NCCAM) includes therapies that involve the manipulation and movement of body parts. Three large groups of therapies comprise this category: chiropractic, osteopathy, and massage. Other therapies in this category are reflexology, Trager body work, acupressure, and Rolfing. Nurses may use some of the other therapies in this group such as hydrotherapy, diathermy, light and color, heat, acupressure, and alternate nostril breathing. Acupressure was placed in Part III because of its tie with the flow of energy.

Massage, in the form of back rubs, is a basic skill included in nursing curricula over the years. In recent years back rubs have been largely abandoned by nurses with "too busy" being the reason cited for the decline in use. However, a substantial number of nurses have pursued education to become massage therapists; the practice of massage therapy is often separate from their practice of nursing although some nurses who are massage therapists use this modality in nursing homes and in independent practice as advanced practice nurses.

While many of the therapies in this group are routinely administered by other therapists such as chiropractors and massage therapists, a number of therapies in this group can be used by nurses. There is increasing evidence documenting the use of light for seasonal affective disorders. Acupressure points can be used to decrease pain. It is also important for nurses to increase their knowledge about therapies in this category in order to be knowledgeable about the therapies their patients are using.

20

Massage

Mariah Snyder and Yueh-hsia Tseng

According to Ellis, Hill, and Campbell (1995), Hippocrates developed his "wheel of health essentials" in the fifth century B.C. and identified rubbing or massage as his favorite wheel spoke. Many people are seeking holistic care. Current nursing practice is embracing more holistic approaches to working with clients in which the clients' physical, psychological, and spiritual aspects of health are included. Massage is one holistic approach that promotes the mind-body-spirituality connection, and it has been part of nursing's armamentarium for centuries. At a time when the public is increasing its use of massage, it is ironic that nursing is abandoning one of its traditional interventions as nurses rarely administer back rubs or other types of massage.

DEFINITION

Massage involves the manipulation of soft tissues for therapeutic purposes (Barr & Taslitz, 1970). Dunn, Sleep, and Collett (1995) defined massage as the application of various systematic and usually rhythmic hand movements performed on the soft tissues of the body. These movements produce different effects, depending on a number of factors: type and speed of movements; pressure exerted by the hands, fingers, or thumbs; and area of the body treated.

A number of different types of massage exist: Swedish (a more vigorous massage with long, flowing strokes); Esalen (a meditative massage with a light touch, and a highly variable style); deep tissue or neuromuscular (an intense kneading of the body); sports massage (a vigorous massage to loosen and ease sore muscles); Shiatsu (a Japanese pressure-point technique to relieve stress); and reflexology (a deep foot massage stimulating all parts of the body).

The various types of massage incorporate different strokes and procedures. Massage may be to the entire body or to specific areas of the body such as the back, feet, or hands (Cochrane, 1993).

SCIENTIFIC BASIS

The use of massage is a natural healing process that helps to connect the body, mind, and spirit. Massage produces therapeutic effects on multiple body systems: integumentary, musculoskeletal, cardiovascular, lymph, and nervous. Manipulating the skin and underlying muscle makes the skin more supple. Massage increases or enhances movement in the musculoskeletal system by reducing swelling, loosening and stretching contracted tendons, and aiding in the reduction of soft-tissue adhesions. Friction to the skin and underlying tissues releases histamines that in turn produce vasodilation of vessels and enhance venous return.

Massage, particularly back massage (Corley, Ferriter, Zeh, & Gifford, 1995; Fraser & Kerr, 1993; Meek, 1993), has been found to produce a relaxation response. Investigators reported that massage resulted in a decrease in physiological parameters (systolic and diastolic blood pressure, heart rate, and skin temperature) indicative of the relaxation response in patients with cancer, institutionalized older adults, hospice clients, and persons with dementia (Ferrell-Torry & Glick, 1993; Fraser & Kerr, 1993; Meek, 1993; Snyder, Egan, & Burns, 1995a).

In some instances, however, arousal rather than a relaxation response has occurred during massage. Barr and Taslitz (1970) found that sympathetic arousal occurred during massage as opposed to the control period. Longworth (1982) used a 6-minute back-massage intervention and found that the heart and electromyogram readings of female subjects increased compared to the baseline period, though the systolic and diastolic blood pressure readings decreased. Likewise, subjects' responses indicated that they felt relaxed following the back massage. Tyler, Winslow, Clark, and White (1990) administered a 1-minute back rub to patients who were critically ill. Findings included increases in the heart rate and decreases in the SVo_2; these gradually returned to the baseline after 4 minutes. However, the investigators noted that although these changes were statistically significant, the changes were not clinically significant as the heart rate only increased by four beats per minute.

The results from studies on the use of massage do not provide conclusive physiological evidence to support that it produces relaxation. Longworth (1982) suggested that the relaxation response occurs through the habituation to tactile stimuli and the inhibition of the muscle spindle by the passive stretch on the tendinous insertion of the muscles. Habituation occurs as the result of repetitive, monotonous stimuli. After a period of time the frontal lobe no longer perceives the stimuli originating from the muscles as threatening and arousal disappears. Stretching the tendon insertions temporarily relaxes the muscle. One factor that may contribute to arousal responses is the short duration of massage that may initially cause stimulation of the sympathetic nervous system before the relaxation response occurs (Ferrell-Torry & Glick, 1993; Tyler et al., 1990). However, in the majority of studies reviewed, subjective indexes for relaxation (anxiety inventories and self-reports) suggested that subjects felt relaxed after the massage intervention.

The impact of massage on the psychoneuroimmunological functions of the body and mind is beginning to be explored. Groer and colleagues (1994) reported that administering a 10-minute back massage stimulated the production of antibodies (salivary secretory immunoglobulin A, s-IgA). Anecdotal reports have suggested that massage has produced positive results in persons with AIDS.

In addition, massage promotes holistic care. Wilkinson, Aldridge, Salmon, Cain, and Wilson (1999) used massage to improve the quality of life in patients with cancer in a palliative care setting. Hernandez-Rief, Field, Fielt, and Theakston (1998) reported that a 45-minute massage twice a week improved self-esteem and enhanced social functional status in patients with multiple sclerosis.

INTERVENTION

Many types of massage exist, applicable to the entire body or to specific body areas such as back, hands, or feet. The techniques for hand and foot massage will be presented.

The environment in which massage is administered and the oils or lotion used add to the therapeutic effects. Room temperature is very important; the room must be warm enough so the person is comfortable. Shivering would negate the effects of the massage. In addition, privacy needs to be ensured.

Adding music and aromatherapy to massage sessions may enhance the effectiveness of massage (Dunn et al., 1995). Chapter 6 details the intervention of music, and aromatherapy is described in chapter 22.

TECHNIQUES

Massage Strokes

The various types of massage involve several stroke techniques. Commonly used strokes include effluerage, friction, pressure, petrissage, vibration, and percussion. *Effluerage* is a slow, rhythmic stroking with light skin contact. Effleurage may be applied with varying degrees of pressure depending on the part of the body being massaged and the outcome desired. The palmar surface of the hands is used for larger surfaces with the thumbs and fingers used for smaller areas. On large surfaces, long, gliding strokes about 10 to 20 inches in length are applied.

In *friction* movements, moderate, constant pressure to one area is made with the thumbs or fingers. The fingers may be held in one place or moved in a small circumscribed area. The *pressure stroke* is similar to the friction stroke, except pressure strokes are made with the hands.

Petrissage, or kneading, involves lifting a large fold of skin and the underlying muscle and holding the tissue between the thumb and fingers. The tissues are pushed against the bone, then raised and squeezed in circular movements. The grasp on the tissues is alternately loosened and tightened. Tissues are supported by one hand while kneading is done with the other hand. Variations of kneading include pinching, rolling, wringing, and kneading with fists or fingers. Petrissage is limited to tissues having a significant muscle mass.

Vibration strokes can be administered with either the entire hand or with the fingers. Rapid, continuous strokes are used. Because administering vibration strokes requires much energy, mechanical vibrators are often used.

For *percussion* strokes, the wrist acts as a fulcrum for the hand, with the hand hitting the tissue. Strokes are made with a rapid tempo over a large body area. Tapping and clapping are variants of percussion strokes.

Foot Massage

Foot massage is a technique that can be easily implemented by nurses and others. For patients with breathing problems, arthritic conditions, or abdominal surgery who may have difficulty maintaining the prone position for a full body massage, a foot massage is an alternative to use.

The foot massage may be combined with foot care. Soaking the feet in a basin of water before massaging is found to be enjoyable. Using heated towels and covering the massaged foot with a warm towel is also pleasurable. It is important to use firm strokes when massaging the feet as light strokes may tickle. The nurse needs to be alert to the facial expressions of the patient, as some areas of the foot may be painful or highly sensitive to touch. A technique for implementing foot massage is provided in Table 20.1.

Hand Massage

A technique for implementing hand massage is presented in Table 20.2. The technique is easy to implement with many populations including older adults (Cho & Snyder, 1996; Snyder, Egan, & Burns, 1995a, 1995b). The

TABLE 20.1   Technique for Foot Massage

The client may be either recumbent or sitting in a chair. The entire foot and ankle areas are rubbed with oil. While holding the foot firmly, the nurse makes circular strokes around the ankle area and over the entire ventral area of the foot. A finger is used to trace a space between the tendons on the foot, starting at the toes and moving toward the ankle. A tapping, squeezing movement is used to massage the four sides of each toe. At the conclusion of massaging the individual toe, the tip of the toe is squeezed. A fist is used to make circular movements on the sole of the foot. Many patients enjoy the effects of a pounding motion made with the fist on the sole proceeding from the toes to the ankle. The sides of the foot are massaged by moving the tissue between the index and third fingers. Firm, sweeping motions over the top and bottom of the foot are used to conclude the massage of the first foot before moving to the second foot.

time noted in the technique for administering massage is 2½ minutes per hand. In an initial study, Snyder and colleagues (1995b) administered hand massage for 5 minutes to each hand. In a subsequent study, when hand massage was administered for 2½ minutes to each hand (Snyder et al., 1995a), the level of relaxation was not as great as that found in the first study. However, in a subsequent study, Burns, Egan, and Teshima (1995) found no differences in the relaxation achieved when massage was administered for 5 versus 10 minutes.

MEASUREMENT OF OUTCOMES

Both physiological and psychological outcomes have been used to measure the effectiveness of massage. Indices of relaxation (heart rate, blood pressure, skin temperature, and muscle tension) have been used in many studies. Anxiety inventories and visual analogue scales to measure pain have also been used to determine the efficacy of massage. It is important that both short- and long-term effects be measured.

PRECAUTIONS

The nurse should obtain the permission of the patient before administering massage because some people do not like to be touched. Although some persons may be sensitive to touch, increasing the pressure of the strokes may overcome their discomfort. A good assessment of patients is needed prior to

TABLE 20.2   Technique for Hand Massage

Each hand is massaged for 2½ minutes. Do not massage if hand is injured, reddened, or swollen.

1. Back of hand
   (a) Short medium-length straight strokes are done from the wrist to the finger tips; moderate pressure is used (effluerage).
   (b) Large half-circle stretching strokes are made from the center to the side of the hand using moderate pressure.
   (c) Small circular strokes are made over the entire hand using light pressure (make small O's with the thumb).
   (d) Featherlike straight strokes are made from the wrist to the fingertips using very light pressure.

2. Palm of hand
   (a) Short, medium length straight strokes are made from the wrist to the fingertips using moderate pressure (effleurage).
   (b) Gentle milking and lifting of the tissue of the entire palm of the hand is done using moderate pressure.
   (c) Small circular strokes are made over the entire palm using moderate pressure (making little O's with index finger).
   (d) Large half-circle stretching strokes are used from the center of the palm to the sides using moderate pressure.

3. Fingers
   (a) Gently squeeze each finger from the base to the tip on both sides and the front and back using light pressure.
   (b) Gentle range of motion of finger.
   (c) Gentle pressure on nail bed.

4. Completion
   (a) Place client's hand on yours and cover it with your other hand. Gently draw your top hand toward you several times. Turn the client's hand over and gently draw the other hand toward you several times.

---

administering massage. Care is needed when areas of the body are reddened, bruised, or a rash is presented.

Patients with post-thrombotic venous edema may not be appropriate candidates for foot massage based on findings of Eliska and Eliskova (1995). In their study, patients with post-thrombotic venous edema appeared to have greater focal damage of lymphatics than control subjects when pressure was applied for 3 to 5 minutes.

Several investigators tried to determine if back rubs produced deleterious effects in specific populations, such as persons who have had a myocardial infarct (Bauer & Dracup, 1987; Tyler et al., 1990). Bauer and Dracup concluded that massage can be safely used with patients with cardiac conditions.

USES

The pleasant experience of massage with aromatherapy allows relationships to develop between receiver and giver. Nurses need to be aware that massage can help release emotions and should be prepared for subjects talking about personal issues during the massage. Multisensory massage can enhance the pleasure effect for people with more profound and multiple learning disabilities. Sometimes a client may wish to return the experience and massage the nurse's hands. This is actively encouraged in interactive massage where improvement in relationships and decrease in stress is sought (Sanderson, Harrison, & Price, 1991).

A list of the numerous conditions for which massage has been used is found in Table 20.3. Use of massage to produce relaxation and reduce pain will be discussed.

RELAXATION

Many people use a massage therapist to ameliorate their stress. The majority of studies that have been conducted on the use of massage have measured the relaxation response. Conley (1996) used foot massage on older adults with dementia to produce relaxation and promote comfort. In another study (Hayes & Cox, 1999), patients who were critically ill received a 5-minute foot massage. Decreased heart rate, mean arterial blood pressure, and respiratory rates were reported indicating relaxation responses.

A short massage given to family members often enables the family to cope more effectively with the stress of the hospitalization of a loved one. Massage also assists patients and families alike to communicate more openly and facilitate disclosure (Ellis et al., 1995). Lloyd (1995) suggested that nurses could give quick massages to colleagues to promote relaxation.

PAIN

Several mechanisms have been proposed to explain the efficacy of massage in decreasing pain. Day, Mason, and Chesrown (1987) hypothesized that massage stimulates the production of endogenous opiates resulting in the modulation of pain. Another possible mechanism for decreasing pain is that

TABLE 20.3   Uses for Massage

Promote relaxation
- Decrease aggressive behaviors (Snyder et al., 1995a, 1995b)
- Produce sleep (Field, Grizzle, Scafidi, & Schanberg, 1996; Richards, 1998)
- Lessen fatigue (Ahles et al., 1999)
- Lessen pain (Hulme, Waterman, & Hillier, 1999; Ferrell-Torry & Glick, 1993; Nixon, Teschendorff, Finney, & Karnilowicz, 1997; Weinrich & Weinrich, 1990)

Reduce edema (Wozniewski, 1991)

Improve mobility (Smith, Stallings, Mariner, & Burrall, 1999)

Decrease need for episiotomy (Mynaugh, 1991; Shipman, Boniface, Tefft, & McCloghry, 1997)

Increase communication (Conley, 1996; Fraser & Kerr, 1993)

Increase sense of well-being (Wells-Federman et al., 1995)

Lessen depression (Field, Peck, et al., 1998; Kite et al., 1998)

Lessen anxiety (Dunn et al., 1995; Johnson, Frederick, Kaufman, & Mountjoy, 1999)

massage reduces muscle spasms and tension, particularly of large muscle groups, and thus modifies the myofascial and muscle tension types of pain and other forms of cancer pain. Ferrell-Torry and Glick (1993) used a 30-minute therapeutic massage on two consecutive evenings to promote relaxation and to alleviate the perception of pain and anxiety in hospitalized cancer patients. In working with cancer patients, Weinrich and Weinrich (1990) found that a 10-minute back massage decreased pain. Meek (1993) found that slow stroke back massage administered to hospice patients produced relaxation; she recommended use of back massage to promote the comfort of hospice patients. Hulme and colleagues (1999) reported that foot massage decreased postoperative pain, and a similar finding was reported by Nixon et al. (1997).

FUTURE RESEARCH

Minimal research has been done on the use of massage. This is particularly true of the techniques for hand and foot massage. Studies that use adequate sample sizes and that control for confounding variables and incorporate psychophysiological parameters are needed. The following are a few of the areas in which further research is needed:

1. Snyder et al. (1995a) reported an increase in aggressive behaviors in males with dementia after the administration of hand massage while a decrease had occurred in the female subjects. Weinrich and Weinrich (1990) reported that males responded more positively. Van der Riet (1995) noted that male students found massage to be more heavily laden with implicit sexual meanings than did female students. Thus, exploration is needed of the impact of gender on the results obtained from use of massage. Both the gender of the client and of the person administering massage need to be examined.

2. Eliska and Eliskova (1995) reported that massage using 70–100 mmHg pressure resulted in focal damage of lymphatics after a 10-minute massage. Further studies are needed to explore the appropriate massage pressure to use for persons with various underlying conditions. In addition, the rate of massage movements, types of movement, and direction of massage may contribute to whether there is a relaxation or arousal response during massage. This needs to be explored so that guidelines can be developed.

3. Few studies on massage have investigated the impact it has on pyschoneuroimmunologcial functions. Such studies would help validate its effects on health conditions such as AIDs and cancer.

REFERENCES

Ahles, T. A., Tope, D. M., Pinkson, B., Walch, S., Hann, D., Whedon, M., Dain, B., Weiss, J. E., Mills, L., & Silbarfarb, P. M. (1999). Massage therapy for patients undergoing autologous bone marrow transplantation. *Journal of Pain and Symptom Management, 18,* 157–163.

Barr, J., & Taslitz, N. (1970). The influence of back massage on autonomic functions. *Journal of Physical Therapy, 50,* 1679–1689.

Bauer, W. C., & Dracup, K. A. (1987). Physiologic effects of back massage in patients with acute myocardial infarction. *Focus on Critical Care Nursing, 14*(6), 42–46.

Burns, K. R., Egan, E. C., & Teshima, M. (1995, April). Testing hand massage protocols for persons with dementia. Paper presented at the meeting of the Midwest Nursing Research Society Conference, Kansas City, MO.

Cho, K., & Snyder, M. (1996). Use of hand massage with presence to increase relaxation in Korean-American elderly. *The Journal of Academy of Nursing, 26,* 623–631.

Cochrane, F. S. (1993). Psychological effects of massage. *International Journal of Alternative and Complementary Medicine, 11*(9), 21–24.

Conley, D. M. (1996, August 30). Biobehavioral responses of individuals with dementia to tactile stimulation (foot massage) intervention. Presentation at Gerontological Nursing Interventions Research Conference, Iowa City, IA.

Corley, M. C., Ferriter, J., Zeh, J., & Gifford, C. (1995). Physiological and psychological effects of back rubs. *Applied Nursing Research, 8*, 39–43.

Day, J. A., Mason, R. R., & Chesrown, S. E. (1987). Effect of massage on serum level of B-endorphin and B-lipotropin in healthy adults. *Physical Therapy, 67*(6), 926–930.

Dunn, C., Sleep, J., & Collett, D. (1995). Sensing an improvement: An experimental study to evaluate the use of aromatherapy, massage, and periods of rest in an intensive care unit. *Journal of Advanced Nursing, 21*, 34–40.

Eliska, O., & Eliskova, M. (1995). Are peripheral lymphatics damaged by high pressure manual massage? *Lymphology, 28*(1), 21–30.

Ellis, V., Hill, J., & Campbell, H. (1995). Hospice techniques: Strengthening the family unit through the healing power of massage. *The American Journal of Hospice and Palliative Care, 12*(5), 19–21.

Ferrell-Torry, A. T., & Glick, O. J. (1993). The use of therapeutic massage as a nursing intervention to modify anxiety and the perception of cancer pain. *Cancer Nursing, 16*, 93–101.

Field, T., Grizzle, N., Scafidi, F., & Schanberg, S. (1996). Massage and relaxation therapies' effects on depressed adolescent mothers. *Adolescence, 31*, 903–911.

Field, T., Peck, M., Krugman, S., Tuchel, T., Schanberg, S., Kuhn, C., & Burman, I. (1998). Burn injuries benefit from massage therapy. *Journal of Burn Care and Rehabilitation, 19*, 241–244.

Fraser, J., & Kerr, J. R. (1993). Psychophysiological effects of back massage on elderly institutionalized patients. *Journal of Advanced Nursing, 18*, 238–245.

Groer, M., Mozingo, J., Droppleman, P., Davis, M., Jolley, M., Boynton, M., Davis, K., & Kay, S. (1994). Measures of salivary immunoglobulin A and state anxiety after a nursing back rub. *Applied Nursing Research, 7*(1), 2–6.

Hayes, J., & Cox, C. (1999). Immediate effects of a five-minute foot massage on patients in critical care. *Intensive and Critical Care Nursing, 15*, 77–82.

Hernandez-Rief, M., Field, T., Fielt, T., & Theakston, H. (1998). Multiple sclerosis patients benefit from massage therapy. *Journal of Bodywork and Movement Therapies, 2*, 168–174.

Hulme, J., Waterman, H., & Hillier, V. F. (1999). The effect of foot massage on patients' perception of care following laparoscopic sterilization as day case patients. *Journal of Advanced Nursing, 30*, 460–468.

Johnson, S. K., Frederick, J., Kaufman, M., & Mountjoy, B. (1999). A controlled investigation of bodywork in multiple sclerosis. *Journal of Alternative and Complementary Medicine, 5*, 237–243.

Kite, S. M., Maher, E. J., Anderson, K., Young, T., Young, J., Wood, J., Howells, N., & Bradburn, J. (1998). Development of an aromatherapy service at a cancer centre. *Palliative Medicine, 12*, 171–180.

Lloyd, K. (1995). The power to colleagues and clients with a two-minute massage. *The Lamp, 51*(22), 30.

Longworth, J. C. (1982). Psychophysiological effects of slow back massage in normotensive females. *Advances in Nursing Science, 4*(4), 44–61.

Meek, S. S. (1993). Effects of slow back massage on relaxation in hospice patients. *Image: Journal of Nursing Scholarship, 25*, 17–21.

Mynaugh, P. A. (1991). A randomized study of two methods of teaching perineal massage: Effects on practice rates, episiotomy rates, and lacerations. *Birth, 18*(3), 153–159.

Nixon, M., Teschendorff, J., Finney, J., & Karnilowicz, W. (1997). Expanding the nursing repertoire: The effect of massage on post-operative pain. *Australian Journal of Advanced Nursing, 14*(3), 21–26.

Richards, K. C. (1998). Effect of a back massage and relaxation intervention on sleep in critically ill patients. *American Journal of Critical Care, 7*, 288–299.

Sanderson, H., Harrison, J., & Price, S. S. (1991). *Aromatherapy and massage for people with learning difficulties.* Birmingham, AL: Hands On.

Shipman, M. K., Boniface, D. R., Tefft, M. E., & McCloghry, F. (1997). Antenatal perineal massage and subsequent perineal outcomes: A randomized controlled trial. *British Journal of Obstetrics and Gynecology, 104*, 787–791.

Smith, M. C., Stallings, M. A., Mariner, S., & Burrall, M. (1999). Benefits of massage therapy for hospitalized patients: A descriptive and qualitative evaluation. *Alternative Therapies in Health and Medicine, 5*(4), 64–71.

Snyder, M., Egan, E. C., & Burns, K. R. (1995a). Efficacy of hand massage in decreasing agitation behaviors associated with care activities in persons with dementia. *Geriatric Nursing, 16* (2), 60–63.

Snyder, M., Egan, E. C., & Burns, K. R. (1995b). Interventions for decreasing agitation behaviors in persons with dementia. *Journal of Gerontological Nursing, 21*(7), 34–40.

Tyler, D. O., Winslow, E. H., Clark, A. P., & White, K. M. (1990). Effects of a 1-minute back rub on mixed venous oxygen saturation and heart rate in critically ill patients. *Heart and Lung, 19*, 562–565.

van der Riet, P. (1995). Massage and sexuality in nursing. *Nursing Inquiry, 2*, 149–156.

Weinrich, S. P., & Weinrich, M. C. (1990). The effect of massage on pain in cancer patients. *Applied Nursing Research, 3*, 140–145.

Wells-Federman, C. L., Stuart, E. M., Deckro, J. P., Mandle, C. L., Baim, M., & Medich, C. (1995). The mind-body connection: The psychophysiology of many traditional nursing interventions. *Clinical Nurse Specialist, 9*(1), 59–66.

Wilkinson, S., Aldridge, J., Salmon, I., Cain, E., & Wilson, B. (1999). An evaluation of aromatherapy massage in palliative care. *Palliative Medicine, 13*, 409–417.

Wozniewski, M. (1991). Value of intermittent pneumatic massage in the treatment of upper extremity lymphedema. *Polski Tygodnik Lekarski, 46*, 550–552.

21

Tai Chi

Kuei-Min Chen

D ue to the pressures of work, many people do not have proper exer-cise, which may lead to mental strain, nervous breakdown, or ineffi-ciency in their daily work (Cheng, 1994). Health is essential to an individual and how to acquire a strong and healthy body is an important task that an individual needs to be concerned with. It is commonly recognized that proper physical exercise is the best method of keeping our body fit and healthy (Cheng, 1994). However, it is not easy to find one that suits people of all ages although many exercises are available to us nowadays (such as golf, tennis, football, etc.) (Cheng, 1994).

Manual therapy, such as tai chi, is one of the interventions that is widely recommended across different professions, including nurses, physicians, occupational therapists, and recreational therapists. The utilization of man-ual therapy can heighten individuals' awareness of their bodies and take advantage of their body structure for expressing feelings and ideas. Gradually, individuals become more aware of their total being which promotes harmony within themselves and leads to an enhanced well-being (Lange, 1975). The purpose of this chapter is to introduce and describe tai chi.

DEFINITION

Tai chi, which means "supreme ultimate," is a traditional Chinese martial art (Koh, 1981) and a mind-body exercise (Forge, 1997). It involves a series of fluid, continuous, graceful, dance-like postures, and the performance of movements known as forms (Perry, 1982; Smalheiser, 1984). The graceful body movements are integrated by mind concentration, the shifting balance of body weight, muscle relaxation, and breathing control. It is performed in a slow, rhythmic, and well-controlled manner (Plummer, 1983).

There are several styles of tai chi that are currently practiced: *chen* (quick and slow large movements), *yang* (slow large movements), *wu* (mid-paced compact), and *sun* (quick compact) (Jou, 1983). Each style has its own distinctive features, yet the basic principles are the same (Koh, 1981). Yang style is the most popular tai chi practiced by older adults (Jou, 1983). There are a few simplified, Westernized forms of the ancient tai chi. The most common one is called tai chi chih, which was developed by an American, Justin Stone. Tai chi chih consists of 20 simple, repetitive, nonstrenuous movements and an ending pose. It emphasizes a soft, flowing, continuous motion and is easier for beginners to learn. Most tai chi movements were named after animals, such as "white crane spreads its wings" and "grasp the bird's tail" (Koh, 1981).

SCIENTIFIC BASIS

Tai chi practice is closely linked to Chinese medical theory, in which the vital life energy, *Chi* (or *qi*), is thought to circulate throughout the body in discrete channels called meridians. Using correct postures and adequate relaxation, the principle of tai chi is to promote the free flow of chi throughout the body, which promotes the health of an individual (Kirsteins, Dietz, Frederick, & Hwang, 1991). In 1992, Tse and Bailey reported that regular tai chi practice significantly improved balance control in three of five tests and advocated the following factors as an explanation for the improvements:

1. All tai chi movements are circular, slow, continuous, even, and smooth. Patterns of movement flow from one to the next. The even, slow tempo facilitates a sensory awareness of the speed, force, trajectory, and execution of movement throughout the exercise.
2. Because movements are well controlled, all unnecessary exertion is avoided, and only sufficient effort is used to overcome gravity. Muscle coordination instead of rigid contraction can therefore be promoted.
3. Throughout the exercise, the body is constantly shifted from one foot to the other. This is likely to facilitate improvement of dynamic standing balance.
4. Throughout the exercises, different parts of the body take turns in playing the role of stabilizer and mover, allowing smooth movements to be executed without compromising the balance and stability of the body (p. 297).

The performance of tai chi looks like a classical dance with graceful movements and attentive actions, which is regulated by the timing of deep breathing and the movement of the diaphragm. It offers a balanced exercise to the muscles and joints of the various parts of the body (Cheng, 1994). In addition, a peaceful state of mind and spiritual dedication to each movement during the exercise ensure that the central nervous system is given sufficient training and is consequently toned up with time as the exercise continues (Cheng, 1994). A strong central nervous system is the basic condition of a healthy body and the various organs depend largely on the soundness of the central nervous system (Cheng, 1994).

INTERVENTION

In Eastern countries such as Taiwan, it is common and popular for older adults to practice tai chi as a group in parks or the athletic grounds of elementary schools in the early morning. Tai chi practice groups are usually led by masters who are pleased to share the essence of tai chi with others. People who are interested in tai chi are welcome to join the groups and learn the movements from tai chi masters. In Western countries there is a growing interest in the practice of tai chi. Various tai chi clubs are available to the public through community centers, health clinics, or private organizations. General information on tai chi is widespread through Web sites, books, and videos. Tai chi is an easy exercise, which can be practiced in any place, at any time, and without any equipment.

TECHNIQUES

Although various styles of tai chi are currently practiced, the underlying practice principles are the same. In Schaller's study (1996), five principles of movement essential to tai chi were identified:

1. Hand and leg movement should be synchronous.
2. The emphasis should be on a soft, relaxed position, rather than a hard, tense position.
3. Moves should be practiced with a quiet and open mind.
4. The soles of the feet should be rooted to the ground with the knees bent in a low stance, and the primary focus of awareness within the lower abdomen.
5. The physical force should be rooted in the feet, passed up through the legs as weight is shifted, and distributed by the pivoting of the waist.

In the physical performance, an individual must relax and think of nothing else before starting. The movements should be slow and according to natural breathing. Every action becomes easy and smooth, the waist turns freely, and the feelings of comfort and relaxation will be gradually developed (Cheng, 1994). In the spiritual aspect, tai chi is an exercise that produces harmony of body and mind. Each movement should be guided by thought instead of concentrating on physical strength. For instance, to lift up the hands an individual must first have the necessary mental concentration, then the hands can be raised slowly in a proper manner. Hence, the breathing will become deeper and the body will be strengthened (Cheng, 1994).

GUIDELINES

The prototype for performing the movement called "around the platter" is presented in Table 21.1. Various videotapes on tai chi are also available through local video rental stores. Welsch (1998) identified the following books as being useful for learning about tai chi:

1. *Tai Chi Chuan for Health and Self-defense* by T. T. Liang is an introduction and reflection on the art of tai chi.
2. *Tai Chi: A Practical Introduction to the Therapeutic Effects of the Discipline* by P. Crompton provides a basic introduction to tai chi as a martial art and as a way to achieve better health.
3. *Tai Chi: Transcendent Art* by T. H. Cheng demonstrates each tai chi movement through pictures and graphs.

Additional information can be found through several useful Web links: (a) www.supply.com/lee/tcclinks.html, which provides links to more than a hundred other Web sites on tai chi and related topics; and (b) http://sunflower.signet.com.sg/~limttk/index.htm, which is a valuable site with complete historical and background information on tai chi.

MEASUREMENT OF OUTCOMES

According to Plummer (1983), mind concentration and breathing control are two of the major tenets of tai chi practice. When practicing tai chi with a peaceful, focused mind and incorporating smooth breathing into each movement, a person will experience physical and psychological relaxation, which leads to an enhanced well-being, both physically and psychologically (Plummer, 1983). With this conceptual framework in mind, the measurement of the effects of tai chi could be in both physical and psychological well-being. Based on the literature, which will be discussed in detail later, more studies were done to measure the physical outcomes of tai chi practice

TABLE 21.1   Prototype for Performing "Around the Platter"

1. Hands are held at chest level, wrists slightly bent and elbows close to sides. Fingers are spread apart. Legs are slightly apart and bent with the left in front of the right. Weight is equally distributed between legs.

2. Begin to rock forward, shifting weight to the left leg with hands moving to the left. (Imagine a round platter at the chest level, and the hands circling around the platter from left to right.)

3. As most of the weight shifts to the left leg and the hands are directly in front of the body, the left heel comes off the ground. As the hands move right of midline, the weight begins to shift to the right leg. When the hands have completed a full circle (held at chest level), most of the weight is on the right leg and the right toe is off the ground.

4. This movement can be repeated 6–9 times and then repeated again going from right to left.

Note: Adapted from *Tai Chi Chih: Joy Through Movement*, by J. F. Stone, 1994, Fort Yates, ND, Good Karma.

(such as physical and cardiovascular functioning) and little emphasis was placed on psychological well-being outcomes (such as mood states).

PRECAUTIONS

Tai chi is unique for its slow graceful movements with low impact, low velocity, minimal orthopedic complications, and is a suitable conditioning exercise for older adults (Lai, Lan, Wong, & Teng, 1995). Although many research studies have shown the benefits of tai chi, there are some limitations to practicing tai chi, such as angina, ventricular arrhythmia, and myocardial ischemia. The instructor and the learner have to be aware of those limitations, and an initial assessment is necessary to determine an individual's exercise tolerance and other contraindications (Forge, 1997). In learning tai chi, a novice should be periodically evaluated on the progress and on program adherence, cognitive response, muscular strength, balance, and flexibility at 4-week intervals for the first 60 to 90 days and at 6-month intervals thereafter (Forge, 1997). It is strongly recommended that one learn tai chi from an experienced master who is able to teach the movements based on individual needs and physical tolerance. Recommendations for choosing a class are provided in Table 21.2.

TABLE 21.2   Choosing a Tai Chi Class

1. If possible find a studio or organization which specializes in tai chi.

2. Find an experienced teacher (6–10 years of experience) who demonstrates and verbally explains the movements. Ask to observe a class before joining.

3. Find a class with less than 20 students.

4. Avoid purchasing any special clothing or equipment.

Note: Adapted from "Tai Chi," by L. B. Downs, 1992, *Modern Maturity,* 35, pp. 60–64.

USES

Tai chi is especially appropriate for older adults or for patients with chronic diseases because of its low intensity, steady rhythm, and low physical and mental tension (Xu & Fan, 1988). It has been shown to enhance cardiovascular and respiratory functions, improve health-related fitness, and promote positive health status (Brown, Mucci, Hetzler, & Knowlton, 1989; Lai et al., 1995; Lan, Lai, Chen, & Wong, 1998; Lan, Lai, Wong, & Yu, 1996). In addition, practicing tai chi has been effective in lowering blood pressure (Channer, Barrow, Barrow, Osborne, & Ives, 1996; Jin, 1989, 1992; Wolf et al., 1996). However, in a pretest-posttest study on the effects of a 10-week, short-term tai chi training program, there were no significant improvements of health status or blood pressure of the community-dwelling elders as compared to their baseline data (Schaller, 1996). Schaller explained that these nonsignificant results might be attributed to the fact that the health status measures may not have been sensitive or specific enough to detect changes in a short-term exercise program.

Falls are common in the older population, and they often cause severe physical trauma (Tideiksaar, 1989). Most studies have shown that tai chi increases postural stability and enhances balance (Jacobson, Chen, Cashel, & Guerrero, 1997; Shih, 1997; Tse & Bailey, 1992; Wolf et al., 1996), which lead to a reduction in the risk of falls (Shih, 1997). Furthermore, several studies found that tai chi enhanced positive mood states and decreased mood disturbances (Brown et al., 1995; Jin, 1992). However, one study showed that it had no significant impact on mood states in community-dwelling elders (Schaller, 1996).

Recently, Chen (2000) found that tai chi practitioners had better physical and mental health status, lower systolic and diastolic blood pressure, fewer falls within the past year, less mood disturbance, and better mood states when compared to nonpractitioners. Researcher suggested that tai chi could be incorporated into community programs or senior center activities to promote well-being of community-dwelling elders. It could also be included as one of the activities in nursing homes or in rehabilitation programs in hospital settings.

FUTURE RESEARCH

Overall, practicing tai chi appropriately has various benefits as evidenced in the literature, and it is highly recommended for the appropriate populations. As nurses, we need to study more about the effects of tai chi from a nursing perspective in order to make it more beneficial as a nursing intervention (Chen & Snyder, 1999). Some questions for further research include:

1. What are possible benefits and harms of practicing tai chi?
2. Which populations can most benefit from practicing tai chi and are there conditions which would preclude its use?
3. What is the nature of stability or change in the well-being status of elders who practice tai chi?
4. What are the differences on well-being outcomes of beginners (people who are just starting to learn tai chi movements), practitioners (people who have practiced tai chi regularly for more than a year), and masters (people who have practiced tai chi regularly for more than a decade and are licensed by the National Tai Chi Association to be instructors)?

REFERENCES

Brown, D. D., Mucci, W. G., Hetzler, R. K., & Knowlton, R. G. (1989). Cardiovascular and ventilatory responses during formalized tai chi chuan exercise. *Research Quarterly for Exercise and Sport, 60*(3), 246–250.

Brown, D. R., Wang, Y., Ward, A., Ebbeling, C. B., Fortlage, L., Puleo, E., Benson, H., & Rippe, J. M. (1995). Chronic psychological effects of exercise and exercise plus cognitive strategies. *Medicine and Science in Sports and Exercise, 27,* 765–775.

Channer, K. S., Barrow, D., Barrow, R., Osborn, M., & Ives, G. (1996). Changes in haemodynamic parameters following tai chi chuan and aerobic exercise in patients recovering from acute myocardial infarction. *Postgraduate Medical Journal, 72*(848), 347–351.

Chen, K. M. (2000). The effects of tai chi on the well-being of community-dwelling elders in Taiwan (Doctoral dissertation, University of Minnesota, 2000). *Dissertation Abstracts International, 61,* 1319.

Chen, K. M., & Snyder, M. (1999). A research-based use of tai chi/movement therapy as a nursing intervention. *Journal of Holistic Nursing, 17*, 267–279.

Cheng, T. H. (1994). *Tai chi: Transcendent art.* Hong Kong: The Hong Kong Tai Chi Association.

Downs, L. B. (1992). Tai chi. *Modern Maturity, 35*(4), 60–64.

Forge, R. L. (1997). Mind-body fitness: Encouraging prospects for primary and secondary prevention. *Journal of Cardiovascular Nursing, 11*(3), 53–65.

Jacobson, B. H., Chen, H. C., Cashel, C., & Guerrero, L. (1997). The effect of tai chi chuan training on balance, kinesthetic sense, and strength. *Perceptual and Motor Skills, 84*(1), 27–33.

Jin, P. (1989). Changes in heart rate, noradrenaline, cortisol and mood during tai chi. *Journal of Psychosomatic Research, 33*, 197–206.

Jin, P. (1992). Efficacy of tai chi, brisk walking, meditation, and reading in reducing mental and emotional stress. *Journal of Psychosomatic Research, 36*(4), 361–370.

Jou, T. H. (1983). *The tao of tai chi chuan: Way to rejuvenation* (3rd ed.). Piscataway, NJ: Tai Chi Foundation.

Kirsteins, A. E., Dietz, F., & Hwang, S. M. (1991). Evaluating the safety and potential use of a weight-bearing exercise, tai-chi chuan, for rheumatoid arthritis patients. *American Journal of Physical Medicine and Rehabilitation, 70*(3), 136–141.

Koh, T. C. (1981). Tai chi chuan. *American Journal of Chinese Medicine, 9*, 15–22.

Lai, J. S., Lan, C., Wong, M. K., & Teng, S. H. (1995). Two-year trends in cardiorespiratory function among older tai chi chuan practitioners and sedentary subjects. *Journal of the American Geriatrics Society, 43*(11), 1222–1227.

Lan, C., Lai, J. S., Chen, S. Y., & Wong, M. K. (1998). 12-month tai chi training in the elderly: Its effect on health fitness. *Medicine and Science in Sports and Exercise, 30*, 345–351.

Lan, C., Lai, J. S., Wong, M. K., & Yu, M. L. (1996). Cardiorespiratory function, flexibility, and body composition among geriatric tai chi chuan practitioners. *Archives of Physical Medicine and Rehabilitation, 77*(6), 612–616.

Lange, R. (1975). *The nature of dance.* Macdonald & Evans.

Perry, P. (1982). Sports medicine in China: A group philosophy of fitness. *The Physician and Sports Medicine, 10*, 177–178.

Plummer, J. P. (1983). Acupuncture and tai chi chuan (Chinese shadow boxing): Body/mind therapies affecting homeostasis. In Y. Lau & J. P. Fowler (Eds.), *The scientific basis of traditional Chinese medicine: Selected papers* (pp. 22–36). Hong Kong: Medical Society.

Schaller, K. J. (1996). Tai chi chih: An exercise option for older adults. *Journal of Gerontological Nursing, 22*(10), 12–17.

Shih, J. (1997). Basic Beijing twenty-four forms of tai chi exercise and average velocity of sway. *Perceptual and Motor Skills, 84*(1), 287–290.

Smalheiser, M. (1984). Tai chi chuan in China today. *Tai Chi Chuan: Perspectives of the Way and Its Movement, 1*, 3–5.

Stone, J. F. (1994). *Tai chi chih: Joy through movement.* Fort Yates, ND: Good Karma.

Tideiksaar, R. (1989) *Falling in old age: Its prevention and treatment* (Springer series on adulthood and aging, Vol. 22). New York: Springer.

Tse, S., & Bailey, D. M. (1992). Tai chi and postural control in the well elderly. *American Journal of Occupational Therapy, 46*(4), 295–300.

Welsch, C. (1998, January 25). Tai chi. *Star Tribune*, pp. G6, G7, Minneapolis, MN.

Wolf, S. L., Barnhart, H. X., Kutner, N. G., McNeely, E., Coogler, C., & Xu, T. (1996). Reducing frailty and falls in older persons: An investigation of tai chi and computerized balance training. *Journal of American Geriatrics Society, 44*(5), 489–497.

Xu, S. W., & Fan, Z. H. (1988). Physiological studies of tai ji quan in China. *Medicine Sport Science, 28*, 70–80.

PART V

Biological-Based Therapies

OVERVIEW

Biological-based therapies are the most popular of the complementary therapies. More than 90 million Americans used at least one herbal preparation during the past year. Additionally, "nutraceuticals" (additives, vitamins, and special diets) are used by many Americans. It is difficult to page through a magazine or watch television without encountering a reference to nutraceuticals or dietary supplements. (The authors have placed aromatherapy in this category because it uses essential oils, which are naturally occurring plant substances.) The National Center for Complementary/Alternative Medicine also places therapies such as laetrile and shark cartilage in the biological-based therapies category.

While research on herbs is relatively sparse in the United States, a significant amount has been conducted in other countries, particularly Germany. The chapter on herbal preparations details concerns about the use of herbal preparations here in this country, but suggestions are given to increase the safety in the use of herbs. Because of the growing percentage of Americans who use herbal preparations, it is incumbent on nurses to have knowledge about common preparations and to assess for a patient's use of herbs.

While nurses ordinarily will not be in a position to prescribe or recommend specific nutraceuticals to patients, the wide use of this group of biological-based therapies requires that nurses have knowledge about them. Much information is available to the public about food additives, vitamins, and special diets, and knowing about a patient's use of these products will assist the health care team in devising a safe plan of care.

As with many of the other biological-based therapies, the essential oils found in aromatherapy have a much wider use in other countries than in the United States. Much of the research on essential oils has been conducted in France and England, and it is only within recent years that aromatherapy has been introduced into health facilities in the United States. Essential oils can be taken internally, but the focus in this book is on their use as aromatic substances or topical applications.

Many of the lists of herbal preparations and other biological-based therapies refer to products common in the Western world. Most give little attention to herbal preparations and biological-based therapies used in other health systems such as traditional Chinese medicine and health care systems of indigenous cultures. The increasing number of first-generation Americans from countries that have traditionally had a more extensive use of biological-based therapies requires that health professionals expand their knowledge about herbs and other biological-based therapies used in other cultures.

22

Aromatherapy

Jane Buckle

Aromatherapy is the use of essential oils, which are steam distillates obtained from aromatic plants. Aromatherapy is a recent addition to nursing care in the United States although it has been accepted as part of nursing care in Switzerland, Germany, Australia, Canada, and the United Kingdom for many years. Aromatherapy is particularly useful in nursing because it addresses patient care through smell and touch. This chapter will introduce the potential uses of aromatherapy in nursing care by drawing on published research.

Aromatherapy is an offshoot of herbal medicine, which is the origin of conventional medicine. Herbal medicine dates back 6,000 years and was used in India, China, North and South America, Greece, the Middle East, and Europe. The renaissance of modern clinical aromatherapy occurred in France just prior to World War II. Physician Jean Valnet, chemist Maurice Gattefosse, and nurse Marguerite Maury were key figures. They each used essential oils in clinical ways, to help wounds heal and to fight infection. The first antiseptic, thymol, which was discovered by Lister, was obtained from the essential oil of thyme. In France, physicians use essential oils as an alternative, or to enhance antibiotics. The use of synthetic scents, which has only appeared in the last few decades, does not have anything to do with aromatherapy.

Aromatherapy was not mentioned in the landmark study on complementary therapies conducted by Eisenberg, Kessler, et al. (1993). However, in the second study conducted by Eisenberg, Davis, et al., (1998), aromatherapy *was* listed with 5.6% of the 2,055 adults surveyed indicating that they used aromatherapy. Although aromatherapy is not considered part of herbal medicine, it clearly has its roots in plant medicine, as the essential oils used in aromatherapy come from plants.

DEFINITIONS

Aromatherapy is the use of essential oils for therapeutic purposes that encompass mind, body, and spirit (Styles, 1997). The name leads people to think the therapy is purely about smelling scents (Schnaubelt, 1999) but this is incorrect. Although there are many facets of aromatherapy, when it is used clinically by nurses it is something very concise and targets clinical outcomes that are measureable. Thus, the definition of clinical aromatherapy is very specific: the use of essential oils for their expected outcomes that are measurable (Buckle, 2000).

The definition of essential oils is also very specific. According to Tisserand and Balacs (1995), essential oils are the steam distillate of aromatic plants. Any extract not obtained by steam distillation is not an essential oil and should not used in aromatherapy. Essential oils are found in the flowers, leaves, bark, wood, roots, seed, and peels of many plants and are stored in microscopic cellular containers of the plant, the cells, glands, ducts, and hairs. Essential oils are highly volatile, complex mixtures of chemical constituents known as terpenes, terpenoids, and phenylpropane derivatives. The proportions of these constituents vary according to plant, climate, and the distillation process used. It is the chemistry of an essential oil that determines its therapeutic properties; therefore, knowing the part of the plant, the country of origin, and the method of extraction is important in giving an indication of the essential oil's chemical constituents.

SCIENTIFIC BASIS

The pharmacologically active components in essential oils work at psychological, physical, and cellular levels. The effects of aroma can be rapid, and sometimes just thinking about a smell can have a powerful impact on a person. The effect can be relaxing or stimulating depending on the individual's previous experiences as well as the chemistry of the essential oil used. Essential oils are absorbed rapidly through the skin; some are being used to help the dermal penetration of orthodox medications. Essential oils are lipotrophic (fat soluble) and are excreted through respiration, kidneys and insensate loss.

Essential oils produce documented therapeutic effects on the mind, body, and spirit. A small selection of research papers that target nursing diagnoses is shown in Table 22.1. The asterisk indicates that the nursing diagnosis "altered levels of comfort" could be used but as this is so broad a more specific target has also been given. A small selection of other scientific studies of interest to nurses is shown in Table 22.2.

TABLE 22.1   Research on Essential Oils for Specific Nursing Diagnoses

Nursing Diagnosis	Essential Oil	Research
Altering pain perception	Roman chamomile	Wilkinson (1995)
	Peppermint	Gobel (1995); Krall & Krause (1993)
	Lavender	Woolfson & Hewitt (1992)
Alleviating depression	Sandalwood, lavender	Moate (1995)
Enhancing conventional analgesia*	Lemongrass	Seth, Kokate, & Varma (1975)
Reducing anxiety	Neroli, lavender	Stevensen (1995)
Relaxing	Lavender, rose	Buchbauer et al. (1991); Manly (1993)
Enhancing immune function	Citrus (lemon)	Komori et al. (1995)
Reduction of seizures*	Ylang-ylang	Betts (1996)
Enhancing concentration	Lemon, lemongrass, peppermint, basil	Manly (1993)

Essential oils are composed of many different chemical components or molecules. These olfactory stimulants travel via the nose to the olfactory bulb, and from there nerve impulses travel to the limbic system of the brain, an inner, complex ring of brain structures that are arranged into 53 regions and 35 associated tracts below the cerebral cortex. Of these regions, the amygdala and the hippocampus are of particular importance in the processing of aromas.

The amygdala governs emotional responses. Diazepam (Valium) is thought to reduce the effect of external emotional stimuli by increasing gamma aminobutyric acid (GABA) that inhibits neurons in the amygdala. *Lavandula angustifolia* (true lavender) is thought to have a similar effect on the amygdala, producing a sedative effect similar to diazepam (Tisserand, 1988). The hippocampus is involved in the formation and retrieval of explicit memories. This is where the chemicals in an aroma trigger learned memory. Smell is very important in our lives, beginning with the newborn baby's identification of its mother and continuing into old age; studies have shown that depression in residential older adults was reduced with the use of fruit and flower aromas.

TABLE 22.2   Research on Essential Oils for Specific Pathogens

Targeted Pathogen	Essential Oil	Research
MRSA	Tea tree, lavender, peppermint	Nelson (1997)
Pseudomonas	Lemon, melissa	Larrondo, Agut, & Calco-Torras (1995)
Ringworm	Lemongrass ·	Wannisorm et al. (1996) Lorenzetti et al. (1991)
Candida albicans	Tea tree	Carson et al. (1995)

The effect of odors on the brain has been mapped using computer-generated topographics. Brain electrical activity maps (BEAMs) may indicate how subjects psychometrically rated odors presented to them when linked to an electroencephalogram (EEG). Smells can have a psychological effect even when the aroma is below the level of human awareness.

INTERVENTION

Essential oils can be absorbed into the body through olfaction, topical application, or ingestion. Table 22.3 provides methods for using essential oils. The compounds within an essential oil find their way into the bloodstream however they are applied (Tisserand & Balacs, 1995). Inhaled aromas have the fastest effect, although compounds absorbed through massage can be detected in the blood within 20 minutes (Jager, Bauchbauer, Jirovetz, & Fritzer, 1979). The choice of the method of application depends on the nurse, the available time for the action to occur, desired outcome, the chemical components within the essential oil, and the psychological needs of the patient. It would appear that the effects of inhaled essential oils do not last as long as topically applied essential oils. However, it is difficult to analyze exactly what impact touch has in outcomes of aromatherapy.

One of the simplest methods is through direct inhalation or olfaction, where an essential oil is directly targeted to the patient: 1 to 5 drops of essential oil is placed on a tissue (or floated on hot water in a bowl) and inhaled for 5 to 10 minutes.

Indirect inhalation includes the use of burners, nebulizers, and vaporizers that can be operated by heat, battery, or electricity and may or may not

TABLE 22.3   Methods of Use for Essential Oils

Inhalation: useful for depression, insomnia, sinusitis, upper respiratory tract
  infection. Inhale directly from tissue or float 2 drops on steaming bowl of water.

Topical: useful for contusions, skin complaints, muscle strain, and scar tissue.
  Compresses, baths and massage, the 'm' technique®.

Vaginal: useful for yeast infections or cystitis. Use diluted in carrier oil on tampon.
  Only use essential oils high in alcohols, such as tea tree.

include the use of water. Larger, portable aroma systems are available to control the release of essential oils on a commercial scale into rooms up to 1,500
square feet. This is similar to environmental fragrancing (using synthetics)
that is common practice in hotels and department stores. Indirect inhalation
can be useful for mood enhancement and stress reduction.

When used in a bath, 4 to 6 drops of the essential oil are dissolved first in
a teaspoon of milk, rubbing alcohol, or carrier oil (cold-pressed) and then
placed in the bath water. Because essential oils are not soluble in water, they
would float on the top of the water if used undiluted, giving an uneven treatment. The water is vigorously agitated before a person relaxes in the bath for
10 minutes.

Research has indicated that the chronically ill can suffer from "skin
hunger," a longing to be touched (Ingham, 1989). When people are ill the
sense of smell can be heightened or altered and familiar pleasant aromas
make a person feel more secure. Another method for using essential oils is in
a compress. To prepare a compress, add 4 to 6 drops of essential oil to warm
water. A soft cotton cloth is soaked in the mixture, wrung out, and applied to
the affected area (contusion or abrasion). The compress is covered with plastic wrap to retain the moisture, and a towel is placed over the plastic wrap
and kept in place for 4 hours.

Essential oils are absorbed through the skin by diffusion, with the dermis
and fat layer acting as a reservoir before the components of the essential oils
reach the dermis and the bloodstream. There is some evidence that massage
or hot water enhances the absorption of at least some of the components of
essential oils.

Aromatherapy using touch enhances communication with patients. One
to two drops of an essential oil are diluted in a teaspoon (5 ml) of cold-pressed
vegetable oil, cream, or gel. Gentle friction and hot water enhance absorption of essential oils through the skin to the bloodstream. The amount of oil
absorbed from a massage using essential oils will normally be 1.125 ml–1 ml
(Tisserand & Balacs, 1995).

Another touch technique using essential oils is the "m" technique® (Buckle, 2000). This method is different from traditional massage. Some of the important aspects of the "m" technique are:

- A recognized, registered method of touch is used.
- A structured stroking sequence with a set pattern and set pressure are used.
- The massage can be used on the hands and face.
- It is a gentle technique and appropriate for critically ill and dying persons, children, and during painful procedures.
- It is easy to learn and can be taught to family caregivers.

MEASUREMENT OF OUTCOMES

The measurements used will depend on the problem for which essential oils are used. For example, if lavender is used to promote sleep, outcomes would be chosen to determine if insomnia decreased.

PRECAUTIONS

Aromatherapy is a very safe complementary therapy if it is used within set guidelines. Nurses should not administer essential oils orally as this is outside a nurse's scope of practice, and poisoning (and in some circumstances fatalities) have been documented. If an essential oil gets into the eyes, nurses should rinse it out with milk or a carrier oil and then water (essential oils do not dissolve in water). A list of contraindicated essential oils can be found in training manuals; novices should consult these lists. Essential oils that are high in phenols tend to be aggressive and should not be used undiluted on the skin or for long periods of time. They should not be used during early pregnancy. Extra care is needed when using them with patients receiving chemotherapy because essential oils may affect the absorption rate of certain chemotherapeutic drugs. Nurses need to be aware of which essential oils are photosensitive, such as bergamot.

Most essential oils have been tested by the food and beverage industry as many are used as flavorings (Opdyke, 1977), and other research has been carried out by the perfume industry. Most of the essential oils commonly used in clinical aromatherapy have been given GRAS (generally regarded as safe) status. However, they are very concentrated and potent compounds and are usually diluted in carrier oils for topical use. Clove and cinnamon, for example, are high in phenols and should not be used undiluted on the skin.

Some essential oils are contraindicated in persons with estrogen-dependent tumors, hypertension, seizures, or pregnancy. Other essential oils can potentiate (or decrease) the effects of barbiturates or antibiotics, may cause dermal irritation, or are contraindicated in the presence of ultraviolet light.

Essential oils should not be confused with herbal extracts, which are completely different chemical mixtures, and the two substances cannot be used interchangeably. Another important distinction is that herbal extracts and teas are usually taken internally while essential oils are not. Essential oils are volatile and herbal extracts are not.

Perhaps one of the greatest risks in aromatherapy is using an incorrect essential oil for a particular health outcome. This could stem from a nurse's lack of knowledge about plant taxonomy, a system that classifies plants according to their similarities. The taxonomy divides plants into family, genus, species, and variety, and, in aromatherapy, the part of the plant that is used in the extraction process: e.g., flos = flower, fol = leaf.

Many essential oils have familiar common names such as lavender, rose, and rosemary, but it is important to know the full botanical name. For example, lavender is a common name that covers three different kinds of lavender and countless synthetic hybrids. The botanical name will give the genus and the species (rather like a surname and a first name, respectively. The genus of lavender is *Lavandula*, and all lavenders begin with this word. *Lavandula angustifolia* is possibly the most widely used and researched essential oil and is recognized as a relaxant. However, the other two species have very different properties. *Lavandula latifolia* (spike lavender) is a stimulant and expectorant; *Lavandula stoechas* is antimicrobial and not safe to use for long periods of time because it contains a large percentage of ketones that can build up toxicity. Another common herb with potential for confusion is marjoram, which is the common name for *Thymus mastichina* (actually a thyme) and *Origanum marjoranum* (the "real" marjoram). For nurses to use aromatherapy clinically it is very important for them to know the full botanical name of an essential oil. Table 22.5 provides examples of plant identification and Table 22.4 lists the botanical names of essential oils discussed in this chapter.

GUIDELINES

There are some general guidelines for use of essential oils:

- Store away from an open flame; essential oils are volatile and highly flammable.
- Store in a cool place away from sunlight; use amber or blue colored containers.

TABLE 22.4   Common and Botanical Names of Essential Oils

Common Name	Botanical Name
Aniseed	*Pimpinella anisum*
Basil	*Ocimum basilicum*
Chamomile, German	*Matricaria recutita*
Chamomile, Roman	*Chamaemelum nobile*
Clary sage	*Salvia sclarea*
Coriander seed	*Coriandrum sativum*
Eucalyptus	*Eucalyptus globulus*
Fennel	*Foeniculum vulgare*
Geranium	*Pelargonium graveolens*
Ginger	*Zingiber officinale*
Hyssop	*Hyssopus officinalis*
Lavender, true	*Lavandula officinalis*
Lemongrass	*Cymbopogon citratus*
Neroli	*Citrus aurantium* var. *amara*
Palmarosa	*Cymbopogon martinii*
Parlsey	*Petroselinum sativum*
Pennyroyal	*Mentha pulegium*
Peppermint	*Mentha piperita*
Rose	*Rosa damascena*
Rosewood	*Aniba rosaeodora*
Sage	*Salvia officinalis*
Sandalwood	*Santalum album*
Tarragon	*Artemesia dracunculus*
Wintergreen	*Gaultheria procumbens*
Ylang-ylang	*Cananga odorata*

- Essential oils can stain clothing—beware!
- Keep away from children and pets.
- Use essential oils from reputable suppliers.
- Close the container immediately after use.
- Care is needed when using with persons who have a history of severe asthma or who have multiple allergies.

TABLE 22.5   Examples of Taxonomy in Plant Identification

Example 1:	Common name	neroli
	Botanical name	*Citrus aurantium* var. *amara flos*
	Family	Rutaceae
	Genus	*Citrus*
	Species	*aurantium*
	Variety	amara
	Part	flos (flower)
Example 2:	Common name	lavender
	Botanical name	*Lavandula angustifolia*
	Family	Lamiaceae (was Labiatae)
	Genus	*Lavandula*
	Species	*angustifolia*
	Part	flowering plant

USES

Essential oils can be used for a myriad of symptoms. These symptoms may be physiological, psychological, or spiritual. They can help alleviate many physiological problems such as infection, pain, respiratory distress, wounds, and poor skin integrity. Psychological problems such as insomnia and depression can also be helped with aromatherapy. Essential oils have been used for thousands of years for spiritual comfort and are useful towards the end of life or when spiritual comfort is needed. Suggestions for using essential oils for a variety of conditions and populations are provided in Table 22.6.

FUTURE RESEARCH

A large volume of unpublished research exists, but there is a dearth of published, randomized, controlled studies. This discrepancy may be because much of the research has been dissertation research. Also, little funding for aromatherapy has been available. As with herbal medicine, research into aromatherapy is fraught with methodological problems. What is the control condition for aroma? Should aroma and touch be evaluated separately when both are used? Should only single essential oils be used? Should standardized oils be used? (Essential oils contain between 100 and 400 different

TABLE 22.6   Suggestions for Use of Essential Oils with Patients*

Pain Relief

Migraine: peppermint, lavender (T)*

Osteoarthritis: eucalyptus, black pepper, ginger, spike lavender, Roman chamomile, rosemary, myrrh (T)

Rheumatoid arthritis: German chamomile, lavender, peppermint, frankincense (T)

Low back pain: lemongrass, rosemary, lavender, sweet marjoram (T)

Cramps: Roman chamomile, clary sage, lavender, sweet marjoram (T)

General aches and pains: rosemary, lavender, lemongrass, clary sage, black pepper, lemon eucalyptus, spike lavender.

Gynecological

Menopausal symptoms: clary sage, sage, fennel, aniseed, geranium, rose, cypress (I**, T)

Menstrual cramping: Roman chamomile, lavender, clary sage (T)

Premenstrual syndrome: Clary sage, geranium, rose (T)

Infertility with no physiological cause: clary sage, sage, fennel, aniseed, geranium, rose (T)

Cardiovascular

Borderline hypertension: ylang-ylang, lavender

Transient hypotension caused by some antidepressants: rosemary, spike lavender

Urinary

Cystitis: tea tree, palma rosa (T especially sitz bath)

Water retention: juniper, cypress, fennel (T)

Gastrointestinal

Irritable bowel syndrome: Roman chamomile, clary sage, mandarin, cardamon, peppermint, mandarin, fennel, lavender

Constipation: fennel, black pepper (T)

Indigestion: peppermint, ginger (I)

Infection

Bacterial including MRSA, VRSA: tea tree, lavender, peppermint (I, T)

Other bacteria: eucalyptus, naiouli, sweet marjoram, oregano, tarragon, savory, German chamomile, thyme, manuka (I, T)

Viral: ravansara, palma rosa, lemon, eucalyptus smithii, melissa, rose, bergamot (I, T)

Fungal: lemongrass, black pepper, clove, caraway (T); geranium, tea tree (particularly good for toenail fungus; apply undiluted daily to nailbed for several months)

TABLE 22.6   (Continued)

Pediatrics
  Behavioral problems: mandarin, lavender, Roman chamomile, rose (I, T)
  Colic: Roman chamomile, mandarin (T)
  Diaper rash: lavender
  Sleep problems: lavender, rose, mandarin
  Autism: rose can help multihandicapped children interact socially

Respiratory
  Bronchitis: ravansara, eucalyptus globulus, eucalyptus smithi, tea tree, spike
    lavender (I)
  Sinusitis: eucalyptus globulus, lavender, spike lavender, rosemary (I)
  Mild asthma: lavender, clary sage, Roman chamomile (I)

Dermatology
  Mild acne: tea tree, juniper, cypress, naiouli (T)
  Mild psoriasis: lavender, German chamomile (T)
  Diabetic ulcers: lavender, frankincense, myrrh (T)

Oncology
  Nausea: peppermint, ginger, mandarin
  Post-radiation burns: lavender, German chamomile, Tamanu carrier oil

Older Adults
  Memory loss: rosemary, rose, peppermint, basil
  Dry flaky skin: geranium, frankincense
  Alzheimer's disease: rosemary, lavender, pine, frankincense

Palliative Care
  Spiritual: rose, angelica, frankincense
  Physical: lavender, peppermint, lemongrass, rosemary
  Emotional: geranium, pine, sandalwood
  Relaxation: lavender, clary sage, mandarin, frankincense, ylang-ylang
  Pressure ulcers: lavender, tea tree, sweet marjoram, frankincense

Care of the Dying
  Rites of passage: choose selection of patient's favorite aromas or frankincense,
    rose
  Bereavement: rose, sandalwood, patchouli, angelica, frankincense, myrrh

*T = topical application
**I = inhalation
If no designation, can be administered either topically or by inhalation.

components, and each component varies slightly according to the climatic growing conditions, harvesting methods, and distillation process.) Because essential oils are herbal derivatives, they act as adaptogens. This means they may react differently from one person to the next, depending on the needs of the person. How can research methods accommodate this?

CREDENTIALING

Currently there is no recognized national certification exam for aromatherapists. Nurses and health professionals wishing to use aromatherapy to enhance their practice should check with their licensing bodies for a list of acceptable courses. There are many different courses available and health professionals should choose one that is relevant to their clinical practice. At present, there is no governing body for aromatherapy. In the United States, the Aromatherapy Registration Council, a nonprofit entity, was established in 2000. It administers a national exam and can provide the public with a list of registered practitioners. The largest professional organization is the National Association of Holistic Aromatherapy (NAHA). There are no requirements at this time for a person administering aromatherapy to be certified or accredited. The length of training in aromatherapy ranges from one weekend to several years. Any person, not necessarily just health professionals, can enroll in the educational programs. The American Holistic Nurses Association can provide a list of accredited courses.

REFERENCES

Betts, T. (1996). The fragrant breeze: The role of aromatherapy in treating epilepsy. *Aromatherapy Quarterly, 51,* 25–27.

Buchbauer, H., Jirovetz, L., Jager, W., Dietrich, H., & Plank, C. (1991). Aromatherapy: Evidence for sedative effect of the essential oil of lavender after inhalation. *Zeitschrift fur Naturforschung Teil C., 46,* 1067–1072.

Buckle, J. (2000). The "m" technique. *Massage and bodywork,* 52–64.

Carson, C., Cookson, B., Farrelly, H., & Riley, T. (1995). Susceptibility of methicillin-resistant *Staphylococcus aureus* to the essential oil of *Melaleuca alternifolia. Journal of Antimicrobial Chemotherapy, 35,* 421–424.

Eisenberg, D., Davis, R., Ettner, S., Applel, S., Wilkey, S., VanRompay, M., & Kessler, R. (1998). Trends in alternative medicine in the USA, 1990–1997. *Journal of the American Medical Association, 280,* 784–787.

Eisenberg, D., Kessler, R., Foster, C., Norlock, F., Calkins, D., & Delbanco, T.

(1993). Unconventional medicine in the United States. *New England Journal of Medicine, 328,* 246–252.

Gobel, H., Schmidt, G., & Soyka, D. (1994). Effect of peppermint and eucalyptus oil preparations on neurophysiological and experimental algesimetric headache parameters. *Cephalalgia, 14,* 228–234.

Gobel, H., Schmidt, G., Dworschak, M., Stolze, H., & Heuss, D. (1995). Essential plant oils and headache mechanisms. *Phytomedicine, 2*(2), 93–102.

Ingham, A. (1989). A review of the literature relating to touch and its use in intensive care. *Intensive Care Nursing, 5,* 65–75.

Jager, W., Bauchbauer, G., Jirovetz, L., & Fritzer, M. (1979). Percutaneous absorption of lavender oil from a massage oil. *Journal of Social Cosmetology Chemistry, 43*(1), 49–54.

Komori, T., Fujiwara, R., Tanida, M., Nomura, J., & Yokoyama, M. (1995). Effects of citrus fragrance on immune function and depressive states. *Neuroimmunomodulation, 2,* 174–180.

Krall, B., & Krause, W. (1993). *Efficacy and tolerance of Mentha arvensis aethoreleum.* Paper presented at the 24th International Symposium of Essential Oils, Berlin, Germany.

Larrondo, J., Agut, M., & Calco-Torras, M. (1995). Antimicrobial activity of essences of labiates. *Microbios (Cambridge), 82,* 171–172.

Lorenzetti, B., Souza, G., Sarti, S., Santos, S., Filho, D., & Ferreira, S. (1991). Myrcene mimics the peripheral analgesic activity of lemongrass tea. *Ethnopharmacology, 34,* 43–48.

Manly, C. H. (1993). Psychophysiological effects of odor. *Critical Review of Food Science Nutrition, 33*(1), 57–62.

Moate, S. (1995). Anxiety and depression. *International Journal of Aromatherapy, 7*(1), 18–21.

Nelson, R. (1997). In vitro activities of five plant essential oils against MRSA and vancomycin-resistant *Enterococcus faecium. Journal of Anticrobial Chemotherapy, 40,* 305–306.

Opdyke, D. L. J. (1977). Safety testing of fragrances: Problems and implications. *Clinical Toxicology, 19*(1), 61–67.

Seth, G., Kokate, C. K., & Varma, K. C. (1975). Effect of essential oil of *Cymbopogon citratus* on central nervous system. *Journal of Experimental Biology, 14,* 370–371.

Schnaubelt, K. (1999). *Medical aromatherapy.* Berkeley, CA: Frog Ltd.

Stevensen, C. (1995). Aromatherapy. In D. Rankin-Box (Ed.), *Nurses handbook of complementary therapies* (p. 55), London: Churchill Livingstone.

Styles, J. (1997). The use of aromatherapy in hospitalized children with HIV. *Complementary Therapies in Nursing, 3,* 16–20.

Tisserand, R., & Balacs, T. (1995). *Essential oil safety.* London: Churchill Livingstone.

Tisserand, R. (1988). Lavender beats benzodiazepines. *International Journal of Aromatherapy, 1*(2), 1–2.

Wannisorm, B., Jarikasem, S., & Soontormtanasart, T. (1996). Antifungal activity of lemongrass oil and lemongrass oil cream . *Phytotherapy Research, 10,* 551–554.

Wilkonson, S. (1995). Aromatherapy and massage in palliative care. *International Journal of Palliative Nursing, 1*(1), 21–30.

Woolfson, A., & Hewitt, D. (1992). Intensive aromacare. *International Journal of Aromatherapy, 4*(2), 12–14.

23

Herbal Medicines

Gregory A. Plotnikoff

Despite herbal medicine's being the oldest and most widely used form of medicine in the world, and despite the wide use of coffee, cocaine, heroin, and tobacco for their physiologic effects, until recently the medicinal properties of plant-derived substances have been overlooked by American health professionals. Of the best-selling 150 prescription drugs, 86 contain at least one major active compound from natural sources. In addition to aspirin, digoxin, and antibiotics, plant-derived medications include numerous anticholinergic agents, anticoagulants, antihypertensives, and antineoplastic agents. Surprisingly, of the top 150 pharmaceuticals, only 35 plant species are represented (Grifo, 1997).

The most recent national survey documented that 44.6 million Americans use herbal remedies on a regular basis and that more than 90 million Americans had used an herbal remedy in the past 12 months. Of those who use herbal medicines 36% do so in lieu of prescription medicines and 31% do so in combination with prescriptions. The leading reason for substitution is preference for a natural or organic product. Sources for information are, in order of preference, friends, magazines, product labels, and advertising. Health professionals are the least frequently consulted for information (Johnson, 2000).

DEFINITION

Herbal medicines, or plant-based therapies, continue to occupy a central importance in the world's many healing traditions. These include the use of single herbs in many Western traditions and the use of multiple-herb combinations

259

in traditional Asian medical systems. Often herbs are part of an overarching belief system that may involve spiritual or metaphysical components. Herbal medicines are often included in the work of shamans and other traditional healers who serve as intermediaries with the spirit world. Herbal medicines are also one tool in traditional Asian medicine for acupuncturists who help open blocked channels (meridians) for the free flow of *qi* (life spirit or force).

Herbal medicines, also known as botanicals or phytotherapies, are one component of the range of natural products sold in the United States as dietary supplements. These include fungi-based products (mycotherapies), essential oils (aromatherapies), and vitamin, mineral, and nutritional therapies (nutraceuticals). Since the passage of the Dietary Supplement Health and Education Act of 1994 (DSHEA), these biological modifiers have been available over the counter as dietary supplements. Though neither food nor drug, these substances are still regulated by the Food and Drug Administration (FDA) but with less stringent requirements. Unlike food and drugs, dietary supplements can be sold based on evidence of safety in the possession of the manufacturer and can only be removed from the market if the FDA can prove them unsafe under ordinary conditions of use.

Under DSHEA, herbal medicines can be sold for "stimulating, maintaining, supporting, regulating and promoting health" rather than for treating disease. As dietary supplements rather than drugs, herbal medicines may not claim to restore normal or to correct abnormal function. Additionally, herbs may not claim to "diagnose, treat, prevent, cure, or mitigate" (DSHEA, 1994). Herbal medicine companies can assert that their product supports cardiovascular health but not that it lowers cholesterol. To do so would suggest that the product is for treating a disease (hypercholesterolemia) and is therefore subject to FDA pharmaceutical regulations.

This has raised questions about what constitutes a disease. The FDA originally suggested that disease is any deviation, impairment, or interruption of the normal structure or function of any part or organ or system of the body that is manifested by a characteristic set of one or more signs and symptoms. This generated many concerns. "Normal structure" appeared to be normed to a 30-year-old male and therefore did not account for gender or aging. For example, are menstrual cramps or menopause diseases? With no signs or symptoms, is hypercholesterolemia a disease or a risk factor? After significant public outcry, the FDA adopted the definition of disease found in the Nutrition Labeling and Health Act of 1990. Disease is currently considered damage to an organ, part, structure, or system of the body such that it does not function properly (e.g., cardiovascular disease) or a state of health leading to such (e.g., hypertension).

SCIENTIFIC BASIS

Significant research has been done using Western biomedical/scientific models on numerous single herbal agents. Beginning in 1978, the German government's *Bundesgesunheitsamt* (Federal Health Agency) began evaluating the safety and efficacy of phytomedicines. The health professionals charged with doing so, named the Commission E, met until 1994 and evaluated 300 herbal medicines. They recognized 190 herbal medicines as suitable for medicinal use. The complete reports have been translated and are available from the American Botanical Council (1997).

Beginning in 1996, significant meta-analyses and review articles of single herb products began appearing on a regular basis in leading Western medical journals. These are readily accessible via the National Library of Medicine's PubMed Web site (*http://www.ncbi.nlm.nih.gov/PubMed/*). Compiling data from similar studies for analysis (meta-analysis) is complicated by the fact that many studies published to date have left out important information including naming the specific plant species studied (e.g., echinacea versus *Echinacea purpurea, E. pallida*, or *E. augustofolia*), the parts used (stems, leaves, or roots), the form (pressed juice, powdered whole extract, aqueous extract, ethanol extract, or aqueous-ethanol extract), and the formulation (stated proportions of water to alcohol or specifically extracted fractions and concentrations).

Standardization of herbal medicines is crucial for both scientific study and consumer protection. Standardization is equated with reproducibility, guaranteed potency, quality, and documentable effectiveness. However, with herbal medicines, standardization presents several problems. First, the active ingredient may not be known. Second, there may be more than one active ingredient, and third, both content and activity of an herbal medicine may be related to the means of extraction and processing. This complicates significantly both research and counseling for health professionals and consumers.

INTERVENTION

TECHNIQUE

Herbal medicines and dietary supplements need to be addressed in clinical settings in the same manner one addresses pharmaceutical agents. This includes attention to interviewing and anticipating complications. Both of these will be discussed.

Every health professional needs to be aware of the wide use of herbal medicines and other dietary supplements. Efficient and effective patient advocacy means including questions on alternative therapies as a standard part of each patient interview. Reasonable questions include, Are you using any herbs? Vitamins? Dietary supplements? Follow up questions include, What dose? What source? What directions are you following? Why are you taking it? Additionally, asking about the source of information can be quite helpful as in, "Are you working with any other health professionals?" As with all good interviewing, listening for understanding rather than agreement or disagreement enhances the therapeutic alliance.

Unfortunately, professionals often are not asking such questions and patients are not volunteering such information. This "don't ask, don't tell" policy makes no sense in patient care. All health professionals need to create a safe and conducive environment where patients can share such important information without fear of ridicule or other negative responses. "Ask, then ask again" is a policy which lends itself to effective and efficient patient care.

PRECAUTIONS

Ascertaining the herbal medicines that are being used is crucial for identifying those patients at risk for interactions with prescription medications or for excessive bleeding in surgery. Patients with special risks of drug interactions include those on the following pharmaceutical agents: anticoagulants, hypoglycemics, antidepressants, sedative-hypnotics, and medications with narrow therapeutic windows such as digoxin and theophylline. Patients at risk for bleeding complications include those using anti-platelet herbs such as *Gingko biloba* and high doses of garlic or cayenne. The use of many herbs are contraindicated in pregnancy and breast feeding. In the vast majority of cases, no scientific documentation exists on actual risk.

Nursing skills include the ability to counsel. Table 23.1 lists key teaching points regarding herbal medicines. Because many herbs have theoretical or actual risks worth recognizing, Table 23.2 cites leading reputable herbal references. All serious adverse reactions should be reported to the FDA through the MedWatch program at 1-800-332-1088 or at http://www.fda.gov/medwatch.

USES

Herbal medicine knowledge for nurses cannot be summarized quickly. This chapter will now address three leading herbs from an evidence-based perspective. The reader will note that there is a significant range in scientific data available on each and that theoretical risks are present that should be acknowledged by both patients and health professionals.

TABLE 23.1 Five Key Patient Learning Points

Just because it is natural does not mean it is safe.

Just because it is safe does not mean it is effective.

Labels may not equal contents.

Self-diagnosis and self-treatment can result in self-malpractice.

Herbs are never a replacement for an emergency room.

Chronic illness, surgery, and use of prescription medications are three situations where herbal medicine reviews by nurses are important. Echinacea does stimulate the immune system, but this is not necessarily a positive effect. *Gingko biloba's* pharmacologic activity places people at risk in surgery. Saint John's-wort is effective for mild to moderate depression but can render many prescription medications ineffective. Every reader should be aware that many herbs have a sufficient evidence base and represent alternative tools. Additionally, every reader should be aware that clinical resources are readily available for informed decision making (see Table 23.2).

Echinacea (*Echinacea augustofolia, E. pallida, E. purpurea*): Echinacea, grown in North American gardens commonly known as the purple coneflower, was used by Native Americans and early settlers as a remedy for infections and for healing wounds. In vitro research has documented that echinacea species contain inulin and increase circulating properdin, both of which activate the alternate complement pathway (Bauer & Wagner, 1991). Echinacea enhances T-cell replication, natural killer cell activity, macrophage phagocytosis, as well as production of tumor necrosis factor-alpha (TNF), interferon beta-2, and interleukin-1, -6, and -10 (Burger, Torres, Warren, Caldwell, & Hughes, 1997; Luettig, Steinmuller, Gifford, Wagner, & Lohmann-Matthes, 1989; Roesler et al., 1991a, 1991b).

Echinacea is promoted in the United States for the prevention and treatment of the common cold. In Europe, it is used topically for wound healing and intravenously for immunostimulation. A 1994 review of 26 controlled trials (18 randomized and 11 double-blind) of echinacea extracts used for cold prevention and treatment, reduction of chemotherapy side effects, and general immune enhancement found positive results in most groups studied. The authors noted, however, that most of the studies were of such poor methodological quality that clear recommendations could not be made regarding the use of echinacea, including dosages (Melchart & Linde, 1994). Since then, two methodologically valid clinical studies have been published.

TABLE 23.2   Herbal References

American Botanical Council: *www.herbalgram.org*

Herb Research Foundation: *www.herbs.org*

Herbal Medicine—The Expanded Commission E Monographs edited by
   Blumenthal, Goldberg, and Brinckmann. Austin, TX: American Botanical
   Council, 2000.

The Professional's Handbook of Complementary and Alternative Medicine edited by
   Fetrow and Avila. Philadelphia: Springhouse, 1999.

*Tyler's Honest Herbal: A Sensible Guide to the Use of Herbs and Related Remedies
   4th Edition* edited by Foster and Tyler. New York: Haworth Press, 1999.

101 Medicinal Herbs: An Illustrated Guide by Foster. Loveland, CO: Interweave
   Press, 1998.

HerbalGram magazine. Published quarterly by the American Botanical Council
   and the Herb Research Foundation. Fax 512-926-2345

First, a double-blind, three-armed, placebo-controlled trial of *E. augustofolia*
and *E. purpurea* prophylaxis of upper respiratory infections in 302 volunteers demonstrated no protective effect when compared with placebo
(Melchart, Walther, Linde, Brandmeaier, & Lersch, 1998). Second, a
double-blind, randomized, placebo-controlled study of 160 patients using
E. pallida for both bacterial and viral upper respiratory infections demonstrated clinically significant reductions in length of illness ($P < 0.0001$),
overall symptom scores ($P < 0.0004$), and whole clinical scores ($P < 0.001$)
(Dorn, Knick, & Lewith, 1997).

Echinacea is not recommended for persons with allergies to members of
the *Asteraceae* family (formerly termed *Compositae*), which includes rag-
weed, daisies, thistles, and chamomile. More importantly, nonspecific
immunostimulation is not always beneficial. Tumor necrosis factor-alpha
and interleukin-1 are pro-inflammatory cytokines and recent evidence
demonstrates that anti-TNF and anti-interleukin-1 therapies are effective for
Crohn's disease and rheumatoid arthritis. Because echinacea increases TNF
production, it cannot be recommended for people with other chronic
immunologic diseases, including multiple sclerosis, lupus, and HIV.

The LD_{50} of intravenously administered echinacea juice is 50 ml/kg in
mice and rats. Regular oral administration to mice at levels greater than proposed human therapeutic doses has failed to demonstrate toxic effects.
(Mengs, Clare, & Poiley, 1991). However, one study has suggested that repeated daily doses suppress the immune response (Coeugniet & Elek, 1987).
Commission E recommends that use be limited to 8 weeks.

TABLE 23.3 Three Popular Herbs: Indications, Actions, Contraindications

Herb	Indications	Actions	Contraindications/Side Effects
Echinacea	Common cold/URIs	Activates alternative complementary pathway; enhances macrophage phagocytosis, T-cell replication, and cytokine production	Not for use with autoimmune diseases—may cause immune suppression with prolonged use
Gingko biloba	Memory problems including dementia; peripheral vascular disease	Antioxidant and vasodilatory properties; antagonizes platelet activating factor (PAF)	Caution required with anticoagulation and/or antiplatelet agents; may rarely cause GI upset, headache, and dizziness
Saint John's Wort	Mild to moderate depression	Inhibits uptake of serotonin, norepinephrine, and dopamine; inhibits binding to GABA receptors	Reduces serum levels of theophylline, digoxin, cyclosporine, idinavir. Reduces INR. Associated with increased photosensitivity. Theoretical risk of serotonergic crisis when used with other agents

Gingko (*Gingko biloba*): Ginkgo is the number one selling herb in Europe, where it is used for circulatory problems such as intermittent claudication (Letzel & Schoop, 1992), impotence (Sikora et al., 1989), and cerebral insufficiency (Kleijnen & Knipschild, 1992a). Commission E also approves its use for dementia syndromes with memory deficits, disturbances in concentration, depressive emotional condition, dizziness, tinnitus, and headaches. A 1992 review of 40 clinical studies found only eight methodologically valid, placebo-controlled trials, of which seven demonstrated that ginkgo was more effective than placebo for memory and concentration problems, headaches, depression, and dizziness (Kleijnen & Knipschild, 1992b). European studies published in 1994 and 1996 demonstrated its effectiveness in slowing or reversing dementia (Hofferberth, 1994; Kanowski, Herrmann, Stephan, Wierich, & Horr, 1996). Recently, these findings were confirmed for patients with Alzheimer's disease and multi-infarct dementia in an American trial with 309 subjects (LeBars et al., 1997).

Ginkgo's mechanism of action is believed to be its in vitro antioxidative, vasodilatory, and antiplatelet properties. It is more effective than beta-carotene and vitamin E as an oxidative scavenger and inhibitor of lipid peroxidation of cellular membranes (Pietschmann, 1992) and stimulates the release of nitric oxide (Chen, Salwinski, & Lee, 1997). Ginkgo is also a potent antagonist of platelet activating factor (Braquet, 1987) and thus inhibits platelet aggregation and promotes clot breakdown. These properties may result in neuroprotective and ischemia re-perfusion protective effects (Oyama, Chikahisa, Ueha, Kanemaru, & Noda, 1996; Fuchs, Katayama, & Noda, 1994; Shen & Zhou, 1995).

Side effects with ginkgo are extremely uncommon. They include gastrointestinal discomfort, headache, and dizziness (Tyler, 1996). Because of the antiplatelet effect, however, there is a risk of significant bleeding when ginkgo is used with anticoagulants and other antiplatelet agents (Matthews, 1998; Rosenblatt & Mindel, 1997; Rowin & Lewis, 1996). Gingko should be discontinued 10 days prior to surgery and not restarted until the surgical wound has healed sufficiently to allow for aspirin use.

Saint John's wort (*Hypericum perforatum*): Saint John's wort has been the subject of innumerable reports on television and radio, and in newspapers and magazines as a "wonder drug" for depression or as "nature's Prozac." Saint John's wort is now the fifth best selling herb in Europe, surpassing fluoxetine by a large margin in Germany, where it is licensed for the treatment of anxiety, depression, and insomnia.

In vitro studies demonstrate that *Hypericum* extract is active at numerous neurotransmitter receptors, including serotonin, adenosine, monoamine oxidase (MAO-A and MAO-B), as well as GABA-A and GABA-B (Cott, 1997). The result is modulated synaptosomal uptake of the neurotransmitters serotonin, norepinephrine, and dopamine as well as GABA receptor binding. Components of the extract appear to inhibit MAO-A and -B weakly. No in vivo inhibition has been demonstrated, however (Bladt & Wagner, 1994; Thiede & Walper, 1994). *Hypericum* extract may inhibit serotonin uptake by postsynaptic receptors (Muller, Rolli, Schafer, & Hafner, 1997).

A 1996 review of 23 randomized trials involving 1,757 patients with mild to moderate depression documented that *Hypericum* extracts are significantly better than placebo and similarly effective as tricyclic antidepressants. Overall, 55.1% of subjects responded to Saint John's wort and 22.3% responded to placebo. (Linde, et al., 1996). These studies have been criticized for not standardizing the diagnosis of depression or the dose of the herb's presumed active ingredient, hypericin. Additionally, the studies were short in duration and enrolled small numbers of subjects. It should be noted, however, that hypericin may not be the active ingredient in Saint John's wort; several constituents such as pseudohypericin and hyperforin have pharmacologic effects.

Saint John's wort has a more favorable side-effect profile than tricyclic antidepressants. In the above meta-analysis, side effects were noted in 19.8% of patients taking Saint John's wort, compared with 35.9% of those who received tricyclic antidepressants. Withdrawal from studies due to side effects occurred in 4% of Saint John's wort patients, compared with 7.7% of those receiving standard antidepressants. A comparison study with fluoxetine funded by NIH is underway. One 6-week randomized, double-blind comparison study of fluoxetine and Saint John's wort in 161 geriatric patients demonstrated nearly identical response rates and declines in the Hamilton Depression Scale scores (Harrer, Schmidt, Kuhn, & Biller, 1999). The Institute of Clinical Pharmacology in Berlin noted that even in high doses, Saint John's wort was well tolerated (Kerb et al., 1996). No in vivo MAO-inhibiting activity has been demonstrated with *Hypericum*; therefore, no dietary precautions are indicated at this time (American Botanical Council, 1997). A direct toxicity concern is the risk of hypericism, a photosensitivity found in animals that graze on large amounts of Saint John's wort. Because of the risk of causing a serotoninergic crisis, there is no indication for using Saint John's wort with prescription antidepressants.

The most serious toxicity associated is the negative interactions with prescription drugs. Saint John's wort is a potent ligand for the nuclear receptor that regulates the expression of cytochrome P450 (CYP) 3A4, the hepatic enzyme involved in the metabolism of more than 50% of all prescription drugs (Moore et al., 2000). These include oral contraceptives, idinavir, cyclosporine, theophylline, digoxin, and warfarin. Hence, the use of Saint John's wort can be life-threatening for people requiring prescription medications.

FUTURE RESEARCH

Before herbal medicines are more widely accepted by the conventional allopathic medical system, more randomized, double-blind, placebo-controlled trials are needed in the United States. The NIH National Center for Complementary and Alternative Medicine (NCCAM) has and will continue to fund such clinical trials of herbal therapies. The most promising and most understudied herbs include the following:

1. Ginseng for restoration of homeostasis under stressful conditions
2. Milk thistle for hepatoprotection in the setting of hepatotoxic agents
3. Feverfew for migraine prophylaxis
4. Garlic for cancer chemoprevention

Additionally, significant efforts are needed to identify the most promising herbal supports for chemotherapy and radiation therapy as well as for asthma and heart disease.

Western medicine has yet to explore the potential benefits from the world's many healing traditions that use customized combinations of herbs. To research these will require a new paradigm, one that accounts for potential synergy and counterbalancing activities of multiple ingredients. Although intriguing preliminary data exists for many dietary supplements, the historic paucity of funding mechanisms in these areas has meant that the scientific support for use of many commercial products lags significantly behind the consumer marketing efforts.

REFERENCES

American Botanical Council (1997). St. John's wort [Monograph], *Herbal Gram, 40*, S28.

Bauer, R., & Wagner, H. (1991). Echinacea species as potential immunostimulatory drugs. *Economics and Medicinal Plant Research, 5*, 253–321.

Bladt, S., & Wagner, H. (1994). Inhibition of MAO by fractions and constituents of hypericum extract. *Journal of Geriatric Psychiatry and Neurology, 7*, S57–59.

Braquet, P. (1987). The gingkolides: Potent platelet activating factor antagonists isolated from *Gingko biloba* L: Chemistry, pharmacology and clinical applications. *Drug Future, 12,* 643–699.

Burger, R. A., Torres, A. R., Warren, R. P., Caldwell, V. D., & Hughes, B. G. (1997) Echinacea-induced cytokine production by human macrophages. *International Journal of Immunopharmacology, 19,* 371–379.

Chen, X., Salwinski, S., & Lee, T. J. (1997) Extracts of *Gingko biloba* and ginsenosides exert cerebral vasorelaxation via a nitric oxide pathway. *Clinical Experimental Pharmacology and Physiology, 24,* 958–959.

Coeugniet, E. G., & Elek, E. (1987). Immunomodulation with *Viscum album* and *Echinacea purpurea* extracts. *Onkologie, 10*(Suppl. 3), 27.

Cott, J. M. (1997). In vitro receptor binding and enzyme inhibition by *Hypericum perforatum* extract. *Pharmocopsychiatry, 30,* 30, 108–112.

Dorn, M., Knick, E., & Lewith, G. (1997). Placebo-controlled, double-blind study of *Echinacea pallidae radix* in upper respiratory tract infections. *Complementary Therapies Medicine, 5,* 40–42.

Fuchs, P. A., Katayama, N., & Noda, K. (1994). Myricetin and quercetin, the flavanoid constituents of *Gingko biloba* extract, greatly reduce oxidative metabolism in both resting and Ca(2+)-loaded brain neurons. *Brain Research, 635,* 125–129.

Grifo, F. (1997). *Biodiversity and human health.* Washington, DC: Island Press.

Harrer, G., Schmidt, U., Kuhn, U., & Biller, A. (1999). Comparison and equivalence between the Saint John's wort extract LoHyp-57 and fluoxetine. *Arzneimittelforschung, 49,* 289–296.

Hofferberth, B. (1994). The efficacy of Egb 761 in patients with senile dementia of the Alzheimer's type: A double-blind, placebo-controlled study on different levels of investigation. *Human Psychopharmacology, 9,* 215–222.

Johnson, B. A. (2000). Prevention magazine assesses use of dietary supplements. *HerbalGram, 48,* 65.

Kanowski, S., Herrmann, W. M., Stephan, K., Wierich, W., & Horr, R. (1996). Proof of efficacy of the *Gingko biloba* extract Egb 761 in outpatients suffering from mild to moderate primary degenerative dementia of the Alzheimer's type of multi-infarct dementia. *Pharmacopsychiatry, 29,* 47–56.

Kerb, R., Brockmoller, J., Staffeldt, B., et al. (1996). Single-dose and steady state pharmacokinetics of hypericin and pseudohypericin. *Antimicrobial Agents Chemotherapy, 40,* 2097–2093.

Kleijnen, J., & Knipschild, P. (1992a). *Gingko biloba* for cerebral insufficiency. *British Journal of Pharmacology, 34,* 352.

Kleijnen, J., & Knipschild, P. (1992b). Gingko biloba. *Lancet, 340,* 1136–1139.

LeBars, P. L., Katz, M. M., Berman, N., Itil, T. M., Freedman, A. M., & Schatzberg, A. F. (1997). A placebo-controlled, double-blind, randomized trial of an extract of *Gingko biloba* for dementia. *Journal of the American Medical Association, 278,* 1327–1332.

Letzel, H., & Schoop, W. (1992). *Gingko biloba* extract Egb 761 and pentoxifylline in intermittent claudication. Secondary analysis of the clinical effectiveness. *Vasa, 21,* 403–410.

Linde, K., Ramirez, G., Mulrow, C. D., Pauls, A., Weidenhammer, W., & Melchart, D. (1996). St. John's wort for depression—An overview and meta-analysis of randomized clinical trials. *British Medical Journal, 3132,* 253–258.

Luettig, B., Steinmuller, C., Gifford, G. E., Wagner, H., & Lohmann-Matthes, M. L. (1989). Macrophage activitation by the polysaccharide arabinogalactan isolated from plant cell cultures of *Echinacea purpurea. Journal National Cancer Institute, 81,* 669.

Matthews, M. K., Jr. (1998). Association of *Gingko biloba* with intracerebral hemorrhage. *Neurology, 50,* 1933–1934.

Melchart, D., & Linde, K. (1994). Immunomodulation with Echinacea—a systematic review of controlled clinical trials. *Phytomedicine, 1,* 245–254.

Melchart, D., Walther, E., Linde, K., Brandmeaier, R., & Lersch, C. (1998). Echinacea root extracts for the prevention of upper respiratory tract infections. *Archives of Family Medicine, 7,* 541–545.

Mengs, U., Clare, C. B., & Poiley, J. A. (1991). Toxicity of *Echinacea purpurea.* Acute, subacute and genotoxicity studies. *Arzneitmittel-Frosch, 41,* 1076–1081.

Moore, L. B., Goodwin, B., Jones, S. A., Wiselg, C. B., Serabjit-Singh, C. J., Wilson, T. M., Collins, J. L., & Kiewer, S. A. (2000). Saint John's wort induces hepatic metabolism through activation of the pregnane x receptor. *Proceedings of the National Academy of Science, 97,* 7500–7502.

Muller, W. E., Rolli, M., Schafer, C., & Hafner, U. (1997) Effects of Hypericum extract (LI60) in biochemical models of antidepressant activity. *Pharmopsychiatry,* 30(Suppl. 2), 102–107.

National Library of Medicine http://www.ncbi.nlm.nih.gov/Pubmed.

Oyama, Y., Chikahisa, L., Ueha, T., Kanemaru, K., & Noda, K. (1996). *Gingko biloba* extract protects brain neurons against oxidative stress induced by hydrogen peroxide. *Brain Research, 712,* 349–352.

Perovic, S., & Muller, W. E. G. (1995). Pharmacological profile of Hypericum extract: Effect on serotonin uptake by postsynaptic receptors. *Arzneim-Frosch, 45,* 1145–1148.

Roesler, J., Emmendorffer, A., Steinmuller, C., Luettig, B., Wagner, H., & Lohmann-Matthes, M. L. (1991). Application of purified polysaccharides from cell cultures of the plant *Echinacea purpurea* to test subjects mediates activation of the phagocyte system. *International Journal of Immunopharmcacology, 13,* 931–941.

Roesler, J., Steinmuller, C., Kiderlen, A., Emmendorffer, A., Wagner, H., & Lohmann-Matthes, M. L. (1991). Application of purified polysaccharides from cell cultures of the plant *Echinacea purpurea* to mice mediates protection against systemic infections with *Listeria monocytogenes* and *Candida albicans. International Journal of Immunopharmacology, 13,* 27–37.

Rosenblatt, M., & Mindel, J. (1997). Spontaneous hyphema associated with ingestion of *Gingko biloba* extract. *New England Journal of Medicine, 336,* 1108.

Rowin, J., & Lewis, S. L. (1996). Spontaneous bilateral subdural hematomas associated with chronic *Gingko biloba* ingestion have also occurred. *Neurology, 46,* 1775–1176.

Shen, J. G., & Zhou, D. Y. (1995). Efficiency of *Gingko biloba* extract (Egb 761) in antioxidant protection against myocardial ischemia and re-perfusion injury. *Biochemical Molecular Biological Institute, 35,* 125–134.

Thiede, H. M., & Walper, A. (1994). Inhibition of MAO and COMT by Hypericum extracts and hypericine. *Journal of Geriatric Psychiatry and Neurology, 7,* S54–56.

Tyler, V. E. (1996). What pharmacists should know about herbal remedies: Pharmacists can help patients differentiate the useful herbs from the harmful ones. *Journal of the American Medical Association, 36,* 29–37.

U. S. Government Printing Office. (1990). Nutrition Labeling and Education Act of 1989. Washington, DC: Author.

U. S. Government Printing Office (1999). Dietary Supplement Health and Education Act: Is the FDA Trying to Change the Intent of Congress. Washington, DC: Author.

U. S. House of Representatives. Hearing before the Committee on Government Reform House of Representatives. First Session, March 25, 1999. Serial No. 106-13.

U. S. Senate. Hearing before the Committee on Labor and Human Resources United States Senate. First Session on S. 1425. (November 13, 1989).

Wagner, B. H., & Bladt, S. (1994). Pharmaccutical quality of Hypericum extracts. *Journal of Geriatric Psychiatry and Neurology, 7*(Suppl. 1), 65–68.

24

Functional Foods and Nutraceuticals

Bridget Doyle

I n the 21st century the focus of the relationship between our eating habits and our health is changing from an emphasis on health maintenance through recommended dietary allowances of nutrients, vitamins, and minerals to an emphasis on the use of foods to provide better health, increase vitality, and to aid in preventing disease and many chronic illnesses. The connection between food and health is not new. Indeed, the adage "Let food be your medicine and medicine your food" was supported by Hippocrates around 400 B.C.E. (Jones, 1932). Now, the philosophy that supports the paradigm of nutraceuticals as functional foods is once again at the forefront.

Despite this ancient wisdom, the use of nutraceuticals and functional foods remains in its infancy in the Western world. It was not until the late 1970s that the trend toward improved physical fitness and overall well-being began. At that time, scientific evidence began to stress the importance of a balanced diet low in saturated fat, sodium, and cholesterol and higher in fiber. Currently, the use of nutraceuticals, including additives to certain conventional foods, phytochemicals, functional foods, dietary foods and supplements, and medical foods is growing at an astronomical rate. In the past several years, the Food and Drug Administration has worked to examine the possible connections between nutritional products and disease states, including calcium and osteoporosis, sodium and hypertension, lipids and cardiovascular disease, lipids and cancer, and dietary fiber and cardiovascular disease (Gardner, 1994).

Today, with the developing market of functional foods, it is estimated that consumers in the United States spent over $6.5 billion on dietary supplements (Kurtzweil, 1999). One can find calcium added to juices, pasta, rice, dry cereals, and in chocolate and caramel candy products. Many companies are using soy protein isolates in foods ranging from candy bars and salad dressings to infant formulas; the contents of margarine-like spreads are altered to reduce cholesterol and LDL levels. Common nutraceuticals receiving broad attention include calcium-fortified fruit drinks (Tropicana or Florida's Natural Orange Juices) and candy (Viactin chews); soy protein bars fortified with whey protein (Rass Nutrition Bars); soy protein products and high-fiber cereals (Kellog's Ensemble Foods); and bars providing L-arginine, which improves vascular functioning (Pharma's HeartBar). Coverage of all nutraceuticals is beyond the scope of this chapter; however, several selected products are covered in depth, including sitostanol ester margarine, glucosamine chondroitin sulfate and collagen hydrolysate, and soy protein. It is important that nurses know about nutraceuticals and the intended beneficial effects, as well as their potential unintended effects and precautions.

DEFINITIONS

To understand the terms functional food and nutraceuticals, one must understand the definition of foods. The Food and Drug Administration (FDA) defines foods as "articles used primarily for taste, aroma, or nutritive value" (FDA, 1938, p. 210). Historically, the FDA has made several attempts to regulate these products and remove selected products from the market (Kottke, 1998). Functional foods are defined as manufactured foods for which scientifically valid claims can be made. They may be produced by food-processing technologies, traditional breeding, or genetic engineering. Functional foods should safely deliver a long-term health benefit. Accordingly, a functional food may be one of the following:

- A known food to which a functional ingredient from another food is added
- A known food to which a functional ingredient new to the food supply is added
- An entirely new food that contains one or more functional ingredients (Pariza, 1999).

The term nutraceutical has been defined as "a blend word of nutrition and pharmaceutical, for a substance that may be considered a food or part of a food and that provides medical or health benefits, including the prevention or treatment of disease" (Marshall, 1994, p. 24). These substances pose problems for official medicine regulators. The Japanese, who were among the first to utilize functional foods, have highlighted three conditions that define a functional food:

- It is a food (not a capsule, tablet, or powder) derived from naturally occurring ingredients.
- It can and should be consumed as part of a daily diet.
- It has a particular function when ingested, serving to regulate a particular body process, such as enhancement of the biological defense mechanism; prevention of a specific disease; recovery from a specific disease; control of physical and mental conditions; and slowing of the aging process (PA Consulting Group, 1990).

Some nutritional products and the conditions for which they are suggested are presented in Figure 24.1.

A major impediment to the maturation of the functional foods category in the United States is the vocabulary used to describe it (Hasler, 2000). Pharmaceutical firms tend to prefer the terms medical foods, nutraceuticals, and nutritional foods, whereas food companies prefer to call them functional foods and nutritional foods (Hasler, 2000).

SCIENTIFIC BASIS

During the past century there have been many changes in the types of foods people eat. This reflects the application of scientific findings and technological innovations in the food industry. Although much research has been conducted on nutrition and health and disease, scientific research on the use of nutraceuticals is more limited.

Interest in foodstuffs has generated research to link nutrient and food intake with improvements in health or prevention of disease. More than 200 studies in the epidemiological literature have been reviewed and consistently show an association between a low consumption of fruits and vegetables and the incidence of cancer. The quarter of the population with the lowest dietary intake of fruits and vegetables has roughly twice the rate of cancer compared to those with the highest intake (Shibamoto, Terao, & Osawa 1997).

In addition to the examples in Figure 24.1 of natural nutrients that are beneficial for disease prevention, much scientific research has been completed on the role of the various products added to normal foods to enhance their ability to inhibit or prevent diseases. Many regard dietary intake as the best means of acquiring necessary nutrients (Kottke, 1998). However,

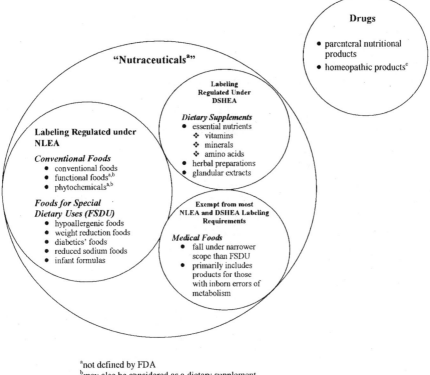

"not defined by FDA
"may also be considered as a dietary supplement
"registered, but not approved as drugs by FDA

FIGURE 24.1   Categorization of nutrition-related products.

Note: From "Scientific Regulatory Aspects of Nutraceutical Products in the United States," by M. K. Kottke, 1998, *Drug Development & Industrial Pharmacy, 24*(12), p. 1179. Copyright 1998 by Marcel Dekker, Inc. Reprinted by permission.

supplementation of nutrients is common. The findings of selected scientific research focused on selected nutraceuticals are summarized below.

Dietary Sitostanol Ester Margarine

Reduction of serum cholesterol decreases mortality in primary and especially in secondary prevention. Gylling and Miettinen (1999) studied postmenopausal women with a previous myocardial infarction to determine whether the use of sitostanol ester rapeseed-oil margarine, alone and in combination with statins, could reduce serum cholesterol. The results of this study demonstrated that sitostanol ester margarine effectively inhibited cholesterol absorption and reduced the LDL cholesterol levels in 32% of the patients. A combination of sitostanol ester margarine and simvastatin therapy further reduced serum total cholesterol and LDL cholesterol.

Glucosamine, Chondroitin Sulfate, and Collagen Hydrolysate

These are another combination of nutraceuticals that are receiving a great deal of scientific review, particularly their use in the symptomatic treatment of osteoarthritis. A meta-analysis by McAlindon and colleagues (2000) and Towheed and Hochberg (1997) reviewed clinical trials of glucosamine and chondroitin in the treatment of osteoarthritis. McAlindon et al. included 13 double-blind placebo-controlled trials of greater than 4 weeks' duration, testing oral or parenteral glucosamine or chondroitin for treatment of hip or knee arthritis. All 13 studies were classified as positive, demonstrating substantial benefits in treating arthritis when compared with the placebo. Towheed and Hochberg reviewed nine randomized, controlled studies of glucosamine sulfate in osteoarthritis. Glucosamine was superior when compared to the placebo in seven random trials. Two of the random trials compared glucosamine sulfate to ibuprofen. In these two trials, glucosamine was superior in one and equivalent in the other.

The literature reflects concern about these specific products. Deal and Moskowitz (1999) underscore the importance that investigators utilizing glucosamine and chondroitin carefully monitor the product manufacturing process because some of the preparations claiming to contain certain doses of these nutraceuticals have significantly less (or none) of the dosages described.

Cost is a factor in the use of these nutraceuticals. The average cost ranges from $35 to $60 per month (Deal & Moskowitz, 1999). In their reviews, the authors emphasize that these agents are not FDA-evaluated or recommended for the treatment of osteoarthritis.

Soy Protein Powder

Certain soy phytoestrogens (isoflavones and lignans) have been suggested to be anticarcinogenic. Xu, Duncan, Wangen, and Kurzer (2000) examined the effects of soy isoflavones on estrogen and phytoestrogen in premenopausal women. They studied specific isoflavones and lignans that had been suggested to be anticarcinogenic. The results of their study indicated that soy isoflavone consumption may exert cancer preventive effects by decreasing estrogen synthesis and altering metabolism away from genotoxic metabolites toward inactive metabolites. In another study by Duncan, Merz-Demlow, Xu, Phipps, and Kurzer (2000), it was determined unlikely that isoflavones or soy exert clinically important estrogenic effects on vaginal epithelium or endometrium. They concluded that more studies are needed before dietary recommendations involving soy and or isoflavones can be made to postmenopausal women looking for an alternative to hormone replacement therapy.

INTERVENTION

Many persons are using nutraceuticals. Therefore, it is important that nurses include nutraceuticals when they obtain the health history of the patient. Table 24.1 presents guidelines for nurses to use in assessing patients. Numerous Web sites provide information about nutraceuticals. The FDA Consumer Information Line (http://www.fda.gov) contains helpful information.

MEASUREMENT OF OUTCOMES

Outcomes of therapy can be assessed in a number of ways depending on the nutraceutical and the intent of the therapy. For example, blood levels of the nutrient or effect on the target organ (e.g., bone with the use of calcium) could be monitored over time. Also, it is important that potential side effects of the therapy be assessed in periodic physical assessments and comprehensive histories. Positive or negative changes in subjective health, energy and symptoms, or subsequent to changes in nutraceutical use can also be assessed in individuals as data for tolerance as part of cost-benefit evaluation. Good teaching of nutraceutical principles, intended purpose, and dose and effects of functional foods can result in informed use by clients and greater awareness of intended and adverse effects.

PRECAUTIONS

The use of nutraceuticals by clients should be assessed as part of health history and nutritional assessment. Safe use must be carefully considered (Zeisel, 1999); safe dosage, drug interaction, toxic side effects due to overdose, or ineffective clearance should be determined.

USES

A variety of nutraceuticals have been used to promote health, and to prevent and treat illness. The broad range of conditions and products used are illustrated in Table 24.2.

TABLE 24.1   Guideline: General Nutraceutical Assessment Guide for Nurses

1. Determine client's current use of nutraceuticals.

2. Determine nutritional needs and potential nutritional deficiencies, especially according to medical conditions and other results of physical assessment, signs and symptoms, activities, body types, or developmental stages (e.g., perimenopausal, extensive athletic training, obesity).

3. Provide information about available suitable nutraceutical products that could provide nutritional benefits, according to most current guidelines, published standards, dosages, and toxicities.

4. Determine client interest in the products.

5. Offer resources for client regarding nutraceuticals in general and 2 or 3 products of potential benefit.

6. Arrange for follow-up to determine therapeutic effects or toxicities; answer questions and discuss perceived cost and benefits with client.

Nutraceuticals can be used to target deficiencies, establish optimal nutritional balance, or to treat diseases. Because heart disease, cancer, and stroke are leading causes of death in the United States, nutraceuticals that have been shown to improve risk-factor profiles would be desirable. Furthermore, people in the U.S. and worldwide could benefit from nutraceuticals when there are deficiencies of specific nutrients.

FUTURE RESEARCH

Although nutraceuticals have longstanding historical usage, increased interest in these substances to promote health, prevent disease, and treat specific medical conditions is reflected in heightened attention to nutritional science and increased consumption. While nurses may not be the "experts" in this area, it is important for them to have some knowledge about common nutraceuticals, their uses, and where information can be obtained. Interdisciplinary research teams may explore

1. Which of the current nutraceuticals should be incorporated as part of the regular routine to promote health
2. Whether nutraceuticals are cost-effective
3. The side effects associated with short- and long-term use of specific nutraceuticals.

TABLE 24.2 Selected Research-based Uses of Nutraceuticals for Medical Conditions and Health Purposes

Product	Use	Research Reference
Calcium additive	Osteoporosis prevention	Gardner (1999); Nelson (1999); Stark & Madar (1994); Beattie et al. (1988)
Dietary fiber supplement (psyllium)	Cholesteral lowering; glucose regulation	
Soy protein isolates	Atherosclerosis and cancer prevention	Xu, Duncan, Wangen, & Kurzer (2000); Wiseman et al. (1998)
Antioxidants (e.g., dietary sitostanol ester) Margarine (benecol)	Secondary prevention in cardiovascular disease, serum cholesterol	Gylling & Miettinen, 2000
Glucosamine and chondroitin	Osteoarthritis	McAlindon, LaValley, Gulin, & Felson (2000); Towheed & Hochberg (1997)
Guar gum	Diabetes; glucose metabolism	LeBlanc, Nadeau, Mercier, McKay, & Sampson, 1991
Pre-pro-biotics in fermented milk	Reduction of plasma cholesterol; improves malabsorption problems from GI function	Richelsen (1996); Gibson & Wang (1994)
Hydrolyzed whey Protein peptides	Anticarcinogenic effects	Bounous, Batist, & Gold (1991)

REFERENCES

Beattie, V. A., Edwards, C. A., Hosker, J. P., Cullen, D. R., Ward, J. D., & Read, N. W. (1988). Does adding fiber to a low-energy, high-carbohydrate, low-fat diet confer any benefit to the management of newly diagnosed overweight type II diabetics? *British Medical Journal Clinical Research Education, 296*, 1147–1149.

Bounous, G., Batist, G., & Gold, P. (1991). Whey proteins in cancer prevention. *Cancer Letters, 57*(2), 91–94.

Deal, C. L., & Moskowitz, R. W. (1999). Nutraceuticals as therapeutic agents in osteoarthritis. The role of glucosamine, chondroidin sulfate, and collagen hydrolysate. *Rheumatic Disease Clinics of North America, 25*(2), 379–953.

Duncan, A. M., Merz-Demlow, B. E., Xu, Z., Phipps, W., & Kurzer, M. (2000). Premenopausal equol excretors show plasma hormone profiles associated with lowered risk of breast cancer. *Cancer Epidemiology, Biomarkers & Prevention, 9*, 581–586.

Federal Food, Drug and Cosmetic Act, 52 Stat. 111. 21 U.S.C. § 210 et seq. (1938).

Gardner, J. (1994). The development of the functional food business. In I. Goldberg (Ed.), *Functional foods: Designer foods, pharmafoods, and nutraceuticals* (pp. 472–473). New York: Chapman & Hall.

Gibson, G., & Wang, X. (1994). Regulatory effects of bifidobacteria on the growth of other colonic bacteria. *Journal of Applied Bacteriology, 77*, 412–420.

Gylling, H., & Miettinen, T. A. (1999). Cholesterol reduction by different plant stanol mixture with variable fat intake. *Metabolism: Clinical and Experimental, 48*(5), 575–580.

Hasler, C. M. (2000). The changing face of functional foods. *Journal of the American College of Nutrition, 19*(5 Suppl), 4995–5065.

Hippocrates. (1923). *Hippocrates* (W. H. S. Jones, Trans.). Cambridge, MA: Harvard University Press.

Kottke, M. K. (1998). Scientific and regulating aspects of nutraceutical products in the United States. *Drug Development and Industrial Pharmacy, 24*(12), 1177–1195.

Kurtzweil, P. (1999). *An FDA Guide to Dietary Supplements* [on-line]. Available: http://vm.cfsan.fda.gov/~dms/fdsupp.html

LeBlanc, J., Nadeau, A., Mercier, I., McKay, C., & Sampson, P. (1991). Effect of guar gum on insulinogenic and thermogenic response to glucose. *Nutritional Research, 11*, 133–139.

Marshall, W. E. (1994). Amino acids, peptides and proteins. In I. Goldberg (Ed.), *Functional foods: Designer foods, pharmafoods, and nutraceuticals* (pp. 242–260). New York: Chapman & Hall.

McAlindon, T. E., LaValley, M. P., Gulin, J. P., & Felson, D. T. (2000). Glucosamine and chondroitin for treatment of osteoarthritis: A systematic quality assessment and meta-analysis. *Journal of the American Medical Association, 283*(11), 1483–1484.

Nelson, N. J. (1999). Purple carrots, margarine laced with wood pulp? Nutraceuticals move into the supermarket. *Journal of the National Cancer Institute, 91*(9), 755–757.

PA Consulting Group. (1990). *Functional foods: A new global added value market?* London: PA Consulting Group.

Pariza, M. (1999). Functional foods: Technology, functionality and health benefits. *Nutrition Today, 34,* 150–151.

Pennsylvania Consulting Group. (1990). *Functional foods: A new global added-value market?* London: PA Consulting Group.

Richelsen, B., Kristensen, K., & Pedersen, S. B. (1996). Long-term (6 months) effect of a new fermented milk product on the level of plasma lipoproteins—a placebo-controlled and double blind study. *European Journal of Clinical Nutrition, 50,* 811–815.

Shibamoto, T., Terao, J., & Osawa, T. (1997). ACS Symposium Series 701. *Functional foods for disease prevention I: Fruits, vegetables, and trees.* Washington, DC: American Chemical Society.

Stark, A., & Madar, Z. (1994). Dietary fiber. In I. Goldberg (Ed.), *Functional foods: Designer foods, pharmafoods, and nutraceuticals* (pp. 187–189). New York: Chapman & Hall.

Thomas, P. R., & Earl, R. (Eds.). (1994). *Enhancing the food supply. Opportunities in the nutritional and food sciences.* Washington, DC: National Academy Press.

Towheed, T. E., & Hochberg, M. C. (1997). A systematic review of randomized controlled trials of pharmacological therapy in osteoarthritis of the hip. *Journal of Rheumatology, 24,* 349–357.

Xu, X., Duncan, A. M., Wangen, K. E., & Kurzer, M. S. (2000). Soy consumption alters endogenous estrogen metabolism in post-menopausal women. *Cancer Epidemiology, Biomarkers and Prevention, 9,* 781–786.

Zeisel, S. H. (1999). Regulation of "nutraceuticals." *Science, 285*(5435), 1853–1855.

PART VI

Lifestyle and Disease Prevention Therapies

OVERVIEW

In its 1999 classification system, the National Center for Complementary/ Alternative Medicine (NCCAM) included a category dedicated to therapies used in lifestyle changes, disease prevention, and health promotion. We elected to retain this category as a section for this book because of the large role nurses play in health promotion and disease prevention. NCCAM had included therapies for stress management and addiction control in this category. Another major therapy was exercise. The goal of these therapies is to promote changes in behaviors that place a person at risk for major health problems such as cardiovascular disease. Many of the therapies included in the earlier sections can also be used to bring about changes in behaviors and promote overall well-being. The holistic philosophy that underpins many of the complementary therapies supports their use to help achieve healing and promote well-being.

Increasing exercise in the lives of all Americans continues to be a major health goal. The value of exercise for everyone from young children to older adults has been documented. Nurses need to give attention not only to instructing patients on the value of exercise, but also on ways to incorporate exercise into their own lives.

25

Exercise

Diane Treat-Jacobson and Daniel L. Mark

Exercise is rapidly becoming recognized as a lifelong endeavor that's essential for energetic, active, and healthy living. The research supporting the benefits of exercise is substantial. The effects and benefits of exercise have been linked to many physiological and psychological responses from reduction in the stress response and to an increased sense of well-being (Pender, 1996; Crews & Landers, 1987). Surprisingly, despite its tremendous benefits exercise is largely ignored by the general population. Indeed, the U.S. Surgeon General (1996) has issued a report identifying millions of inactive Americans as being at risk for a wide range of chronic diseases and ailments including coronary heart disease (CHD), adult onset diabetes, colon cancer, hip fractures, hypertension, and obesity.

It is important to recognize the role of exercise as a component of health. Exercise *must* be an integral part of personal lifestyle if it is to have optimum effects on health. Maintaining physical fitness can be enjoyable and rewarding for people of all ages and can contribute significantly to extending longevity and improving quality of life. Knowledge of exercise and its application in multiple populations will assist in the delivery of expert nursing care. This chapter discusses the definition, physiological basis, and application of exercise as a nursing intervention.

DEFINITION

Physical activity is defined as "any bodily movement produced by skeletal muscles that results in caloric expenditure" (Pender, 1996, p. 185). The definitions of exercise are complex and vary according to discipline; however, they all incorporate physical activity.

Exercise is commonly classified according to whether oxygen is consumed during the activity. Exercise is considered aerobic when the energy needed is supplied by the oxygen inspired (Kisner & Colby, 1996). In general, aerobic exercise increases demand on the respiratory, cardiovascular, and musculoskeletal systems. Sustained periods of work require aerobic metabolism of energy at a level compatible with the body's oxygen supply capabilities. Anaerobic exercise is exercise during which the energy needed is provided without utilization of inspired oxygen (Kisner & Colby, 1996). This occurs during short, vigorous bouts of exercise or when the body's oxygen supply capabilities cannot meet the metabolic demands of the exercise.

SCIENTIFIC BASIS

A better understanding of exercise physiology and the body's response to various stages of physical activity will assist in developing exercise programs that are appropriate for the individual and the goal of the exercise. The response of the body to exercise occurs in stages. Eight to ten seconds after the initiation of exercise, a large sympathetic outburst occurs and the heart overshoots the rate needed for increased activity, but then returns to the rate required. Impulses from the muscles being exercised are sent to the brain; an increase in the heart rate is initiated (Fletcher, 1982). During this phase, there is a sluggish adjustment of respiration and circulation, resulting in an oxygen deficit; exercise is fueled by the anaerobic metabolism of creatine phosphate and glucose (Kisner & Colby, 1996).

As exercise continues, oxygen consumption increases (VO_2). Cardiac output (CO) is increased to meet the increased oxygen demands of the working muscle. The increase in CO is due to increased stroke volume (SV) and heart rate (HR), increased myocardial contractibility (from positive inotropic sympathetic impulses to the heart), increased venous return, and a decreased peripheral resistance by the exercising muscles (Fletcher, 1982). In normal individuals, CO can increase 4–5 times, allowing for increased delivery of oxygen to the exercising muscle beds and facilitating removal of lactate, carbon dioxide, and heat. Respiration increases to deliver oxygen and to allow for elimination of carbon dioxide (Shepard, 1992). Blood pressure increases as a result of increased cardiac output and the sympathetic vasoconstriction of vessels in the nonexercising muscles, viscera, and skin. During this "steady state" exercise phase, oxygen uptake equals oxygen tissue requirement, aerobic metabolism of glucose and fatty acids occurs, and there is no accumulation of lactic acid.

As exercise becomes more strenuous, there is a shift toward anaerobic metabolism of glucose, resulting in increased production of lactic acid (Balady & Weiner, 1992). The anaerobic threshold is a point during exercise at which ventilation abruptly increases despite linear increases in work rate. At a given work rate, the oxygen supply does not meet the oxygen requirement. This increases anaerobic glycolysis for energy generation and increases lactate production. Accumulation of lactic acid can lead to symptoms of dyspnea and fatigue. Shortly beyond the anaerobic threshold, fatigue ensues and work ceases. Exercise at a level that allows for aerobic metabolism and reduces the need for anaerobic metabolism reduces the production of lactic acid and may delay the onset of these symptoms.

INTERVENTION

According to the National Institutes of Health (NIH) consensus statement, exercise is considered beneficial to health (NIH, 1995). The Surgeon General (1996) recently released a report detailing the benefits of physical activity, including

- decreased the risk of premature death
- decreased risk of premature death from heart disease
- decreased risk of acquiring Type II diabetes
- decreased risk of incurring high blood pressure
- decreased high blood pressure in hypertensive individuals
- decreased risk of colon cancer
- decreased feelings of uneasiness and despair

Exercise also aids weight control and strengthening and maintaining muscles, joints, and bones; aids older adults with balance and mobility; and fosters feelings of psychological well-being. In addition to these benefits, the American Heart Association's (AHA) scientific statement on the benefits of exercise summarizes evidence confirming physical activity as a significant factor in both primary and secondary prevention of cardiovascular disease (AHA, 1996). There is a relationship between the lack of physical activity and developing coronary artery disease and increased cardiovascular mortality. Furthermore, there is evidence that persons who engage in regular exercise as part of their recovery post–myocardial infarction have improved rates of survival (Fletcher et al., 1996).

Given that the benefits of exercise apply to all age groups across a broad spectrum of health and disease, it is important for nurses to recognize opportunities to promote exercise as a nursing intervention. Finding an activity that suits an individual's capabilities and that meets the purposes for which exercise is prescribed is key to the success of the intervention (Gavin, 1988). When prescribing an intervention, it is important to take into account the recommended exercise intensity for the patient population being served, whether children, older adults, or those with chronic disease.

Evidence suggests that exercise is more likely to be initiated if the individual (a) recognizes the need to exercise, (b) perceives the exercise as beneficial and enjoyable, (c) perceives that the exercise has minimal negative aspects such as expense, time required, and negative peer pressure, (d) feels capable and safe engaging in the exercise, and (e) has ready access to the activity and can easily fit it into the daily schedule (NIH Consensus Statement, 1995).

TECHNIQUE

An exercise session should involve three phases: warm-up, aerobic exercise, and cooling-down. The phases of exercise are designed to allow the body an opportunity to sustain internal equilibrium by gradually adjusting its physiological processes to the stress of exercise and thus maintaining homeostasis.

Warm-Up Phase

The goal of the warm-up is to allow the body time to adapt to the rigors of aerobic exercise. Warming up results in an increase in muscle temperature, a higher need for oxygen in order to meet the increased demands of the exercising muscles, dilatation of capillaries resulting in increased circulation, adjustments within the neural respiratory center to the demands of exercise, and a shifting of blood flow centrally from the periphery, result in increased venous return (Kisner & Colby, 1996). In addition, a good warm-up increases flexibility and decreases or prevents arrhythmias and ischemic ECG changes (Kisner & Colby, 1996). Warming up exercises should be done for 10 minutes, involve all major body parts, and achieve a heart rate within 20 beats per minute of the target heart rate for the ensuing aerobic exercise (Kisner & Colby, 1996). In addition, a good warm-up should incorporate stretching exercises. Stretching exercises are done at a slow, steady pace and help maintain a full range of motion in body joints and strengthen tendons, ligaments, and muscles.

Aerobic Exercise Phase

The aerobic phase of exercise has four components: intensity, frequency, duration, and mode of exercise. The combination of these components determines the effectiveness of the exercise. A balance needs to be achieved to obtain maximal benefit with the least amount of risk and discomfort. Adjustment of intensity is important not only for safety reasons, but also for comfort and enjoyment of the activity (Foster & Tamboli, 1992). If exercise can be kept at a level that is comfortable, the individual is more likely to continue to perform the activity. As tolerance for exercise develops, any or all of the exercise components can be increased to meet the individual's aerobic capacity. For example if an individual is comfortable with the intensity of the exercise, the duration and frequency can be increased to further improve training effect.

Cool-Down Phase

Immediately following the endurance exercises, the person should engage in a cooling down period. This allows the body to adjust to normal conditions and to eliminate the lactic acid that may have accumulated in the muscle tissue during exercise. Five to ten minutes are needed for the body to adjust to a slower pace. Cooling down exercises may include walking slowly and deep breathing, and stretching exercises.

Maintenance

Maintaining the exercise program is the key to the effectiveness of the intervention. Setting both short- and long-term goals helps improve adherence. The individual can experience a sense of accomplishment upon meeting short-term goals while still striving for overall goals. Keeping a record or graph provides a visual demonstration of progress and may provide insight into adjustments to the exercise program that may assist in achievement of goals.

Specific Technique: Walking

Walking is one exercise in which persons of all age groups and with varying levels of disability can engage to improve endurance. A major advantage is that walking requires no special equipment, facilities, or new skills. It is also safer and easier to maintain than many other forms of exercise. Intensity, duration, and frequency are easily regulated and adjusted to accommodate a wide range of physical capabilities and limitations. The initial intensity should be outlined at the start of the program and is dependent on the baseline level of conditioning, physical or disease-related limitations or precautions, and outcome goals.

A walking program can be approached in two ways. The exercise can be completed in one or multiple daily sessions. For example, a previously sedentary individual may wish to begin an exercise program with 2-minute brisk walks throughout the day. This could be increased to 5 minutes, and then 10 minutes as stamina increases. The more traditional alternative would be to engage in one longer session at least 3 times per week. These sessions would include a warm-up session for 5–10 minutes, an aerobic period which could start at 10–15 minutes and gradually increase to 30–60 minutes in length, and a cool-down period of 5–10 minutes (AHA, 1995).

The individual should monitor the body's response to the activity to ensure that the intensity is appropriate. This can be done in several ways:

Monitor Target Heart Rate

The target heart rate should be between 50% and 75% of the maximal heart rate, which is calculated by subtracting one's age from 220 (AHA, 1995). The heart rate should be assessed one third to one half way through the exercise session and immediately after stopping exercise. Exercise intensity can be increased or decreased based on this measurement.

The "Talk Test"

The talk test can replace target heart rate monitoring when an individual is exercising at a moderate intensity. If the exercise prevents the individual from talking comfortably, the intensity should be decreased.

Rating of Perceived Exertion

This is a scale that describes the sense of effort during the exercise. This scale can be ranked from 1 to 10 with 1 indicating no effort and 10 indicating maximal effort (AHA, 1995).

Table 25.1 contains easy-to-follow tips for a walking regimen.

MEASUREMENT OF OUTCOMES

The appropriate measure of the effectiveness of an exercise intervention depends on the specific exercise prescribed and the goals of the intervention. If cardiovascular fitness is the targeted outcome, an aerobic exercise program would be prescribed. Changes in the cardiovascular system such as increased stroke volume and cardiac output, increased anaerobic threshold, and improved local circulation would be used to determine the effectiveness of the intervention (Halfman & Hojnacki, 1981). Exercise prescribed to improve function may use parameters such as improved joint mobility, prevention or reduction of osteoporosis, and improved strength in determining exercise effectiveness (Benison & Hogskel, 1986). Assessment may also include changes in physical functioning and disability, ability to perform ADLs, changes in symptoms and activity tolerance, and other variables that reflect the individual's ability to function in daily life. Lower intensity programs,

TABLE 25.1   Nine Tips for Fitness Walking

1. Warm up by performing a few stretches.

2. Think tall as you walk. Stand straight with your head level and your shoulders relaxed.

3. Your heel should hit the surface first. Use smooth movements rolling from heel to toe.

4. Keep your hands free and let your arms swing naturally in opposition to your legs.

5. When you're ready to pick up the pace, quicken your step and lengthen your stride, but don't compromise your upright posture or smooth, comfortable movements.

6. To increase your intensity, burn more calories, and tone your upper body, bend your arms at the elbows and pump your arms. Keep your elbows close to your body.

7. Breathe in and out naturally, rhythmically, and deeply.

8. Use the "talk test" to check your intensity, or take your pulse to see if you are within your target heart rate.

9. Cool down during the last 3 to 5 minutes by gradually slowing your pace to a stroll.

American Heart Association (1995)

which may not demonstrate great changes in maximal exercise capacity, might produce sufficient changes in these outcome variables to make a difference in the individual's quality of life. Such programs would be appropriate especially in older adults and very sedentary individuals where low-intensity exercise can produce a modest increase in fitness and more significant improvements in function (Belman & Gaesser, 1991; Foster, Hume, Byrnes, Dickenson, & Chatfield, 1989). Development and implementation of programs designed to meet the specific needs of patients can help maximize functional and quality-of-life outcomes.

PRECAUTIONS

To avoid injury, it is important to begin an exercise program slowly, to follow safety guidelines, and to exercise consistently, several times per week. Potential exercise-related injuries include muscle and joint pain, cramps, blisters, shin splints, low back pain, and tendonitis and other sprains or muscle strains.

The AHA (1995) has listed general guidelines to help ensure exercise safety:

1. Stretch the muscles and tendons prior to beginning exercise.
2. Wear appropriate footwear.
3. Exercise on a surface with some "give" to it, especially during high-impact activities.
4. Learn the exercise properly and continue good form even with increased speed or intensity.

Should exercise-related injuries occur, they can usually be treated with one or a combination of the RICE therapies: *rest, ice, compression,* and *elevation* (AHA, 1995).

Previously sedentary older individuals and those with chronic disease, especially heart disease, should consult a physician prior to initiating an exercise program to ensure that an appropriate exercise prescription is given. Warning signs of heart disease should be provided prior to initiating an exercise program, especially to those in high-risk categories.

USES

CONDITIONS/POPULATIONS

Several populations in which exercise is particularly beneficial include older adults, those with affective disorders, with heart disease, and with peripheral arterial disease. The application and demonstrated effects of exercise intervention in each of these populations is discussed below.

Older Adults

Older adults are especially prone to the "hazards of immobility," which affect many of the body's systems. Exercise increases bone strength (Smith & Reddan, 1976) and total body calcium (Dalsky et al., 1988), as well as improving coordination, which may result in a reduction in falls (Bassett, McClamrock, & Schmelzer, 1982). It has also been shown to improve body functioning and overall well-being. Blumenthal, Schocken, Needles, and Hindle (1982) reported that 40% of the older adults in their study who exercised felt healthier, were more satisfied with life, had more self-confidence, and improved mood.

It is particularly important to tailor exercise programs to this population, who may have specific limitations. Exercise needs to be initiated at lower levels and increased gradually. Previously sedentary individuals may be more comfortable starting an exercise program with some supervision, which allows them to become accustomed to this new level of activity in a safe environment. Group exercise may be especially appealing to the older person.

Affective Disorder

Exercise is an effective though underused intervention for individuals with affective disorders. There is considerable evidence supporting the positive effects of exercise in combating depression as well as anxiety (Byrne & Byrne, 1993). There are fewer if any side effects when compared with pharmacotherapy, and exercise is often more cost-effective than psychotherapy and pharmacotherapy (Yaffe, 1981). Although most studies have evaluated the effects of aerobic activity as the intervention, anaerobic activity has also been shown to be beneficial in alleviating depression. This suggests that improvement in mood is associated with exercise in general, rather than with increased aerobic capacity (Doyne et al., 1987).

Heart Disease

Cardiac (exercise) rehabilitation (CR) is a common intervention prescribed for those with coronary heart disease (CHD), providing a safe environment for the initiation of an exercise program. Programs usually have several phases and are tailored to the specific needs, limitations, and characteristics of individual patients, helping them resume active and productive lives (Foster & Tamboli, 1992; Hamm & Leon, 1992).

Exercise training has been shown to improve symptom-limited exercise capacity in CHD patients primarily as a result of peripheral hemodynamic adaptations (Ferguson et al., 1982; Juneau, Geneau, Marchand, & Brosseau, 1991; Wenger, 1993). Patients with CHD have a low skeletal muscle oxidative capacity that is significantly improved with training, despite relatively low workloads and exercise intensities, consistent with other non-heart-disease populations (Ferguson et al., 1982). Prior to training, patients with CHD are often unable to perform activities of daily living (ADLs) without symptoms. Exercise-trained CHD patients function further above the ischemic threshold in performing ADLs and thus require a lower percentage of maximal effort to perform activities. This increases stamina and endurance and helps to maintain independence (Wenger, 1993). Even patients with heart failure, who typically have very poor cardiac function, have found that CR improves their exercise tolerance (Koch, Douard, & Broustet, 1992; Sullivan, 1994).

Peripheral Arterial Disease

Peripheral arterial disease (PAD), a prevalent atherosclerotic occlusive disease, limits functional capacity and is related to decreased quality of life.

Individuals with PAD typically experience exercise-induced ischemic pain in the lower extremities, know as claudication. Exercise training is one of the most effective interventions available for the treatment of claudication due to PAD (Hiatt, Regensteiner, Hargarten, Wolfel, & Brass, 1990; Regensteiner, Steiner, & Hiatt, 1996). Exercise training has been shown to improve walking distance up to 180% (Regensteiner, 1997; Regensteiner & Hiatt, 1995). Prior to initiating a program, an exercise prescription should be generated based on a graded exercise test, and patients should start training at 50% of their functional capacity (Ekers & Hirsch, 1999). During a typical exercise session, patients will exercise at a moderate pace until they experience moderate to severe claudication. At that point they will rest until the pain subsides. This exercise/rest pattern is repeated throughout the exercise session (Hiatt et al., 1990). The most effective exercise programs for the treatment of claudication include the following components: The patient should exercise to the point of almost maximal claudication; the exercise session should be at least 30 minutes in length, with at least 3 sessions per week. The exercise program should continue for at least 6 months, and intermittent walking is the most effective mode of exercise (Gardner & Poehlman, 1995).

FUTURE RESEARCH

There are many gaps in our knowledge about exercise, its measurement, the benefits, and methods to improve exercise adherence. Areas of needed specific research include the following:

- Development of measures of exercise behavior that are valid and reliable in different populations and with various levels of activity
- Development and testing of specific interventions to increase exercise adherence in multiple populations
- Assessment of the impact of exercise interventions in multiple populations through controlled longitudinal studies

REFERENCES

American Heart Association (1995). *Your heart: An owner's manual.* Englewood Cliffs, NJ: Prentice Hall.

Balady, G., & Weiner, D. (1992). Physiology of exercise in normal individuals and patients with coronary heart disease. In N. Wenger & H. Hellerstein (Eds.), *Rehabilitation of the coronary patient* (pp. 103-122). New York: Churchill Livingstone.

Bassett, C., McClamrock, E., & Schmelzer, M. (1982). A 10-week exercise program for senior citizens. *Geriatric Nursing, 3,* 103–105.

Belman, M., & Gaesser, G. (1991). Exercise training below and above the lactate threshold in the elderly. *Medicine and Science in Sports and Exercise, 23*(5), 562–568.

Benison, B., & Hogstel, M. (1986). Aging and movement therapy: Essential interventions for the immobile elderly. *Journal of Gerontological Nursing 12*(12), 8–16.

Blumenthal, J., Schocken, D., Needles, T., & Hindle, P. (1982). Psychological and physiological effects of physical conditioning on the elderly. *Journal of Psychosomatic Medicine 26,* 505–510.

Byrne, A., & Byrne, D. G. (1993). The effect of exercise on depression, anxiety and other mood states: A review. *Journal of Psychosomatic Research, 37,* 565–574.

Crews, D., & Landers, D. (1987). A meta-analytic review of aerobic fitness and reactivity to psychosocial stressors. *Medicine and Science in Sports and Exercise, 19*(Suppl.), S114–S120.

Dalsky, O., Stocke, K., Ehsani, A., Slatopolsky, E., Lee, W., & Birge, S. (1988). Weight-bearing exercise training and lumbar bone mineral content in postmenopausal women. *Annals of Internal Medicine, 108,* 824–829.

Doyne, E. J., Osip-Klein, D. J., Bowman, E. D., Osborn, K. M., McDougall-Wilson, I. B., & Neimeyer, R. A. (1987). Running versus weight-lifting in the treatment of depression. *Journal of Consulting and Clinical Psychology, 55*(5), 748–754.

Ekers, M. A., & Hirsch, A. T. (1999). Vascular medicine and vascular rehabilitation. In V. Fahey (Ed.), *Vascular nursing* (3rd ed., pp. 188–211). Philadelphia: W. B. Saunders.

Ferguson, R., Taylor, A., Cote, P., Charlebois, J., Dinelle, Y., Perionnet, F., Dechamplain, J., & Borassa, M. (1982). Skeletal muscle and cardiac changes with training in patients with angina pectoris. *American Journal of Physiology, 243,* H830–H836.

Fletcher, G. (1982). *Exercise on the practice of medicine.* Mount Kisco, NY: Futura.

Fletcher, G. F., Balady, G., Blair, S., Blumenthal, J., Casperson, C., Chairman, B., Epstein, S., Froelicher, E. S., Froelicher, V. F., Pina, I. L., & Pollock, M. L. (1996). Statement on exercise: Benefits and recommendations for physical activity programs for all Americans. *American Heart Association Scientific Statement* [On-line]. Available: http//www.americanheart.org/Scientific/statements/1996/0815_exp.html.

Foster, V., Hume, G., Byrnes, W., Dickenson, A., & Chatfield, S. (1989). Endurance training for elderly women: Moderate vs. low intensity. *Journal of Gerontology, 44*(6), M184–178.

Foster, C., & Tamboli, H. (1992). Exercise prescription in the rehabilitation of patients following coronary artery bypass graft surgery and coronary angioplasty. In R. Shepard & H. Miller (Eds.), *Exercise and the heart in health and disease.* New York: Marcel Dekker.

Gardner, A. W., & Poehlman, E. T. (1995). Exercise rehabilitation programs for the treatment of claudication pain: A meta-analysis. *Journal of the American Medical Association, 274*(12), 975–980.

Gavin, J. (1988). Psychological issues in exercise prescription. *Sports Medicine, 6,* 1–10.

Halfman, M., & Hojnaki, L. (1981). Exercise and the maintenance of health. *Topics in Clinical Nursing, 3*(2), 1–10.

Hamm, L., & Leon, A. (1992). Exercise training for the coronary patient. In N. Wenger & H. Hellerstein (Eds.), *Rehabilitation of the coronary patient* (pp. 367–402). New York: Churchill Livingstone.

Hiatt, W. R., Regensteiner, J. G., Hargerten, M. E., Wolfel, E. E., & Brass, E. P. (1990). Benefit of exercise conditioning for patients with peripheral arterial disease. *Circulation, 81*(2), 602–609.

Juneau, M., Geneau, S., Marchand, C., & Brosseau, R. (1991). Cardiac rehabilitation after coronary artery bypass surgery. *Cardiovascular Clinics, 12*(2), 25–42.

Kisner, C., & Colby, L. (1996). *Therapeutic exercise: Foundations and techniques* (3rd ed.). Philadelphia: F.A. Davis.

Koch, M., Douard, H., & Broustet, J-P. (1992). The benefit of graded physical exercise in chronic heart failure. *Chest, 101*(Suppl. 5), 231S–235S.

National Institutes of Health Consensus Statement. (1995). *Physical Activity and Cardiovascular Health, 13*(3), 1-17 [on-line]. Available: http://text.nlm.nih.gov/nih/cdc/www/101text.html

Pender, N. (1996). *Health promotion in nursing practice* (3rd ed.). Stamford, CT: Appleton & Lange.

Regensteiner, J. G. (1997). Exercise in the treatment of claudication: Assessment and treatment of functional impairment. *Vascular Medicine, 2*(3), 238–242.

Regensteiner, J. G., & Hiatt, W. R. (1995). Exercise rehabilitation for patients with peripheral arterial disease. *Exercise and Sport Sciences Reviews, 23,* 1–24.

Regensteiner, J. G., Steiner, J. F., & Hiatt, W. R. (1996). Exercise training improves functional status in patients with peripheral arterial disease. *Journal of Vascular Surgery, 23*(1), 104–115.

Smith, E., & Reddan, W. (1976). Physical activity—a modality for bone accretion in the aged. *American Journal of Roentgenology, 126,* 1297.

Sullivan, M. (1994). New trends in cardiac rehabilitation in patients with chronic heart failure. *Progress in Cardiovascular Nursing, 9*(1), 13–21.

U. S. Surgeon General. (1996). *Report on physical activity and health* [On-line]. Available: http//www.cde.800/nccdphd/sgr/mm.htm

Wenger, N. (1993). Modern coronary rehabilitation. New concepts in care. *Postgraduate Medicine, 94*(2), 131–141.

Yaffe, M. (1981). Sport and mental health. *Journal of Biosocial Science—Supplement, 7,* 83–95.

26

Groups

Merrie J. Kaas and Mary Fern Richie

U sing groups as a nursing intervention is congruent with nursing's concern for individuals, families, groups, and communities. Nursing-led groups have been developed to foster independence, promote health, and prevent illness for clients and their families and for community consumers. As an intervention, groups can be cost-efficient treatments with positive therapeutic outcomes. The purpose of this chapter is to provide practitioners with the basics for incorporating group work as an intervention into their practice. In this chapter we will review types of groups and group characteristics and describe techniques for establishing, conducting, and evaluating a group. We will also discuss current issues related to multicultural and computer-based groups, cautions about doing group work, and important research questions.

DEFINITION

What is a group? We all belong to groups, but a group is more than a just collection of people. Forsyth (1990) defines a group as "two or more interdependent individuals who influence one another through social interaction" (p. 23). Groups have a number of common features that can change over time such as interaction among members, a specific group structure, variations in size, shared common goals, and cohesiveness.

Groups are an agent of change, and people join them for a variety of reasons. Some want to learn different skills in managing an illness or lifestyle change; others want to understand their behavior in order make changes in relationships; still others want personal support during a life change or loss of health status. Therapeutic groups help individuals achieve goals they cannot achieve alone by helping members increase their knowledge about themselves and others, clarifying the changes they want to make, and giving them the tools to make the changes (Corey & Corey, 1997). Yalom (1995) identified 11 curative factors that are operative in therapeutic groups: instillation of hope, universality, imparting information, altruism, development of socialization techniques, imitative behavior, learning interpersonal skills, group cohesiveness, and catharsis.

SCIENTIFIC BASIS

Practitioners use groups because they are efficient. Empirical data suggest that groups are as effective as other treatments with certain clients. For example, a Cochrane Review (Stead & Lancaster, 2000) reports evidence from meta-analysis that shows group programs were more effective than self-help groups and other less intensive interventions for smoking cessation with adults. Another review of group work with adult cancer patients reports positive outcomes for both diagnostic measures and well-being (Bottomley, 1997). Although much progress has been made in the empirical demonstration of the efficacy of group interventions, practitioners are still unsure about what evaluation measures best demonstrate the outcomes of their group work; e.g., symptom reduction, short-term behavioral change, satisfaction, or adherence to protocols or programs. The use of research and assessment instruments can document changes in clients' diagnostic and treatment outcomes while patient satisfaction and personal goal measures can also demonstrate the therapeutic response to group interventions (Dies & Dies, 1993).

INTERVENTION

Groups established for the purpose of support and behavioral change will be discussed in this chapter. Establishing, conducting, terminating, and evaluating a group requires specific knowledge and skills.

TECHNIQUES

It is difficult to describe a particular technique for the intervention, group. Because the group leader sets the context of the group and facilitates the group process, having good group leadership skills are important to the success of the group.

Group Leadership

The group leader's behavior and skills have a profound effect on the process of the group. Initial group-leader activities include identifying the objectives and purpose of the group, selecting members, and establishing the parameters of the group sessions, as well as orienting the members to the group's purpose and goals. The group leader also promotes the growth of the group by recognizing and monitoring the stages of group development and summarizing progress toward group and personal goals. To facilitate group cohesion, the group leader identifies and manages group processes such as trust, power, conflict, scapegoating, resistance, decision making, and performance. The reader is referred to Corey and Corey (1997), Forsyth (1990), or Yalom (1995) for specific group-leader functions at various stages of group development and for information on managing problem behaviors.

In some instances the use of a coleadership model is preferable. Having coleaders allows one person to actively lead the group while the other attends to the group process. This model is also useful when a senior leader works with a novice leader who is learning how to do group work. Coleadership also provides for continuity if one person is unable to be present. The disadvantages of coleadership include the possibility of competition and rivalry if group members become attached to one leader or if leadership between the coleaders becomes unbalanced. Therefore, considerable planning and debriefing at the conclusion of each session are needed if coleadership is to be used successfully.

A final consideration with respect to group leadership relates to supervision and consultation. It is recommended that the group leader, particularly the novice, establish a relationship with an experienced person who can assist the group leader in processing the dynamics of the group and provide constructive feedback regarding ways in which group functioning and member outcomes can be improved.

Process of Group Development

Most models of group work include five or six basic stages of group development relating to the beginning, working, and ending aspects of groups. The most noted group development model is Tuckman's 1965 five-stage model. (For a thorough description of this model, the reader is referred to Tuckman, 1965, and Forsyth, 1990.) In this chapter, we have modified Tuckman's model of group work by including a pretreatment stage because the group leader is very involved in facilitating the work of the group before the group actually begins.

Pretreatment Stage

One goal of this stage is the selection of group members and the importance of careful screening and selection for group membership cannot be overemphasized. Ideally, preliminary screening sessions can be held in which both the group leader and potential member can interview one another about the proposed group experience. The group leader can assess the degree to which the group would benefit the potential member, whether he or she understands the purpose of the group, and whether any contraindications for group participation exist. Audiotapes, videotapes, printed material, and interviews can facilitate the selection process and prepare potential members for the group experience, thereby improving member involvement in the group process (Dies & Dies, 1993).

Inclusion and exclusion criteria should be developed to guide the selection of group members. Utilizing research instruments that are brief, easily administered, and valid can assist the group leader in determining whether the potential member is appropriate for the group and can provide a measurement of individual change throughout the group experience.

Homogeneity or heterogeneity of membership is another factor to be considered. In most instances, for a specific population with given needs, a group composed of persons of that population would be more desirable than a heterogeneous group that includes persons with potentially unrelated needs.

The minimum and maximum number of members for a successful group has been debated and depends upon several factors: age of the members, the experience of the leader, the type of group, and the problems to be explored (Corey & Corey, 1997). If the group is too small, interaction and gain from others is limited. On the other hand, a smaller group is desirable with certain populations, like school-age children or cognitively impaired older adults. When the group becomes too large, subgroups tend to form, which mitigates against the cohesiveness of the total group. Therapeutic exchange also is reduced in large groups because there is less time for each member to speak. In all, the group should have sufficient opportunity for interaction, but such that the group leader can maintain control, and at the same time offer an experience in which a sense of the group exists. Declining attendance is not an unusual feature of the group intervention modality. For that reason, some group leaders may choose to start out with a slightly larger number of members. Group leaders may use contracts, postcard reminder mailings, and telephone calls to maintain the attendance of the group members.

The group leader must also decide whether membership will be open or closed. Open groups are marked by a changing membership. Closed groups are typically time-limited and members are expected to attend until the group ends. The disadvantages of open groups include increased difficulty attaining cohesion because membership is in a constant flux and the need to spend more time orienting new members to ground rules and goals. Similarly, groups that have definite objectives to be accomplished in a predetermined time would find it difficult to function as an open group.

The necessary number and frequency of sessions varies according to the purpose for which the group was established. Support groups that are offered to families of patients in intensive care units may be ongoing. Psychotherapy groups, which offer the opportunity for more in-depth insight and behavioral change, often extend over months. Interpersonal learning education and psychoeducation groups typically run for 6 to 12 sessions with predetermined topics for each meeting. Although single group sessions are used infrequently, that do have value. For example, single sessions have been used successfully for preoperative teaching and discharge-planning. The length of time for group sessions is usually 1 to 2 hours although they may run shorter for children or adults whose attention spans are limited or who may grow restless. Beginning and ending each group session on time is critical. With most groups, it is recommended that a termination date be determined at the outset.

Forming Stage

Once the group leader has determined the group structure and selected the members, the place, and measurement tools, the group is ready to meet. Tuckman's model (1965) differentiates the stages of group development based on the processes and tasks associated with each. The first stage, forming, is characterized by members' feeling insecure and ambivalent about being in the group. They question whether they want to be in or out of the group and how much they want to disclose. Orientation occurs during this stage as members exchange information and explore their commonalities. Interactions are tentative and polite. The general goals of the group leader during this stage of development are to teach the group members the basics of group membership, facilitate trust, and model therapeutic communication.

Storming Stage

As group members establish an initial level of trust and openness, resistance to disclosure develops and disagreement between members or with the group leader becomes more overt. Group members struggle with how close they want to get to others in the group and how much control they have in the group (Corey, 1999). It is important to recognize that conflict in groups is inevitable and should not be viewed as negative. Corey and Corey (1997) note that avoiding conflict is what makes it destructive. They urge group leaders to avoid cutting off the expression of conflict and to facilitate a more direct expression of feelings and thoughts among members and the leader.

Norming Stage

As trust develops and conflicts are resolved, a feeling of "we-ness" and cama-raderie increases. When a cohesive group has developed, members feel free enough to express what they think and feel, they relate to others on a deeper level. The group leader promotes cohesion by looking for and sharing com-monalities among members and by positively reinforcing member behaviors that foster cohesion.

Performing Stage

Once cohesion exists, the group moves into the next stage of performing in which there is great emphasis on achieving goals. Members feel hopeful that they can change and are willing to work outside the group to make those changes. Behaviors evident in this stage include personal decision-making, group problem-solving, and mutual cooperation. The group leader provides positive reinforcement for trying new behaviors and encourages members in their efforts.

Adjourning Stage

Because the termination period is vital to a successful group experience and may be difficult for some members, it is important that termination issues be brought up early in the group development. In this stage, members have the opportunity to pull together the information and insight they have gained, clarify the meaning of the group, and make plans for using the experience and learning in their lives (Corey & Corey, 1997). Termination is a time for dealing with feelings of sadness and anxiety, giving and receiving feedback, and practicing new behaviors. Some groups may choose to combine the last session with a social activity such as a potluck meal. The focus of the group leader is on helping the members to separate from the group in a way that encourages them to function independently. It is important for the group leader to administer some type of group evaluation to evaluate both the group process and individual changes.

Table 26.1 provides a guide to assist nurses in developing a proposal for using group as an intervention in their practice. In addition to the questions posed in this guideline, it is recommended that both empirical evidence and the financial cost for using group as the intervention of choice be included in the proposal. This information may be desired or required by insurance payers and by prospective members as well. Once the proposal has been developed, it can serve as the framework for the group including the ses-sion content, objectives, activities, and evaluation. The proposal can also serve as a basis for developing advertising to inform colleagues and recruit potential members.

TABLE 26.1   Guideline for Planning a Group

Rationale:
   What type of group is to be formed?
   Who is the group for?
   Why is there a need for such a group?
   Can the needs best be met via a group experience?
   What are the basic assumptions underlying this experience?
   What are your qualifications to lead the group?

Objectives:
   What are the general goals and purposes of the group?
   Are specific outcomes measurable and attainable?

Practical Considerations:
   What recruitment, screening, and selection procedures for membership will
      be used?
   How many members will be in the group?
   How often and for how long will the group meet?
   Will other new members be allowed to join the group once it has started?
   How will the members be prepared for the group experience?
   What ground rules will be established at the outset?

Procedures:
   What structure will the group have?
   What techniques will be used?
   What topics will be explored in the group?
   Are these appropriate and realistic for the given population?
   To what extent are the topics and structure determined by the group members
      and to what extent by the leader?

Evaluation:
   What evaluation procedures are planned? What follow-up procedures?
   Are the measurement instruments valid and reliable?
   Are the evaluation methods objective, practical, and relevant?
   What do you expect to be the characteristics of the various stages of the group?
   What might the problems be at each stage, and how will these be addressed?

Note: Adapted from *Groups: Process and practice* (4th ed.), pp. 75–77, by M. S. Corey
and G. Corey, 1992, Pacific Grove, CA: Brooks-Cole.

Measurement of Outcomes

Evidence-based practice for group work is slowly emerging. Kahn and Kahn (1992) identified several problem areas with respect to research of group outcomes, including the lack of comparison groups, biased assignment to treatments, lack of standardized treatment techniques, and limitations of the outcome measurement indicators. Wilson (1992) suggests that for outcomes of group interventions to have meaning, groups must meet several standards: (a) the membership of the group must be well defined; (b) the group intervention must be clearly described so that it can be duplicated by others; (c) measurable outcomes of the group intervention must be identified; and (d) there must be meaningful comparison groups.

Nurses are beginning to systematically measure outcomes of group interventions. Nehls (1992) compared various therapist interventions that were related to successful group work. Pollack and Cramer (1999) compared two models of group therapy for adults hospitalized for bipolar disorder and consequently developed a taxonomy for patient satisfaction with such groups. Ritchie et al. (2000) tested the impact on caregiving of a 22-week, telephone peer-support group of parents living with a child or adolescent with significant health problems. Results suggest that formal peer support by telephone was successful. If groups are to be used successfully as an intervention across client populations and clinical settings, further clinical research is needed to validate the group's process and outcomes.

Precautions

Although groups have been used widely, they should not be used with everyone. Loomis (1979) and Adrian (1980) stressed the importance of conducting an adequate assessment before recommending that a person become a member of a group. Some people need extensive one-to-one interaction before they can benefit from group interaction. Not only initial assessment, but ongoing assessment is also necessary to determine if the person is benefitting from participation in the group. (Prior assessment may not always be possible with an on-line group.)

Loomis (1979) identified a number of disadvantages of groups. For one thing, it may be too large for the intended purpose, and the members may become dissatisfied because they are unable to meet their goals for joining the group. Leading a group requires specific knowledge and skills. Too often groups are begun without a leader having the requisite basic skills, particularly in knowing how to resolve problems that may arise. Planning the environment and the number, length, and content of sessions is critical to the success of the group (Heiney & Wells, 1989).

USES

Nurses have incorporated many types of groups into their practice. For example, Lewis, Hepburn, Narayan, Corcoran-Perry, and Lally (1999) used family education/support groups to teach family members of patients with Alzheimer's disease about decision-making. Phoenix, Irvine, and Kohr (1997) developed a 10-week intervention model for using group therapy to treat depression in older women, and Peden, Hall, Rayans, and Beebe (2000) developed an intervention model of cognitive behavioral group therapy for reducing negative thinking and depressive symptoms in college women. Christman and Bingham (1989) discussed how nurse practitioners can influence their clients to stop smoking by developing group therapy programs for smoking cessation. Lovrin (1995) described a support group at a public school for 8-year-old girls who had lost a parent or sibling to AIDS.

Table 26.2 presents a description of various types of groups and examples of specific populations and conditions for which nurses have used groups. Nurses will continue to use groups as an intervention, but in the future we will be required to standardize our group intervention and provide evidence of its effectiveness. We will also need to consider doing group work in a multicultural environment and over the Internet.

As our society becomes more culturally diverse, so too will group membership. Special knowledge and skills are necessary to facilitate group work with culturally diverse group members and leaders. And more research is needed to identify the characteristics of groups and group leaders that are most effective with specific ethnic populations. Corey and Corey (1997) suggest that group leaders understand their own cultural conditioning, that of their group members, and an awareness of the sociopolitical context in which they come together. The literature is beginning to demonstrate that group work is successful with modifications in specific cultural populations; for example, Cambodian women (Nicholson & Kay, 1999) and Hispanic brain-injury patients (Armengol, 1999).

The use of computer-assisted group therapy is beginning to get the attention of researchers and practitioners (Brown et al., 1999; Cudney & Weinert, 2000; Ripich, Moore, & Brennan, 1992). Finfgeld (2000) reviews the usefulness of on-line groups for mental health improvement and lifestyle changes. Potential advantages of on-line groups include accessibility, thoughtfulness instead of impulsivity, unseen physical characteristics that may increase connectedness and cohesion, and a more distributed leadership. Disadvantages may include the lack of nonverbal cues, Internet addiction, the lack of rules and established norms for group conduct and enforcement of those

TABLE 26.2   Types and Uses of Groups

Type of Group	Basic Goal	Examples	Uses
Group therapy	Improve psychological functioning and adjustment of individual members	Psychodynamic and cognitive-behavioral groups, interactional group therapy, behavior therapy	• Negative thinking of college women (Peden et al., 2000) • Depressed elderly women in nursing homes (Phoenix et al., 1997) • Patient satisfaction with bipolar patients (Pollack & Cramer, 1999)
Psychoeducational group	Help members gain self-understanding and change interpersonal skills	Skills-training seminars and workshops; medication groups	• Decision-making with caregivers of Alzheimer's patients (Lewis et al., 1999) • Borderline personality (Nehls, 1992) • Anger management (Dyer, 2000)
Self-help/support group	Help members cope with or overcome specific problems or life crises	Alcoholics Anonymous, Weight Watchers, support groups, smoking cessation	• Parents' telephone support group (Ritchie et al., 2000) • Weight loss groups on the Internet (Lingle, 1999) • Caregiver support groups on-site and by telephone (Brown et al., 1999) • Smoking cessation programs (Stead & Lancaster, 2000)

Note: Adapted from *Group Dynamics* (2nd ed.), p. 462. By D. R. Forsyth, 1990, Pacific Grove, CA: Brooks/Cole.

rules by group members and leaders, and the potential for delay in seeking professional help. There are numerous practice and research implications related to this new mode of delivery for group work.

FUTURE RESEARCH

Clinical research is needed to examine, specify, and expand the use of groups in nursing. Often such interventions such as imagery, music, and dance are used within the context of a group, yet the interactive effects frequently are not examined. There are a number of areas in which nursing research is needed to improve the use of groups as a practice intervention. The following are some areas in which research is needed:

1. Developing culturally specific outcomes for various types of groups and the instruments that measure those outcomes.
2. Determining the most effective delivery method for facilitating behavioral change and providing support through group therapy modality such as in-person, telephone, or Internet.
3. Comparing group treatment models to other nursing interventions (e.g., supportive therapy, medication, home visits) in reducing morbidity and improving quality of life for our clients.
4. Exploring the application and efficacy of complementary therapies that are delivered in a group format to enhance well-being and reduce illness, including music, meditation, and relaxation exercises.

REFERENCES

Adrian, S. (1980). A systematic approach to selecting group participants. *Journal of Psychosocial Nursing, 18*(2), 37–41.

Armengol, C. G. (1999). A multimodal support group with Hispanic traumatic brain injury survivors. *Journal of Head Trauma Rehabilitation, 14*(3), 233–246.

Bottomley, A. (1997). Where are we now? Evaluation of two decades of group interventions with adult cancer patients. *Journal of Psychiatric and Mental Health Nursing, 4*(4), 251–265.

Brown, R., Pain, K., Berwald, C., Hirschi, P., Delehanty, R., & Miller, H. (1999). Distance education and caregiver support groups: Comparison of traditional and telephone groups. *Journal of Head Trauma Rehabilitation, 14*(3), 257–268.

Christman, C., & Bingham, M. (1989). The nurse practitioners' role in smoking cessation. *Journal of American Academy of Nurse Practitioners, 1*(2), 49–54.

Corey, G. (1999). *Theory and practice of group counseling* (5th ed.). Pacific Grove, CA: Brooks/Cole.

Corey, M. S., & Corey, G. (1997). *Groups: Process and practice* (5th ed.). Pacific Grove, CA: Brooks/Cole.

Cudney, S. A., & Weinert, C. (2000). Computer-based support groups: Nursing in cyberspace. *Computers in Nursing, 18*(1), 35–46.

Dies, R. R., & Dies, K. R. (1993). The role of evaluation in clinical practice: Overview and group treatment illustration. *International Journal of Group Psychotherapy, 43*(1), 77–105.

Dyer, I. (2000). Cognitive-behavioral group anger management for out-patients: A retrospective study. *International Journal of Psychiatric Nursing Research, 5*(3), 602–621.

Finfgeld, D. L. (2000). Therapeutic groups online: The good, the bad, and the unknown. *Issues in Mental Health Nursing, 21*(3), 241–255.

Forsyth, D. R. (1990). *Group dynamics* (2nd ed.). Pacific Grove, CA: Brooks/Cole.

Heiney, S. P., & Wells, L. M. (1989). Strategies for organizing and maintaining support groups. *Oncology Nursing Forum, 16,* 803–809.

Kahn, E. M., & Kahn, E. W. (1992). Group treatment assignment for outpatients with schizophrenia: Integrating recent clinical and research findings. *Community Mental Health Journal, 28,* 539–550.

Lewis, M., Hepburn, K., Narayan, S., Corcoran-Perry, S., & Lally, R. (1999). The options, outcomes, values, likelihoods decision-making guide for patients and families. *Journal of Gerontological Nursing, 25*(12), 19–25.

Lingle, V. A. (1999). Weight-loss groups on the Web. *Health Care on the Internet, 3*(1), 19–30.

Loomis, M. (1979). *Group process for nurses.* St. Louis, MO: C. V. Mosby.

Lovrin, M. (1995). Interpersonal support among 8-year-old girls who have lost their parents or siblings to AIDS. *Archives in Psychiatric Nursing, 1*(2), 92–98.

Nehls, N. (1992). Group therapy for people with borderline personality disorder: Interventions associated with positive outcomes. *Issues in Mental Health Nursing, 13,* 255–269.

Nicholson, B. L., & Kay, D. M. (1999). Practice update. Group treatment of traumatized Cambodian women: A culture-specific approach. *Social Work: Journal of the National Association of Social Workers, 44*(5), 470–479.

Peden, A. R., Hall, L. A., Rayans, M. K., & Beebe, L. L. (2000). Reducing negative thinking and depressive symptoms in college women. *Journal of Nursing Scholarship, 32*(2), 145–151.

Phoenix, E., Irvine, Y., & Kohr, R. (1997). Sharing stories: Group therapy with elderly depressed women. *Journal of Gerontological Nursing, 23*(4), 10–15.

Pollack, L. E., & Cramer, R. D. (1999). Patient satisfaction with two models of group therapy for people hospitalized with bipolar disorder. *Applied Nursing Research, 12*(3), 143–152.

Ripich, S., Moore, S. M., & Brennon, P. F. (1992). A new nursing medium: Computer networks for group intervention. *Journal of Psychosocial Nursing and Mental Health Services, 30*(7), 15–20.

Ritchie, J., Stewart, M., Ellerton, M., Thompson, D., Meade, D., & Viscount, P. W. (2000). Patients' perceptions of the impact of a telephone support group intervention. *Journal of Family Nursing, 6*(1), 25–45.

Stead, L. F., & Lancaster, T. (2000). Group behavior therapy programmes for smoking cessation. *Cochrane Library,* Issue 3. Oxford, England: Update Software.

Tuckman, B. W. (1965). Developmental sequence in small groups. *Psychological Bulletin, 63,* 384–399.

Wilson, W. H. (1992). Response to Kahn and Kahn: Group treatment assignment for outpatients with schizophrenia. *Community Mental Health Journal, 28,* 551–560.

Yalom, I. (1995). *The theory and practice of group psychotherapy* (4th ed.). New York: Basic Books.

27

Progressive Muscle Relaxation

Mariah Snyder, Elizabeth Pestka, and Catherine Bly

Progressive muscle relaxation (PMR), a technique developed by Edmund Jacobson (1938), is one of the most widely used therapies in stress management. It is used alone or in combination with other therapies. For example, PMR may be used before instructions for guided imagery are provided. A variety of techniques have been developed for achieving relaxation of muscles and overall relaxation.

DEFINITION

Progressive muscle relaxation is defined as the progressive tensing and relaxing of successive muscle groups. A person's attention is drawn to discriminating between the feelings experienced when the muscle group is relaxed compared to when it was tensed. With continued use of PMR, an individual can sense muscle tension without having to progress through the tensing and relaxing of specific muscle groups.

SCIENTIFIC BASIS

When people perceive an actual or potential event as a threat to their well-being, a sympathetic nervous system response occurs, which is often referred to as the *fight-flight* response. It includes dilation of the pupils, shallowness of respiration, increased heart rate, and tensing of muscles. This response assists humans in handling short-term stressful situations such as moving quickly to avoid a car that appears suddenly. However, if the perceived stressor persists over time, the repeated psychophysiological stress response can have deleterious effects on the body. The desired outcome of relaxation strategies is the mitigation of persisting high levels of stress or the avoidance of high stress levels.

Brown (1977) noted that the stress response is part of a closed feedback loop between the muscles and the mind. Appraisal of stressors results in a tensing of the muscles which send stimuli to the brain, establishing a feedback loop. Relaxation of the muscles interrupts the feedback loop.

Jacobson (1938) reported that PMR decreases the body's oxygen consumption, metabolic rate, respiratory rate, muscle tension, premature ventricular contractions, and systolic and diastolic blood pressure, and it increases alpha brain waves. Subsequent studies (Gift, Moore, & Soeken, 1992; Hahn et al., 1993) have validated Jacobson's findings. Additionally, Teshima, Sogawa, and Mizobe (1991) proposed that relaxation could enhance B-endorphins and potentially enhance cellular immune function.

Although findings from many studies have shown positive outcomes from the use of PMR, the results have been conflicting. Reasons for the differences in outcomes may relate to the type of technique used, the length and type of instruction, subjects not practicing the technique on a regular basis, and lack of a good fit between subject characteristics and PMR.

INTERVENTION

Numerous techniques for PMR have been developed since Jacobson publicized his technique in 1938. These include active muscle relaxation (Bernstein & Borkovec, 1973), passive muscle relaxation (Haynes, Moseley, & McGowan, 1975), self-control relaxation (Lichstein, 1988), and rapid relaxation (Deffenbacher & Snyder, 1976). Differences among techniques include the method for relaxing muscle groups, the groups of muscles to which attention is given, type of instruction (live versus tape), the number of teaching sessions used, and the environment in which the teaching is done.

TECHNIQUE

The technique developed by Bernstein and Borkovec (1973) is the most widely used PMR technique. They combined the 108 muscles and muscle groups of Jacobson's technique and reduced it to 16, thus making it more useable.

Instructions that apply to all PMR techniques will be described before detailing Bernstein and Borkovec's technique. A quiet environment is needed so that the person can concentrate on relaxing the muscles. This includes eliminating interruptions, reducing noises, and dimming the lighting. The instructor also needs to assist in modifying the home environment so that a relaxing environment exists for the person's practice. A comfortable chair that provides support for the body is ideal. A bed or couch may be used, but this position may result in the person's falling asleep. Clothing should be loose and not restrictive; shoes, glasses, and contact lenses should be removed. Since the initial sessions may last 45 to 60 minutes, the patient may wish to use the bathroom before the PMR session.

The scientific basis for use of PMR is provided during the first session. Information about stressors, the impact of stress on the body, and the signs and symptoms of high levels of stress are discussed. Descriptions and demonstrations for achieving tension of each muscle group are given, and patients then practice tensing each of the muscle groups. If difficulty is encountered in achieving tension with the demonstrated method, an alternate method for achieving tension of a muscle group can be tried.

Bernstein and Borkovec's Technique

As noted earlier, this technique initially focuses on tensing and relaxing 16 muscle groups, 14 of which are described in Table 27.1. Although Bernstein and Borkovec included instructions for tensing muscles of the feet, these are not included in Table 27.1 because it often results in spasms in the foot. The 14 muscle groups are subsequently combined into 7 and then 4 groups with the ultimate goal of achieving muscle relaxation without having to tense the specific muscle groups.

After progressing through all the muscle groups, the instructor asks the patient to identify whether tension remains in any of the muscle groups. The instructor observes the patient to assess if general relaxation has occurred. Indicators of relaxation are slowed, shallower breathing; arms relaxed and shoulders forward; and feet apart with toes pointing out. Two or three minutes are provided at the conclusion of the session for the patient to enjoy the feelings associated with relaxation.

Terminating relaxation is done gradually. The instructor counts backward from four to one. On the count of four, patients are instructed to move their hands and feet; on three, the arms and legs; on two, the head and neck; and on the count of one, to open the eyes. An opportunity is provided for the patient to ask questions or discuss the feelings experienced.

Bernstein and Borkovec proposed using 10 sessions to teach PMR. However, in many studies instruction was limited to fewer sessions with positive results (Gift et al., 1992; Peck, 1997; Renfroe, 1988; Sloman, Brown, Aldana, & Chee, 1993). In a review of studies in which PMR was used,

TABLE 27.1   Guidelines for 14-Muscle Group PMR

General Information:
   Instruct persons to tense a specific muscle group when they hear "tense," and
      to release the tension when they hear "relax." Tension is held for 7 seconds.
      Patter is used to draw attention to the feelings of tension and relaxation.
      When muscles are relaxed, attention is drawn to the differences between the
      two states.

Tensing Specific Muscle Groups:
   Dominant hand and forearm: Make a tight fist and hold it.
   Dominant upper arm: Push elbow down against the arm of the chair.
   Repeat instructions for the nondominant arm.
   Forehead: Lift eyebrows as high as possible.
   Central face (cheeks, nose, eyes): Squint eyes and wrinkle nose.
   Lower face and jaw: Clench teeth and widen mouth.
   Neck: Pull chin down toward chest but do not touch chest.
   Chest, shoulders, and upper back: Take deep breath and hold it, pull shoulder
      blades back.
   Abdomen: Pull stomach in and try to protect it.
   Dominant thigh: Lift leg and hold it straight out.
   Dominant calf: Point toes toward ceiling.
   Repeat instructions for nondominant side.

Note: Adapted from *Progressive Relaxation Training,* by D. Bernstein and T. Borkovec,
1973, Champaign, IL: Research Press.

Borkovec and Sides (1979) found that better results occurred when four or
more teaching sessions were used. A critical factor in determining the number of teaching sessions needed is ensuring that persons have mastered relaxing the muscle groups and have integrated PMR into their life styles.

   An essential factor in the effectiveness of PMR is daily practice. At least
one 15-minute practice session a day is necessary to master the technique
and achieve relaxation. Helping patients find a time of day to practice relaxation is an important component of instruction. The time of day PMR is
practiced is not important, but it must become a part of the person's daily
routine. Often an audiotape of the instructions is provided to patients to
guide them as they practice at home.

MEASUREMENT OF OUTCOMES

A variety of outcomes have been used to measure the efficacy of PMR.
Physiological measurements that are often used include blood pressure and

heart rate (Collins & Rice, 1997), body posturing, respiratory rate, and skin temperature (Gift et al., 1992), and dyspnea (Renfroe, 1988). Electromyogram readings are occasionally taken to determine the degree of tension in the specific muscle groups. Practitioners need to be alert to underlying pathology or medications that may interfere with reduction in physiological parameters. Also, if a patient does not have an elevated blood pressure or heart rate, few changes will occur with the use of PMR.

Measurement of anxiety is the variable most frequently measured to determine the efficacy of PMR (Snyder, 1993). The State-Trait Anxiety Self-Questionnaire of Spielberger, Gorsuch, Luschene, Vagg, and Jacobs (1983) has been widely used. State anxiety measures a persons feelings at a particular point in time, and trait captures a person's general feelings. Four items of the state-anxiety inventory have been found to have a good correlation with the 20-item inventory (O'Neil, Spielberger, & Hansen, 1969) and provide a useable measurement for clinical settings. Patient self-report about feelings of relaxation has been included in many studies because satisfaction is a good indicator of whether a person will continue to use PMR.

PRECAUTIONS

Although PMR has been used with multiple populations and has been proven to be an effective therapy for nurses to use, care should be exercised in its use. It is important for practitioners to know if patients practice PMR on a regular basis as this may affect the pharmacokinetics of medications. Trophotropic reactions may occur (Lichstein, 1988), which potentiates the effects of some medications and may result in a toxic level of the medication. Because of a relaxed state, a lower dose of a medication may be indicated. This is particularly true for insulin, in which case a hypoglycemic state results.

Complete relaxation may produce a hypotensive state. People need to be taught to remain seated for a few minutes after practicing PMR. Movement in place and gradual resumption of activities helps overcome the hypotensive state. Taking a person's blood at the conclusion of teaching sessions may help to identify those who are prone to hypotensive states.

Some persons with chronic pain have reported a heightened awareness of pain following PMR. Concentrating on tensing and relaxing of muscles may draw attention to the pain rather than to the muscle sensation. Thus, a good assessment of individuals is needed to determine whether negative outcomes are occurring.

Persons with cardiac conditions should not combine the 14 muscle groups into 7 and 4 muscle groups, as tensing and relaxing these large muscle groups results in large volumes of blood being placed in circulation at one time. This places an undue load on the damaged heart muscles.

USES

PMR has been used to achieve a variety of outcomes in diverse populations. Table 27.2 shows conditions and populations in which PMR has been used. Its use for health promotion, relief of pain, and reduction of stress in specific conditions will be discussed.

HEALTH PROMOTION

Nursing has been at the forefront in teaching patients about health-promotion practices. Studies on PMR in healthy persons have shown that the intervention has little or no effect in lowering blood pressure or reducing heart rate (Glaister, 1982). However, these findings do not negate teaching PMR to healthy persons, as they can use the therapy to maintain their blood pressure within normal limits.

PAIN

PMR has been used extensively in the management of pain: headache, postoperative and labor pain, and chronic pain such as low back pain. Muscle tension increases the perception of pain, so lessening anxiety and tension can reduce it. PMR may provide people with a sense of control over their pain. Carroll and Seers (1998) reviewed studies that had used relaxation for the relief of chronic pain. In the nine studies that met the investigators' inclusion criteria, positive findings were found in only four; however, positive results have been reported in numerous other studies.

PMR is frequently used as an adjunct or complementary therapy in the management of pain, particularly with patients who have cancer. Sloman (1995) found that 92% of the patients with cancer who were taught PMR reported that relaxation occurred, and 90% noted that they would continue to use the therapy.

Tension headaches are a common malady in today's society, and PMR has been shown to be an effective therapy in decreasing tension headache. Blanchard and colleagues (1991) reported that subjects with tension headaches

TABLE 27.2   Conditions for Which PMR Has Been Used

Stress Reduction:
   Insomnia (Borkovec, Kaloupek, & Slama, 1975)
   Asthma (Freedberg, Hoffman, Light, & Kreps, 1987)
   Reduction of seizures (Whitman et al., 1990)
   Hypertension (Hahn et al., 1993)
   Chronic obstructive pulmonary disease (Gift et al., 1992)
   Psychiatric patients (Weber, 1996)
   Functional outcomes following head injury (Lysaught & Bodenhammer, 1990)
   Memory training (Yesavage, 1984)

Pain Reduction:
   Cancer (Sloman, 1995)
   Postoperative (Miller & Perry, 1990)
   Headache (Blanchard et al., 1991)

Health Promotion:
   Decrease of nausea and vomiting (Akakawa, 1994)
   Diagnostic procedures (Rice, Caldwell, Butler, & Robinson, 1986)
   HIV (Eller, 1999)
   Herpes (Burnette, Koehn, Kenyon-Jump, Hutton, & Stark, 1991)

who had received 8 weeks of PMR training had an improvement that was significantly different from subjects in the control group. Those who are prone to tension headaches can be taught to use PMR on a regular basis to avoid their occurring.

REDUCTION OF STRESS

As noted in Table 27.2, PMR has been used to reduce the stress associated with a number of conditions. It has been used as an adjunct therapy in the treatment of hypertension (Larkin, Knowlton, & D'Allesandri, 1991). Although fewer studies have been done on the use of PMR as an antiseizure adjunct therapy, Whitman, Dell, Legion, Eibhlyn, and Staatsinger (1991) found a 54% decrease in seizures in persons who practiced PMR as an adjunct to their anticonvulsant medications. Many of those who have seizures have high levels of stress because they are concerned about having another seizure (others finding out that they have epilepsy). Reducing high levels of stress can have positive effects in the lives of persons who have epilepsy.

FUTURE RESEARCH

PMR has been used singly and in combination with other therapies. A scientific body of knowledge is emerging to guide the use of PMR but considerably more research is needed:

1. Eller (1999) has examined the impact of PMR on the quality of life in persons with HIV. Further studies on the use of PMR with HIV are needed, particularly an examination of its effect on immune function.

2. Compliance with PMR is critical to its success. What factors prompt persons to continue or discontinue use after receiving instruction?

3. Many studies continue to examine only the psychological outcomes such as anxiety or mood. Although these are important variables to study, the inclusion of physiological variables will contribute information about the holistic perspective of complementary therapies.

4. In the majority of studies that have been conducted, the effect of PMR has been evaluated immediately following administration of the intervention. Longitudinal studies are needed to determine if PMR produces ongoing positive results in conditions such as hypertension and dyspnea.

REFERENCES

Arakawa, S. (1995). Use of relaxation to reduce side effects of chemotherapy in Japanese patients. *Cancer Nursing, 18,* 60–66.

Bernstein, D., & Borkovec, T. (1973). *Progressive relaxation training.* Champaign, IL: Research Press.

Blanchard, E. B., Nicholson, N. L., Taylor, A. E., Steffek, B. D., Radnitz, S., & Appelbaum, K. A. (1991). The role of regular home practice of relaxation treatment for tension headache. *Journal of Consulting and Clinical Psychology, 59,* 467–470.

Borkovec, T., Kaloupek, D., & Slama, K. (1975). The facilitative effect of muscle tension-release in the relaxation of sleep disorders. *Behavior Therapy, 6,* 301–309.

Borkovec, T., & Sides, J. (1979). Critical procedural variables related to the physiological effects of progressive muscle relaxation. *Behavior Research and Therapy, 17,* 119–125.

Brown, B. (1977). *Stress and the art of biofeedback.* New York: Bantam.

Burnette, M. M., Koehn, K. A., Kenyon-Jump, R., Hutton, K., & Stark, C. (1991). Control of genital herpes recurrences using progressive muscle relaxation. *Behavior Therapy, 22,* 237–247.

Carroll, D., & Seers, K. (1998). Relaxation for the relief of chronic pain: A systematic review. *Journal of Advanced Nursing, 27,* 476–487.

Collins, J. A., & Hill, V. H. (1997). Effects of relaxation intervention in phase II cardiac rehabilitation: Replication and extension. *Heart and Lung, 26,* 31–44.

Deffenbacher, J., & Snyder, A. (1976). Relaxation and self-control in the treatment of test and other anxieties. *Psychological Reports, 39,* 379–385.

Eller, L. S. (1999). Effects of cognitive-behavioral interventions on quality of life in persons with HIV. *International Journal of Nursing Studies, 36,* 222–233.

Freedberg, P. D., Hoffman, L. A., Light, W. C., & Kreps, M. K. (1987). Effect of progressive muscle relaxation on the objective symptoms and subjective responses associated with asthma. *Heart and Lung, 16,* 24–30.

Gift, A. G., Moore, T., & Soeken, K. (1992). Relaxation to reduce dyspnea and anxiety in COPD patients. *Nursing Research, 41,* 242–246.

Glaister, B. (1982). Muscle relaxation training for fear reduction of patients with psychological problems: a review of controlled studies. *Behavior Therapy Research, 20,* 493–504.

Hahn, Y. B., Ro, Y. J., Song, H. H., Kim, N. C., Sim, H. S., & Yang, S. Y. (1993). The effect of thermal biofeedback and progressive muscle relaxation training in reducing blood pressure of patients with essential hypertension. *Image: Journal of Nursing Scholarship, 25,* 204–207.

Haynes, S., Moseley, D., & McGowan, W. (1975). Relaxation training and biofeedback in the reduction of frontalis muscle tension. *Psychophysiology, 12,* 547–552.

Jacobson, E. (1938). *Progressive relaxation.* Chicago: University of Chicago Press.

Larkin, K. T., Knowlton, G. E., & D'Alessandri, R. (1990). Predicting treatment outcomes to progressive muscle relaxation training in essential hypertensive patients. *Journal of Behavioral Medicine, 13,* 605–618.

Lichstein, K. L. (1988). *Clinical relaxation strategies.* New York: John Wiley & Sons.

Lysaught, R., & Bodenhammer, E. (1990). The use of relaxation training to enhance functional outcomes in adults with traumatic head injuries. *American Journal of Occupational Therapy, 44,* 797–802.

Miller, K. M., & Perry, P. A. (1990). Relaxation training and postoperative pain in patients undergoing cardiac surgery. *Heart and Lung, 19,* 136–146.

O'Neil, H. F., Spielberger, C. D., & Hansen, D. N. A. (1969). The effects of state anxiety and task difficulty on computer-assisted learning. *Journal of Educational Psychology, 60,* 343–350.

Peck, S. (1997). The effectiveness of therapeutic touch for decreasing pain in elders with degenerative arthritis. *Journal of Holistic Nursing, 15*(2), 13–26.

Renfroe, K. (1988). Effect of progressive muscle relaxation in dyspnea and state anxiety in patients with chronic obstructive pulmonary disease. *Heart and Lung, 17,* 408–413.

Rice, V. H., Caldwell, M., Butler, S., & Robinson, J. (1986). Relaxation training and response in cardiac catheterization. *Nursing Research, 35,* 39–43.

Shapiro, S., & Lehrer, P. (1980). Psychophysiological effects of autogenic training and progressive relaxation. *Biofeedback and Self-Relaxation, 5,* 249–255.

Sloman, R. (1995). Relaxation and the relief of cancer pain. *Nursing Clinics of North America, 30,* 697–709.

Sloman, R., Brown, R., Aldana, E., & Chu, E. (1994). The use of relaxation for promotion of comfort and pain relief in persons with advanced cancer. *Contemporary Nurse, 3*(1), 6–12.

Snyder, M. (1993). The influence of interventions on the stress-coping linkage. In J. Barnfather & B. Lyon (Eds.), *Stress and coping: State of the science and implications for nursing theory, research, and practice* (pp. 159–170). Indianapolis, IN: Sigma Theta Tau International.

Spielberger, C., Gorsuch, R., Luschene, R., Vagg, P., & Jacobs, G. (1983). *Manual for STAI.* Palo Alto, CA: Consulting Psychological Press.

Teshima, H., Sogawa, H., & Mizobe, K. (1991). Application of psychoimmunotherapy in patients with alopecia universalis. *Psychotherapy and Psychosomatics, 56,* 235–241.

Weber, S. (1996). The effects of relaxation exercise on anxiety levels in psychiatric inpatients. *Journal of Holistic Nursing, 14,* 196–205.

Whitman, S., Dell, J., Legion, V., Eibhlyn, A., & Staatsinger, J. (1990). Progressive relaxation for seizure reduction. *Journal of Epilepsy, 3,* 17–22.

Yesavage, J. A. (1984). Relaxation training and memory training in 39 elderly patients. *American Journal of Psychiatry, 141,* 778–781.

Index

Index

Active listening, 29
Active presence, 37
Acupressure, 205–220
  acupuncture, 205
  Alzheimer's, wandering behaviors in,
      211
  angina, 211
  auriculotherapy, 205
  breech presentation, 213
  cardiovascular system, effect on,
      211
  chemotherapy, nausea of, 210
  constipation, 211
  definitions, 205–207
  dental procedures, 210
  effectiveness, 211–214
  frozen shoulder, 212
  future research, 217
  gastrointestinal disorders, 215–216
      pain, 215–216
  guidelines for use, 209–214
  intervention, 209–214
  labor, 213
  meridians, 205
  morning sickness, 210
  moxibustion, 206
  nausea, 210, 214–215
      postoperative, 210
  osteoarthritis, 212
  pain, 215–216

  postoperative, 211
  posttraumatic, 212
  patello-femoral pain syndrome, 212
  precautions, 216–217
  pressure points
      large intestine, 215
      pericardium, 214–216
  rheumatoid arthritis, 212
  scientific basis, 207–209
  shiatsu, 205–206
  stimulating point, 214
  traditional Chinese medicine,
      206–207
  use of, 214–217
Acupuncture, 9
Adoration prayer, 116
Aerobic exercise, 288–289; see also
      Exercise
AHNA, see American Holistic Nurses'
      Association
Alternative Medicine Homepage, 12
Alternative systems of care, overview, 7
American Association for Therapeutic
      Humor, 70, 77
American Holistic Nurses'
      Association, 12, 166, 179
American Indian culture, meditation,
      101
Ancient cultures, initiation of healer
      in, 20

Animal-assisted therapy, 152–162
    definition, 153–154
    dogs, companion, 159
    dolphins, 159
    future research, 159–160
    guidelines, 156–157
    hippotherapy, 159
    horseback riding, 159
    intervention, 155–158
    outcome, measurement of, 156–158
    porpoises, 159
    precautions, 158
    in prisons, 159
    psychotherapy, animals to decrease
        anxiety, 159
    rehabilitation units, 159
    scientific basis, 154–155
    use of, 158–159
Aromatherapy, 245–258
    aches, 254
    acne, 255
    Alzheimer's disease, 255
    analgesia, 247
    anxiety, 247
    asthma, 255
    autism, 255
    bacterial uses, 254
    behavioral problems, 255
    bereavement, 255
    botanical names, 252
    bronchitis, 255
    burns, post-radiation, 255
    cancer, 255
    candida albicans, 248
    cardiovascular uses, 254
    colic, 255
    concentration, 247
    constipation, 254
    cramps, 254
    credentialing, 256
    cystitis, 254
    definitions, 246
    depression, 247

dermatologic uses, 255
diabetic ulcers, 255
diaper rash, 255
dying, care of, 255
fungal uses, 254
future research, 253–256
gastrointestinal uses, 254
guidelines, 251–253
gynecological uses, 254
immune function, 247
indigestion, 254
infection, 254
infertility, 254
inhalation, 249
intervention, 248–253
irritable bowel syndrome, 254
low back pain, 254
memory loss, 255
menopausal symptoms, 254
menstrual cramping, 254
migraine, 254
National Association of Holistic
    Aromatherapy, 256
nausea, 255
older adults, 255
osteoarthritis, 254
outcome, measurement of, 250
pain, 247, 254–255
pediatrics, 255
precautions, 250–251
premenstrual syndrome, 254
pressure ulcers, 255
pseudomonas, 248
psoriasis, 255
relaxation, 247, 255
research, 247–248
respiratory system, 255
rheumatoid arthritis, 254
ringworm, 248
rites of passage, 255
scientific basis, 246–248
seizures, 247
simusitis, 255

skin, flaky, 255
sleep problems, 255
spiritual uses, 255
thymol, 245
topical use, 249
urinary system, 254
use of, 253–254
vaginal use, 249
viral uses, 254
water retention, 254
Auriculotherapy, 205
Ayurvedic medicine, 9, 12

Basil, 252, 255
Bencol, 279
Bergamot, 254
Bernstein, Borkovec technique,
    progressive muscle relaxation,
    312–313
Biofeedback, 89–100
    chronic pain, 95
    conditions, 94–96
    definition, 89
    diabetes mellitus, 96
    future research, 97
    hypertension, 94–95
    intervention, 90–94
    outcome, measurement of, 92–94
    parameters, feedback to patient,
        94
    precautions, 96–97
    protocol, 93
    relaxation, biofeedback-assisted, 92
    scientific basis, 89–90
    techniques, 90–92
    urinary incontinence, 95–96
    use of, 94–97
Biological-based therapies, 243–282
    overview, 7
Body-based therapies, 221–242
    overview, 7
Breathing, yoga, 82
Buddhist meditation, 101

Calcium additives, 279
Centering, 29
    meditation, 104–105
    prayer, 102
Chakras, 170–171
Chamomile
    German, 252
    Roman, 252
Chen style, in tai chi, 235
Chinese martial arts, 234
Chinese medicine, traditional, 8–9,
    206–207
Chiron, 20
Chondroitin, 276, 279
Christian contemplation, 101
Chronic pain, biofeedback, 95
Clary sage, 252, 254–255
Classical music, 61
Classification, complementary
    therapies, 7
Clove, 254
Collagen hydrolysate, 276
Colloquial prayer, 116
Colorado Center for Healing Touch,
    179
Companion dogs, in pet therapy, 159
Complicating action, of story, 125
Consciousness, altered states of, 20
Contemplation, Christian, 101
Coriander seed, 252
Cultural aspects, complementary
    therapies, 8–10
Cupping, 9
Cypress, 254–255

Dalai Lama, 21
Dance of Deer Foundation, 12
Dharana, 82
Diabetes mellitus, biofeedback, 96
Dietary fiber supplement, 279
Dietary sitostanol ester, 279
Dietary Supplement Health and
    Education Act of 1994, 260

Directed prayer, 116
Disease prevention therapies, 283–320
Dogs, in pet therapy, 159
Dolphins, in animal therapy, 159
Dreams, 19–20
DSHEA, see Dietary Supplement
    Health and Education Act of
    1994

Echinacea, 263, 265
Effluerage, 226
Energy field
    clearing, 187–188
    human being as, 184
Energy flow imbalance, illness as, 184
Energy therapies, 163–221
    National Center for
        Complementary/Alternative
        Medicine, 163
    overview, 7
Ethnic humor, 72
Eucalyptus, 252, 254–255
Exercise, 285–296
    aerobic, 288–289
    conditions/populations, 290–293
    cool-down phase, 289
    definition, 285–286
    future research, 294
    heart disease, 292
    intervention, 287–290
    maintenance, 289
    older adults, 290–291
    outcome, measurement of, 293
    perceived exertion, rating of, 290
    peripheral arterial disease,
        292–293
    precautions, 293–294
    scientific basis, 286–287
    target heart rate, 290
    technique, 288–289
    use of, 290–294
    walking, 289–290, 291
    warm-up phase, 288

FDA, see Food and Drug
    administration
Federal Drug Administration
    Consumer Line, 12
Fennel, 252, 254
Food and Drug Administration, 260
Foot massage, 226–227
    technique, 227
Formal humor, 71–72
Frankincense, 254–255
Free flow journaling, 138
Friction movements, in massage,
    226
Full-body techniques, healing touch,
    170
Full presence, 26

Gastrointestinal disorders,
    acupressure, 215–216
Geranium, 252, 254–255
German chamomile, 254–255
Ginger, 252, 254–255
Gingko biloba, 265, 266
Glycosamine, 276, 279
Groups, 297–309
    adjourning stage, 302–303
    definitions, 297–298
    forming stage, 301
    future research, 307
    group development, process of, 299
    group leadership, 299
    group therapy, 306
    intervention, 298–304
    norming stage, 302
    nursing-led groups, 297
    outcome, measurement of, 304
    performing stage, 302
    planning, 303
    precautions, 304
    pretreatment stage, 300–301
    psychoeducational group, 306
    scientific basis, 298
    self-help/support group, 306

storming stage, 301
techniques, 298–303
types, 306
use of, 305–307
Guar gum, 279

Hand massage, 226–227
Healing touch, 165–182
    agitation, 177
    American Holistic Nurses'
        Association, 166, 179
    anxiety, 177
    chakra connection, 170
    chakra spread, 171
    clearing, 174
    Colorado Center for Healing
        Touch, 179
    definition, 165–166
    depression, 177
    full-body techniques, 170
    future research, 176–179
    Healing Touch International, 179
    immune system enhancement, 177
    intervention, 169–174
    laser, 172
    magnetic unruffle, 170
    mana, 168
    medical procedures, 177
    mind clearing, 172
    modulating, 174
    outcome, measurement of, 174–175
    pain drain, 172
    pain relief, 177
    precautions, 175
    procedure, 170–173
    relaxation response, 177
    scientific basis, 167–169
    sending energy, 174
    techniques, 169–174
    therapeutic touch, 170
    universal energy, 168
    unruffling, 174
    use of, 176

well-being, enhancement of, 177
    wound healing, 177
Healing Touch International, 179
Heart disease, exercise and, 292
Heart rate, target, 290
Herbal medicines, 243–282
    definition, 259–260
    Dietary Supplement Health and
        Education Act of 1994, 260
    echinacea, 263, 265
    Food and Drug Administration, 260
    future research, 268
    gingko biloba, 265–266
    intervention, 261–262
    precautions, 262
    Saint John's Wort, 265–266
    scientific basis, 261
    technique, 261–262
    use of, 262–268
Hippocrates, 223
Hippotherapy, 159
Homeopathy, 9
Horseback riding, as therapy, 159
Humor, 69–80
    American Association for
        Therapeutic Humor, 70, 77
    assessment, 74–75
    definition, 70–72
    effectiveness, measurement of,
        75–76
    ethnic humor, 72
    formal humor, 71–72
    future research, 77–78
    Humor and Health Institute, 77
    humor styles, 71–72
    intervention, 74–76
    interview guide, humor assessment,
        75
    Joyful Noiseletter, 77
    on-line humor resources, 77
    precautions, 77
    puns, 72
    rationale for, 70–71

Humor (*continued*)
  release, 71
  scientific basis, 72–74
  self-deprecating humor, 72
  superiority, 71
  surprise, 71
  techniques, 75–76
  use of, 76–77
Humor and Health Institute, 77
Hypertension
  biofeedback, 94–95
  meditation, 108–109
Hyssop, 252

Imagery, 43–57
  asthma, 50
  burn-dressing change, 50
  cancer, 50, 52–53
    pain, 50, 52
  cardiac catheterization, 50
  childbirth, 50
  definition, 44
  depression, 50
  emotional disorders, 50
  future research, 53–54
  immune response, 50
  intervention, 45–49
  lymphoma, 50
  nausea, 50
  outcome, measurement of, 48–49
  pain, 49–52
  phobias, 50
  precautions, 49
  procedural pain, 50
  psoriasis, 50
  scientific basis, 44–45
  techniques, 45–48
  use of, 49–53
Incontinence, urinary, biofeedback,
    95–96
Initiation of healer, in ancient
    cultures, 20
Intensive journaling, 138–139

Intercessory prayer, 116
International Center for Reiki Training,
    197
Interview guide, humor assessment, 75

Journaling, 135–151
  anxiety, 141
  creativity, 141
  critical thinking, 141
  daily log, 139
  definition, 135–136
  depression, 141
  depth dimension, 139
  free flow journaling, 138
  future research, 141
  intensive journaling, 138–139
  intervention, 137–141
  outcome, measurement of, 140
  period log, 139
  personal growth, 141
  precautions, 140
  scientific basis, 136–137
  techniques, 138–139
  topical journaling, 138
  transitions, assisting with, 141
  use of, 140–141
Journey, transformational, 20–21
Joyful Noiseletter, 77
Juniper, 254–255

Ki, 163
Krieger, Dolores, 183
Kunz, Dora, 183

Laughter, 69–80
Lavender, 254–255
  true, 252
Leadership, group, 299
Lemon, 254
Lemon eucalyptus, 254
Lemongrass, 252, 254–255
Lifestyle therapies, 283–320
  overview, 7

Magnetic unruffle, with healing touch, 170
Mana, 168
Mandarin, 254–255
Manipulative therapies, 221–242
  overview, 7
Margarine, 279
  sitostanol ester, 275–276
Martial arts, Chinese, 234; *see also* Tai chi
Massage, 223–233
  definition, 223–224
  effluerage, 226
  foot massage, 226–227
    technique, 227
  friction movements, 226
  future research, 230–231
  hand massage, 226–227
    back of, 228
    palm of, 228
    technique for, 228
  intervention, 225–229
  kneading, 226
  outcome, measurement of, 227
  pain, 229–230
  percussion strokes, 226
  petrissage, 226
  precautions, 227–229
  relaxation, 229
  scientific basis, 224–225
  strokes of massage, 225–226
  techniques, 225–226
  use of, 229–230
  vibration strokes, 226
Meditation, 82, 101–113
  aikido, 101
  American Indian Culture, 101
  anxiety, 109–110
  Buddhist, 101
  centering prayer, 102
  Christian contemplation, 101
  conditions, 107
  definition, 102

future research, 111
  guidelines, 106
  hypertension, 108–109
  intervention, 104–106
  mindfulness meditation, 102
  moving meditations, 101
  outcome, measurement of, 110
  pain, chronic, 107–108
  populations, 107–110
  precautions, 110–111
  relaxation response, 102, 105
  scientific basis, 103
  stress, 109–110
  techniques, 104–106
    centering prayer, 104–105
    mindfulness meditation, 105–106
    transcendental meditation, 104
  transcendental meditation, 102
  use of, 106–111
  walking meditation, 101
  Zen Buddhist, 101
Melissa, 254
Meridians, in acupressure, 205
Mind-body therapies, 41–162
  overview, 7
Mindfulness meditation, 102, 105–106
Movement meditations, 101
Moxibustion, 9, 206
Music intervention, 58–68
  anxiety, 64
    decreasing, 64–65
  classical music, 61
  definition, 58–59
  disruptive behaviors, minimizing, 64
  distraction, 64–65
  frequency, 58
  future research, 65
  guidelines, 62–63
  individual, versus group, 61
  intensity, 58

Music intervention (continued)
    interval, 59
    intervention, 60–63
    listening, 60–61
    new age music, 61
    nontraditional music, 61
    orientation, 64
    outcome, measurement of, 62
    pain, 64
    patriotic songs, 61
    pitch, 58
    popular songs, 61
    precautions, 62–63
    relaxation, 64
    rhythm, 59
    scientific basis, 59–60
    stimulation, 64
    stress reduction, 64
    synthesized music, 61
    techniques, 60–61
    tempo, 59
    timbre, 58
    tone, 58
    types of music, 61–62
    use of, 63–65

NAHA, see National Association of
        Holistic Aromatherapy
Naiouli, 254–255
National Association of Holistic
        Aromatherapy, 256
National Center for
        Complementary/Alternative
        Medicine, 5, 12, 221
National Institutes of Health, 5
NCCAM, see National Center for
        Complementary/Alternative
        Medicine
Neroli, 252
NIH, see National Institutes of Health
Nondirected prayer, 116
North America, Native Americans,
        meditation, 101

Nursing-led groups, 297
Nutraceuticals, 272–284
    antioxidants, 279
    bencol, 279
    calcium additives, 279
    categorization, nutrition-related
            products, 275
    chondroitin, 279
    chondroitin sulfate, 276
    collagen hydrolysate, 276
    definitions, 273–274
    dietary fiber supplement, 279
    dietary sitostanol ester, 279
    future research, 278–279
    glucosamine, 276
    glycosamine, 279
    guar gum, 279
    hydrolyzed whey, 279
    intervention, 277
    margarine, 279
        sitostanol ester, 275–276
    outcome, measurement of, 277
    pre-pro-biotics, in fermented milk,
            279
    precautions, 278
    protein peptides, 279
    psyllium, 279
    scientific basis, 274–277
    soy protein, 276–277, 279
    use of, 277–278
Nutrition-related products,
        categorization of, 275

On-line humor resources, 77
Oregano, 254
Oriental massage, 9

Pain
    acupressure, 215–216
    biofeedback, 95
    chronic, 107–108
    healing touch and, 172, 177
    imagery, 49–52

massage for, 229–230
progressive muscle relaxation,
    315–316
Palma rosa, 254
Palmarosa, 252
Parsley, 252
Partial presence, 26
Patchouli, 255
Pennyroyal, 252
Peppermint, 252, 254–255
Perceived exertion, rating of, 290
Percussion strokes, in massage, 226
Performing stage, of groups, 302
Pericardium, 214–215
Period log, 139
Peripheral arterial disease, exercise
    and, 292–293
Pet assisted therapy, 152–162
    definition, 153–154
    dogs, companion, 159
    dolphins, 159
    future research, 159–160
    guidelines, 156–157
    hippotherapy, 159
    horseback riding, 159
    intervention, 155–158
    outcome, measurement of, 156–158
    porpoises, 159
    precautions, 158
    in prisons, 159
    psychotherapy, animals to decrease
        anxiety, 159
    rehabilitation units, 159
    scientific basis, 154–155
    use of, 158–159
Petrissage, in massage, 226
Pine, 255
Pitta, 9
Plant identification, taxonomy in, 253
Points, in acupressure, stimulating,
    214
Porpoises, in animal therapy, 159
Postpartum care, 50

Postures
    breathing techniques, 83
    yoga, 82
Prana, 163, 168, 184
Pranayama, 82
Pratyahara, 82
Prayer, 114–123
    addictive behaviors, 121
    adoration, 116
    assessment, 118–119
    cancer, 121
    cardiac conditions, 121
    caregivers, 121
    centering, 102
    colloquial, 116
    definition, 115
    depressive symptoms, 121
    derivation of word, 115
    directed, 116
    effectiveness of, 121
    future research, 121
    immunosufficiency syndrome, 121
    intercessory, 116
    intervention, 117–120
    lamentation, 116
    nondirected, 116
    outcome, measurement of, 120
    petition, 116
    praise, 116
    precautions, 120
    ritual, 116
    scientific basis, 115–117
    technique, 119
    thanksgiving, 116
    types of, 116
    use of, 120–121
Presence, 24–32, 129
    accountability, 29
    active listening, 29
    centering, 29
    classifications of, 25
    communication, 29
    components, 29

Presence (continued)
  definition, 24–25
  effectiveness, measurement of, 29
  existential being with patient, 24
  full presence, 26
  future research, 30–31
  intervention, 27–30
    centering, 28
    technique, 28–29
  openness, 29
  partial presence, 26
  physical being with patient, 24
  precautions, 29–30
  presence, intervention, centering,
    28
  psychological being, with patient,
    24
  scientific basis, 25–27
  skills, 29
  transcendent presence, 26
  types of, 26
  use of, 30
Pressure points, in acupressure
  large intestine, 215
  pericardium, 214–216
Pretreatment stage, of groups,
    300–301
Prisons, pet therapy in, 159
Progressive muscle relaxation,
    310–320
  asthma, 316
  Bernstein, Borkovec technique,
    312–313
  cancer pain, 316
  chronic obstructive pulmonary
    disease, 316
  definition, 310
  diagnostic procedures, 316
  future research, 317
  guidelines, 313
  head injury, functional outcome
    following, 316
  headache, 316

health promotion, 315–316
herpes, 316
HIV, 316
hypertension, 316
insomnia, 316
intervention, 311–315
memory training, 316
nausea, 316
outcome, measurement of, 313–314
pain, 315–316
postoperative pain, 316
precautions, 314–315
psychiatric patients, 316
scientific basis, 310–311
seizures, 316
stress, 316
technique, 311–313
use of, 315–316
Psychoeducational group, 306
Psychotherapy, animals to decrease
    anxiety, 159

Qi, 8, 163, 206
Qi gong, 9

Ravansara, 254
Reiki, 163, 197–220
  addiction, 202
  anxiety, 202
  applications, 202
  cancer patients, 202
  dialysis, 202
  full Reiki session, 200
  future research, 201–203
  Hayashi, Chujiro, 197
  hematologic measure improvement,
    202
  immune function, 202
  International Center for Reiki
    Training, 197
  intervention, 199–201
  labor, delivery, 202
  outcome, measurement of, 200–201

pain, 202
precautions, 201
respiratory problems, 202
scientific basis, 199
surgical patients, 202
Takata, Hawayo, 197
techniques, 200
use of, 201
Usui, Mikao, 197
wound healing, 202
Reminiscence, 143–151
    acutely ill, 148–149
    definition, 143–144
    families/staff, 148
    future research, 149–150
    intensive care, 149
    intervention, 145–148
    nurses, 149
    outcome, measurement of, 146–147
    precautions, 147–148
    scientific basis, 144
    technique, 145–146
        group structured, 146–147
        individual unstructured, 145
    use of, 148–149
Rhythm, 59
Ritual prayer, 116
Roman chamomile, 254–255
Rose, 252, 254–255
Rosemary, 254–255
Rosewood, 252

Sage, 252, 254
Saint John's Wort, 265–266
Samadhi, 82
Sandalwood, 252, 255
Savasana, 84
Self as healer, 16–23
    altered states of consciousness, 20
    Chiron, 20
    Dalai Lama, 21
    future research, 21–22
    Greek temples, 19

initiation of healer, in ancient
    cultures, 20
self-care, 17–20
    dreams, 19–20
    spiritual direction, 18–19
shamans, 20
Taoist philosophy, 20
transformational journey, 20–21
Self-care, 17–20
    dreams, 19–20
    spiritual direction, 18–19
Self-deprecating humor, 72
Self-help/support group, 306
Sending energy, with healing touch,
    174
Shamans, 20
Shiatsu, 205–206
Sitostanol ester margarine, 275–276
Soy protein isolates, 279
Soy protein powder, 276–277
Spike lavender, 254–255
Spiritual development, enhancement
    of, with healing touch, 177
Stimulating point, acupressure, 214
Storytelling, 124–134
    abstract, of story, 125
    coda, of story, 125
    community, 130
    complicating action, of story, 125
    definition, 124–125
    empathy, 129
    evaluation, of story, 125
    future research, 131–132
    intervention, 128–131
    listening, 129
    nonjudgment, 129
    orientation, of story, 125
    outcome, measurement and,
        130–131
    precautions, 131
    presence, 129
    research, 126–128
    resolution, of story, 125

Storytelling (continued)
  scientific basis, 125–128
  spontaneity, 129
  talking circle, 128
  techniques, 128–130
  use of, 131–132
Strokes of massage, 225–226
Sun style tai chi, 235
Support group, 306
Sweet marjoram, 254–255
Synthesized music, 61

Tai chi, 101, 234–244
  chen style, 235
  class, choosing, 239
  definition, 234–235
  guidelines, 237
  intervention, 236–239
  martial art, Chinese, 234
  outcome, measurement of, 237–238
  precautions, 238–239
  scientific basis, 235–236
  styles of, 235
  sun style, 235
  techniques, 236–237
  wu style, 235
  yang style, 235
Takata, Hawayo, 197
Talking circle, 128
Tamanu carrier oil, 255
Taoists, meditation, 101
Target heart rate, 290
Tarragon, 252, 254
Tea tree, 254–255
Tempo of music, 59
Thanksgiving prayer, 116
Therapeutic listening, 33–42
  accepting attitude, 37
  active presence, 37
  clarifying statements, 37
  definition, 33–34
  future research, 38
  intervention, 35–38

  guidelines, 36
  outcome, measurement of,
      36–37
  precautions, 37–38
  scientific basis, 34–35
  silence, use of, 37
  techniques, 37
  tone, 37
  use of, 38
Therapeutic touch, 183–196; see also
      Healing touch
  assessing, 187
  balancing, 188
  centering, 185–186
  clearing, mobilizing energy field,
      187–188
  definition, 183
  directing energy, for healing, 188
  human beings, as energy fields,
      184
  illness, as energy flow imbalance,
      184
  intervention, 185–189
  Krieger, Dolores, 183
  Kunz, Dora, 183
  outcome, measurement of, 188–189
  prana, 184
  precautions, 189
  process, 186
  research, 190–194
  scientific basis, 183–185
  technique, 185–188
  use of, 189–190
Thyme, 254
Thymol, in aromatherapy, 245
TM, see Transcendental meditation
Toenail fungus, 254
Tone, in therapeutic listening, 37
Topical journaling, 138
Traditional Chinese medicine, 8–9,
      206–207
Transcendent presence, 26
Transcendental meditation, 102, 104

Transformational journey, 20–21
Twasi of Africa, meditation, 101
Types of music, 61–62

Ultrasound, healing touch, 171
Universal energy, 168
Universal ethical principles, 81
Unruffling, with healing touch, 174
Urinary incontinence, biofeedback, 95–96
Usui, Mikao, 197

Vata, 9
Vibration strokes, in massage, 226
Vital life force, 8
Vomiting, 50

Walking, 289–291
Walking meditation, 101
Wandering behaviors, in Alzheimer's, acupressure, 211
Web sites, information on complementary therapies, 12
Well-being, enhancement of, 177
Wheel of health essentials, of Hippocrates, 223
Whole person, to whole person, interaction, see Presence
Wintergreen, 252

Wound sealing, with healing touch, 172
Wu style tai chi, 235

Yama, see Universal ethical principles
Yang, 8
Yang style tai chi, 235
Yin, 8
Ylang-ylang, 252, 254–255
Yoga, 81–88
    concentration of mind, 82
    control of senses, 82
    definition, 81–82
    future research, 85–86
    intervention, 83–84
    meditation, 82
    outcome, measurement of, 83
    postures, 82
        breathing techniques, 83
    precautions, 83–84
    research findings, 86
    savasana, 84
    scientific basis, 82–83
    universal ethical principles, 81
    use of, 84–85
    yoga breathing, 82

Zen Buddhist meditation, 101